METHODS IN MOLECULAR BIOLOGY

*Series Editor*
John M. Walker
School of Life and Medical Sciences
University of Hertfordshire
Hatfield, Hertfordshire, AL10 9AB, UK

For further volumes:
http://www.springer.com/series/7651

# Drug Target miRNA

## Methods and Protocols

Edited by

**Marco F. Schmidt**

*BEROCEUTICA GmbH, Potsdam, Germany*

Humana Press

*Editor*
Marco F. Schmidt
BEROCEUTICA GmbH
Potsdam, Germany

ISSN 1064-3745 ISSN 1940-6029 (electronic)
Methods in Molecular Biology
ISBN 978-1-4939-6561-8 ISBN 978-1-4939-6563-2 (eBook)
DOI 10.1007/978-1-4939-6563-2

Library of Congress Control Number: 2016956244



Printed on acid-free paper

This Humana Press imprint is published by Springer Nature
The registered company is Springer Science+Business Media LLC
The registered company address is: 233 Spring Street, New York, NY 10013, U.S.A.

# Preface

Only 20 years after the discovery of small non-coding, single-stranded ribonucleic acids, so-called microRNAs (miRNAs), as post-transcriptional gene regulators, the first miRNA-targeting drug Miravirsen for the treatment of hepatitis C has been successful in clinical phase II trials. Addressing miRNAs as drug targets may enable the cure of diseases, which presently seems impossible. However, due to miRNAs' chemical structure, generation of potential drug molecules with necessary pharmacokinetic properties is still challenging. Thus, Miravirsen remains an exception. In conclusion, drug target miRNA requires innovation at the level of drug discovery.

Until today, several approaches have been developed to modulate miRNAs' function in the hope of potential therapeutic use. After a short introduction to the field of miRNA drug discovery (Chapter 1) and to miRNA target identification (Chapter 2), the book summarizes the three strategies to overcome pharmacodynamics and pharmacokinetics challenges: Firstly, due to their poor cell permeability, anti-sense agents targeting miRNA are applied in advanced formulations, or are chemically optimized to increase their delivery (Chapters 3–9). Secondly, efforts were made to develop small molecule miRNA modulators to overcome anti-sense agents' limitations (Chapters 10–11). Especially, DICER-mediated miRNA maturation is a target for small molecules. General enhancers of miRNA maturation, as well specific substrate inhibitors, were identified, thereby demonstrating the potential of adopting the concept of small molecules to target miRNA functions (Chapters 12–14). Thirdly, as miRNA function is executed by the Argonaute 2 protein, new chemical entities, addressing this protein (or its complex with target miRNA of interest) with likely better pharmacokinetic parameters than reported oligonucleotides, may open new perspectives in miRNA drug discovery (Chapters 15–21).

Regarding the enormous potential of miRNAs in drug discovery, my motivation to edit this Methods in Molecular Biology volume was not to give an overview of existing challenges but rather to provide a concise technical manual of recently developed approaches to overcome these challenges in miRNA drug discovery to open new ways in therapies. Therefore, I am thankful to all contributors, leading practitioners from academia and industry, of the chapters in this book for their outstanding effort and commitment to this project. I would also like to thank Prof. John Walker for his encouragement. Additional thanks go to the staff at Springer Science + Business Media for their excellent support.

*Potsdam, Germany* — *Marco F. Schmidt*

## Contents

## Contributors


CHRIS ABELL • *University Chemical Laboratory, University of Cambridge, Cambridge, UK*

JOHN R. ANDROSAVICH • *Regulus Therapeutics Inc., San Diego, CA, USA*

ANDREAS G. BADER • *Mirna Therapeutics Inc., Austin, TX, USA*

MARK A. BEHLKE • *Integrated DNA Technologies Inc., Coralville, IA, USA*

TERESA BELLISSIMO • *Department of Anatomical, Histological, Forensic & Orthopaedic Sciences, Section of Histology & Medical Embryology, Sapienza University of Rome, Rome, Italy*

JULIE BERNAUER • *Inria Saclay-Île de France, 1 rue Honoré d'Estienne d'Orves, Bâtiment Alan Turing Campus de l', École Polytechnique, Palaiseau, France; Laboratoire d'Informatique de l'École Polytechnique (LIX), CNRS UMR 7161, École Polytechnique, Palaiseau, France*

YANGCHAO CHEN • *School of Biomedical Sciences, Faculty of Medicine, The Chinese University of Hong Kong, Shatin, Hong Kong, China; State Key Laboratory of Digestive Disease, Institute of Digestive Disease, The Chinese University of Hong Kong, Shatin, Hong Kong, China; Shenzhen Research Institute, The Chinese University of Hong Kong, Shenzhen, China*

JESSICA L. CHILDS-DISNEY • *Department of Chemistry, The Scripps Research Institute-Scripps Florida, Jupiter, FL, USA*

GIANNI COLOTTI • *IBPM – CNR Institute of Molecular Biology and Pathology, Italian National Research Council, Department of Biochemical Sciences "A. Rossi Fanelli", Sapienza University of Rome, Rome, Italy*

JOHANNES DANNER • *Biochemistry Center Regensburg (BZR), Laboratory for RNA Biology, University of Regensburg, Regensburg, Germany*

MATTHEW D. DISNEY • *Department of Chemistry, The Scripps Research Institute-Scripps Florida, Jupiter, FL, USA*

MARIA DUCA • *Institute of Chemistry of Nice, University of Nice Sophia Antipolis, UMR7272 CNRS, Parc Valrose, Nice, France*

FRANCESCO FAZI • *Department of Anatomical, Histological, Forensic & Orthopaedic Sciences, Section of Histology & Medical Embryology, Sapienza University of Rome, Rome, Italy*

JONATHAN FERRAND • *Centre for Cancer Research, Hudson Institute of Medical Research, Clayton, VIC, Australia; Department of Molecular and Translational Science, Monash University, Clayton, VIC, Australia*

MICHAEL P. GANTIER • *Centre for Cancer Research, Hudson Institute of Medical Research, Clayton, VIC, Australia; Department of Molecular and Translational Science, Monash University, Clayton, VIC, Australia*

XIN GAO • *King Abdullah University of Science and Technology (KAUST), Computational Bioscience Research Center (CBRC), Computer, Electrical and Mathematical Sciences and Engineering (CEMSE) Division, Thuwal, Saudi Arabia*

ILARIA GENOVESE • *CNR-National Research Council of Italy, Institute of Molecular Biology and Pathology, Department of Biochemical Sciences "A. Rossi Fanelli", Sapienza University of Rome, Rome, Italy*

DINA GROHMANN • *Department of Microbiology, Single Molecule Biochemistry Lab, Universität Regensburg, Regensburg, Germany*
CHRISTOPHER L. HAGA • *Department of Molecular Therapeutics, The Scripps Research Institute-Scripps Florida, Jupiter, FL, USA*
ARTEMIS G. HATZIGEORGIOU • *Hellenic Pasteur Institute, Athens, Greece; Department of Electrical & Computer Engineering, University of Thessaly, Volos, Greece*
AMÉLIE HÉLIOU • *Inria Saclay-Île de France, 1 rue Honoré d'Estienne d'Orves, Bâtiment Alan Turing Campus de l', École Polytechnique, Palaiseau, France; Laboratoire d'Informatique de l'École Polytechnique (LIX), CNRS UMR 7161, École Polytechnique, Palaiseau, France*
SUNGCHUL HOHNG • *Department of Physics and Astronomy, Seoul National University, Seoul, Republic of Korea; Institute of Applied Physics, Seoul National University, Seoul, Republic of Korea; National Center of Creative Research Initiatives, Seoul National University, Seoul, Republic of Korea; Department of Biophysics and Chemical Biology, Seoul National University, Seoul, Republic of Korea*
XUHUI HUANG • *Division of Biomedical Engineering, The Hong Kong University of Science and Technology, Clear Water Bay, Kowloon, Hong Kong, China; Department of Chemistry, The Hong Kong University of Science and Technology, Clear Water Bay, Kowloon, Hong Kong, China; Center of Systems Biology and Human Health, School of Science and Institute for Advance Study, The Hong Kong University of Science and Technology, Clear Water Bay, Kowloon, Hong Kong, China*
HANLUN JIANG • *Graduate Program in Biological Physics, Structure and Design, University of Washington, Washington, DC, USA*
MYUNG HYUN JO • *Department of Physics and Astronomy, Seoul National University, Seoul, Republic of Korea; Institute of Applied Physics, Seoul National University, Seoul, Republic of Korea; National Center of Creative Research Initiatives, Seoul National University, Seoul, Republic of Korea*
OLIVER KORB • *Cambridge Crystallographic Data Centre (CCDC), Cambridge, UK*
KIM A. LENNOX • *Integrated DNA Technologies Inc., Coralville, IA, USA*
SILVIA MASCIARELLI • *Department of Anatomical, Histological, Forensic & Orthopaedic Sciences, Section of Histology & Medical Embryology, Sapienza University of Rome, Rome, Italy*
GUNTER MEISTER • *Biochemistry Center Regensburg (BZR), Laboratory for RNA Biology, University of Regensburg, Regensburg, Germany*
BALAGOPAL PAI • *Biochemistry Center Regensburg (BZR), Laboratory for RNA Biology, University of Regensburg, Regensburg, Germany*
GENEVIÈVE PÉPIN • *Centre for Cancer Research, Hudson Institute of Medical Research, Clayton, VIC, Australia; Department of Molecular and Translational Science, Monash University, Clayton, VIC, Australia*
VINITA PERIWAL • *GN Ramachandran Knowledge Center for Genome Informatics, CSIR Institute of Genomics and Integrative Biology, Delhi, India*
DONALD G. PHINNEY • *Department of Molecular Therapeutics, The Scripps Research Institute-Scripps Florida, Jupiter, FL, USA*
ELENA POSER • *CNR-National Research Council of Italy, Institute of Molecular Biology and Pathology, Department of Biochemical Sciences "A. Rossi Fanelli", Sapienza University of Rome, Rome, Italy*
TOBIAS RESTLE • *Institute of Molecular Medicine, Universitätsklinikum Schleswig-Holstein, University of Lübeck, Lübeck, Germany*

ALBERTO DEL RIO • *CNR-National Research Council of Italy, Institute for Organic Chemistry and Photoreactivity, Bologna, Italy; Innovamol Srls, Modena, Italy*
VINOD SCARIA • *GN Ramachandran Knowledge Center for Genome Informatics, CSIR Institute of Genomics and Integrative Biology, Delhi, India*
MARCO F. SCHMIDT • *BEROCEUTICA GmbH, c/o Universität Potsdam, Potsdam, Germany*
JACQUELINE STRIVELLI • *Department of Molecular Therapeutics, The Scripps Research Institute-Scripps Florida, Jupiter, FL, USA*
CHRISTOPHER A. VAKULSKAS • *Integrated DNA Technologies Inc., Coralville, IA, USA*
SAI PRADEEP VELAGAPUDI • *Department of Chemistry, The Scripps Research Institute-Scripps Florida, Jupiter, FL, USA*
IOANNIS S. VLACHOS • *Hellenic Pasteur Institute, Athens, Greece*
DUC D. VO • *Institute of Chemistry of Nice, University of Nice Sophia Antipolis, UMR7272 CNRS, Parc Valrose, Nice, France*
LUDWIG WANKERL • *Biochemistry Center Regensburg (BZR), Laboratory for RNA Biology, University of Regensburg, Regensburg, Germany*
SARAH WILLKOMM • *Institute of Molecular Medicine, Universitätsklinikum Schleswig-Holstein, University of Lübeck, Lübeck, Germany; Department of Microbiology, Single Molecule Biochemistry Lab, Universität Regensburg, Regensburg, Germany*
ZHANGANG XIAO • *School of Biomedical Sciences, Faculty of Medicine, The Chinese University of Hong Kong, Hong Kong, China*
ADRIAN ZANDER • *Department of Microbiology, Single Molecule Biochemistry Lab, Universität Regensburg, Regensburg, Germany*
JANE ZHAO • *Mirna Therapeutics Inc., Austin, TX, USA*
LIZHE ZHU • *Department of Chemistry, The Hong Kong University of Science and Technology, Clear Water Bay, Kowloon, Hong Kong, China; Center of Systems Biology and Human Health, School of Science and Institute for Advance Study, The Hong Kong University of Science and Technology, Clear Water Bay, Kowloon, Hong Kong, China*
DIMITRIOS G. ZISOULIS • *Regulus Therapeutics, San Diego, CA, USA*

# Part I

## Reviews

# Chapter 1

# miRNA Targeting Drugs: The Next Blockbusters?


## Marco F. Schmidt



## Abstract

Only 20 years after the discovery of small non-coding, single-stranded ribonucleic acids, so-called microRNAs (miRNAs), as post-transcriptional gene regulators, the first miRNA-targeting drug Miravirsen for the treatment of hepatitis C has been successfully tested in clinical Phase II trials. Addressing miRNAs as drug targets may enable the cure, or at least the treatment of diseases, which presently seems impossible. However, due to miRNAs' chemical structure, generation of potential drug molecules with necessary pharmacokinetic properties is still challenging and requires a re-thinking of the drug discovery process. Therefore, this chapter highlights the potential of miRNAs as drug targets, discusses the challenges, and tries to give a complete overview of recent strategies in miRNA drug discovery.



**Key words** miRNA, Drug discovery, microRNA-induced silencing complex, Antisense agents, Small-molecule miRNA modulators, Argonaute 2 protein


## 1 miRNAs: Post-transcriptional Gene Regulators

microRNAs (miRNAs), small, non-coding, single-stranded *r*ibo*n*ucleic *a*cid (RNA) molecules, on average only 22–23 nucleotides long, are post-transcriptional gene regulators [1]. miRNAs bind specifically by base pairing to the sequence of their target *m*essenger *r*ibo*n*ucleic *a*cid (mRNA). The binding initiates complex formation of several proteins, the so-called *mi*cro*R*NA-*i*nduced *s*ilencing *c*omplex (miRISC) [2], that results in the decay of the target mRNA. Whereas only approximately 2000 microRNAs exist in humans (www.mirbase.org), compared to 22,000 genes and 200,000 proteins, they regulate 30% of all genes [2, 3]. Thus, microRNAs are a crucial player in gene regulation.

RNA polymerase II/III transcribes miRNAs encoding genes producing the so-called *pri*mary *mi*cro*RNAs* (pri-miRNAs) (Fig. 1). In the nucleus, these transcripts are further processed by the nuclease Drosha forming the *pre*cursor *mi*cro*RNAs* (pre-miRNAs). Those are up to 70–80 nucleotides long and are organized in a double-stranded hairpin conformation. Then, the


Marco F. Schmidt (ed.), *Drug Target miRNA: Methods and Protocols*, Methods in Molecular Biology, vol. 1517,
DOI 10.1007/978-1-4939-6563-2_1,

pre-miRNAs are transported out of the nucleus into the cytosol. There, a complex formed by ribonuclease DICER and two proteins, PACT (*p*rotein *act*ivator of the interferon induced protein kinase) as well TRBP (human immunodeficiency virus (HIV) *t*ransactivating response *R*NA-*b*inding *p*rotein-2), cleaves the double-stranded pre-miRNA yielding the later miRNA. This is also be known as miRNA maturation. Next, the double-stranded miRNA is unwound by *Argo*naute *2* (AGO2) protein. miRNA stays bound to the AGO2 and binds to its target mRNA by sequence-specific complementarity [2, 3]. AGO2 protein itself recruits several other proteins: glycine(*g*)-tryptophan(*w*) repeat-containing protein of *182*kDa (GW182), *p*oly(*A*)*b*inding *p*rotein (PABP), CCR4-NOT, *p*oly(*A*) *n*ucleases *2* and *3* (PAN2-PAN3), and some unknown proteins, forming all together the so-called *micro*RNA-*i*nduced *s*ilencing *c*omplex (miRISC) [3].

Then, miRISC-mediated gene silencing executes through three different molecular actions (Fig. 1): Firstly, as the Argonaute protein is an RNase it catalyzes the cleavage of target mRNA sequence specifically guided by bound miRNA. Secondly, GW182 blocks translation initiation by preventing ribosomal complex formation. Thirdly, CCR4-NOT and PAN2-PAN3 initiate deadenylation of the poly(A) tail (AAA). Thus, mRNA decay is terminated by exonucleases followed by removal of the 5-terminal cap ($m^7G$) [3].

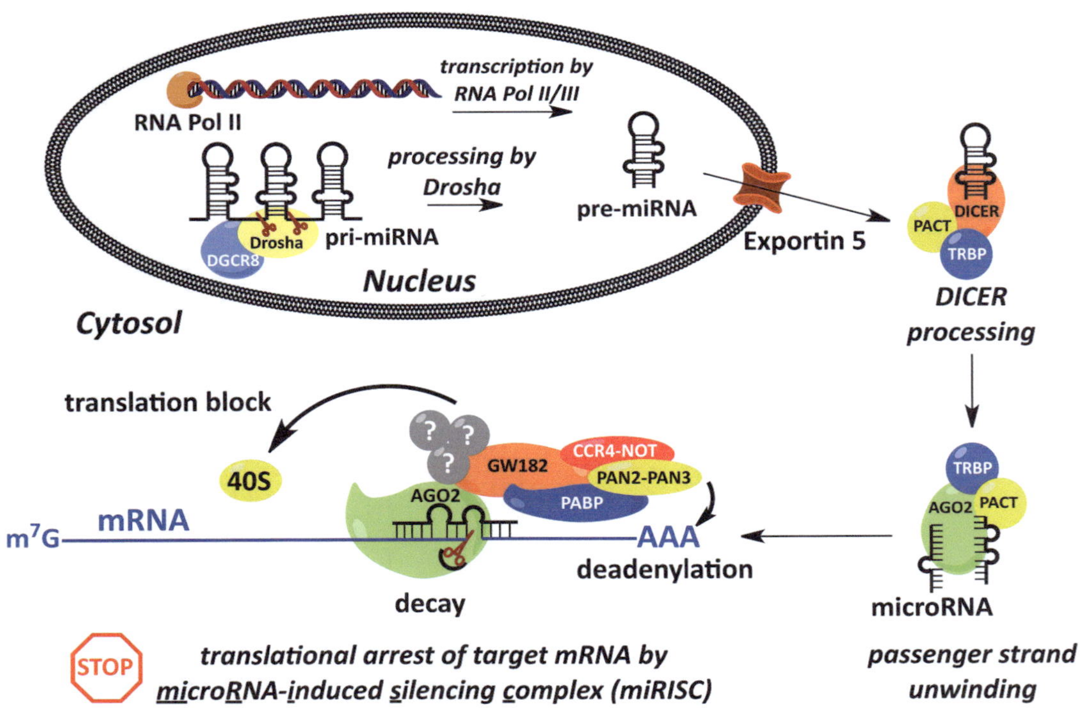


**Fig. 1** Schematic illustration of miRNA-mediated gene silencing with permission from [7]

## 2 Drug Target miRNA

Although it has been described that miRNAs are involved in various diseases and, from there, they are regarded as high-potential drug targets, this does not explain their full potential.

The development of a new drug molecule has become an increasingly expensive and risky business. The average cost per approved new drug molecule from 2002 to 2006 was US $2.8 billion, in contrast from 2007 to 2011, the average cost was US $4.2 billion (www.pwc.com/pharma2020). This may be a result of management mistakes in the pharmaceutical industry and higher regulatory requirements. Nonetheless, one reason of pharmaceutical industry's poor R&D outcome is drug target selection. More than 99% of all approved drugs bind to proteins, most of them (>80%) only to three protein classes: enzymes, receptors, and transporters [4, 5]. Established protocols in the industrial drug discovery process such as compound selection ('Lipinski's Rule of Five') only work for protein drug targets [5]. However, not every protein can be targeted or modulated by a drug molecule. On one hand, a protein needs a binding site—often a deep binding pocket with the ability to accommodate a ligand—to be modulated in its function. On the other hand, the modulation of a single protein does not always affect a clinical effect. These proteins are referred to as being 'undruggable' [6]. Subsequently, the number of protein drug targets is limited. Although the human genome encodes 100,000–200,000 proteins, it has been shown that only 207 proteins are targeted by FDA-approved small-molecule drugs. Furthermore, it is estimated that only 600 disease-modifying protein drug targets exist [4]. Therefore, the focus in target selection has now shifted to other macromolecules, especially such as miRNAs. Due to their involvement in gene regulation, intervention at the miRNA level may allow specific manipulation of every protein population: miRNA inhibitors induce selective upregulation of one protein population, whereas miRNA mimics induce gene silencing, thus resulting in downregulation of the target protein. Consequently, also former 'undruggable' proteins can be modulated via their miRNA gene regulators, enabling the cure of diseases, which, at present, seems impossible. As a result, miRNAs are regarded as high-value targets for therapy [7].

## 3 Strategies in miRNA Drug Discovery

Until now, there is no standard protocol for the development of miRNA modulators as reported for protein targets [7]. The most reasonable strategy in miRNA drug discovery is the use of antisense agents [8].

### 3.1 Antisense Agents in miRNA Drug Discovery

As mentioned before, oligonucleotides can either mimic miRNA, thus inducing gene silencing in a similar manner to RNAi, or bind to a target miRNA and block the translational arrest. Nonetheless, it has been shown that, in practice, single as well double-stranded DNA or RNA oligonucleotides are useless for clinical application. DNA and RNA oligonucleotides are, firstly, not resistant to serum nucleases; secondly, are poorly cell-permeable due to their negatively charged backbone; consequently, they cannot enter the cell by diffusion; and, thirdly, they often show off-target effects due to hybridization to other, similar oligonucleotide sequences or to activation of immune responses. Therefore, due to their pharmacokinetic profile the general application of oligonucleotides in therapy is limited [7, 8]. Only under certain circumstances antisense agents have been successful in clinical trials (Table 1).

#### 3.1.1 Chemical Modifications of Oligonucleotides

Simple oligonucleotides are inappropriate for therapeutic use as naked DNA or RNA moieties are not resistant against serum nucleases [8]. From there, efforts were made to design oligonucleotide derivatives with increased lipophilicity compared to ribonucleic acids, in the hope of overcoming inappropriate PK properties such as missing serum nucleases resistance and cell-permeability.

The most common chemical modification of oligonucleotides to improve the resistance to nucleases and to induce rapid and stable hybridization in vitro and in vivo is a methylation of the 2′-OH group, the so-called 2′-O-methyl (2′-OMe)-modification (Fig. 2). According to this, it has been shown by two independent studies that 2′-OMe-modified RNAs block effectively the slicing activity of miRISC [9, 10]. However, a drawback of 2′-OMe-modified anti-miRs is that they are still susceptible to degradation by serum exonucleases [8–10]. Thus, they are not suitable for in vivo applications. Serum exonucleases cleave the phosphate bonds between nucleotides. Thus, there is a need for modifications that induce resistant to serum exonucleases.

The most feasible synthetic approach is the replacement of non-bridging oxygen in the phosphate backbone by a sulfur atom (sulfurization) to form a phosphorothioate (PS) bond. Consequently, their reported half-life time in the bloodstream is 1 up to 4 weeks [11]. However, the improved stability of PS-containing oligonucleotides against serum exnucleases comes along with reduced hybridization affinity to their target miRNAs [12]. Nonetheless, the most notable aspect is that PS-modification enhances binding affinity to plasma proteins. Thereupon, PS-containing oligonucleotides are absorbed effectively from the injection site into the bloodstream in 1–2 h compared to other modified antisense agents [11, 13]. Eventually, their ability to bind to proteins is not limited to plasma proteins. The binding to tissue or cell surface proteins is much stronger. Therefore, PS-containing oligonucleotides exhibit good uptake behavior in several tissues, such as kidney, spleen, lymph nodes, adipocytes, bone marrow, and especially the liver, but not in skeletal

**Table 1**
**Overview of miRNA targeting drugs in clinical development. *Santaris Pharma has been acquired by F. Hoffmann-La Roche AG in 2014**

| miRNA | Mode of action | Indication | Company | Developmental stage |
|---|---|---|---|---|
| miR-122 | LNA-modified antisense inhibitor | HCV infection | Santaris Pharma* | Successful in phase II |
| miR-34a | miRNA mimic encapsulated in a liposomal nanoparticle formulation | Liver cancer | Mirna Therapeutics | Phase II (2017) |
| miR-122 | GalNAc-conjugated antisense inhibitor | HCV infection | Regulus Therapeutics | Phase I |
| miR-21 | 2′-F and 2′-MOE bicyclic sugar-modified antisense inhibitor | Cancer, fibrosis | Regulus Therapeutics/Sanofi | Phase I |
| miR-29 | miRNA mimic | Fibrosis | miRagen Therapeutics | Phase I |
| miR-101 | miRNA mimic encapsulated in a liposomal nanoparticle formulation | Cancer | Mirna Therapeutics | Phase I (2016) |
| miR-215 | miRNA mimic encapsulated in a liposomal nanoparticle formulation | Cancer | Mirna Therapeutics | Phase I (2016) |
| *let-7* | miRNA mimic encapsulated in a liposomal nanoparticle formulation | Cancer | Mirna Therapeutics | Preclinical |
| miR-16 | miRNA mimic encapsulated in a liposomal nanoparticle formulation | Cancer | Mirna Therapeutics | Preclinical |
| miR-10b | Antisense inhibitor | Glioblastoma | Regulus Therapeutics | Preclinical |
| miR-103/107 | Antisense inhibitor | Insulin resistance | Regulus Therapeutics/AstraZeneca | Preclinical |
| miR-221 | Antisense inhibitor | Hepatocellular carcinoma | Regulus Therapeutics/Sanofi | Preclinical |
| miR-155 | Antisense inhibitor | Amyotrophic lateral sclerosis (ALS), cancer | miRagen Therapeutics | Preclinical |
| miR-92a | Antisense inhibitor | Diabetic wound healing | miRagen Therapeutics | Preclinical |
| miR-15 | Antisense inhibitor | Post-myocardial infarction | miRagen Therapeutics/Servier | Preclinical |
| miR-208 | Antisense inhibitor | Heart failure | miRagen Therapeutics/Servier | Preclinical |

muscles or the brain [11]. In summary, in addition to their resistance against serum exonucleases PS-modified oligonucleotides show unique pharmacokinetic behavior due its capability to bind to proteins enabling them a more efficient distribution in the body through the blood stream and cellular up-take compared to other modified oligonucleotides. From there, PS-modification can be often found in clinically tested anti-miRs (Table 1).

Another nuclease-resistant chemical modification is the introduction of a methoxyethyl group at the 2′-sugar position (2′-MOE) analogously to the 2′-OMe modification (Fig. 2). In contrast to 2′-OMe, 2′-MOE-modified oligonucleotides display higher affinity to their target sequences due to its more lipophilic character and, additionally, comparable serum nuclease resistance as the PS-modified anti-miRs [13]. In conclusion, 2′-MOE-modified antisense agents showed superior efficacy than these with 2′-OMe-modification.

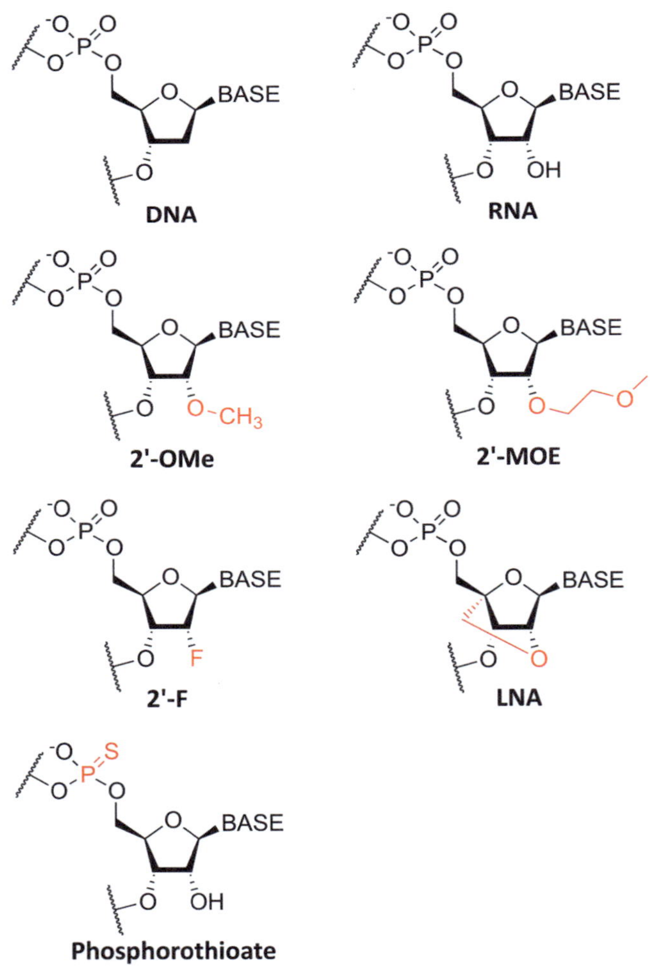


**Fig. 2** Overview of chemical modifications used for the design of miRNA-targeting oligonucleotides

In contrast to 2′-MOE-modified anti-miRs, introduction of a fluorine atom substituent at the C2′-ribose position (2′-F) does not have any effect on serum nuclease resistance. However, the fluorine in the 2′-position induces the sugar ring into a high C3′-endo conformation, that is characteristic for A-form duplexes and results in exceptional affinity for target RNAs (increased melting temperature $T_m$: up to 3 °C per nucleotide) [14]. More important, it has been shown that 2′-F-modified anti-miRs enhance formation of miRISC through protein recruitment [15], possibly due their higher hybridization ability and/or pre-organization in an A-form duplex.

The most successful nucleotide derivative is locked nucleic acid (LNA): Here, the ribose moiety of an LNA nucleotide has an additional methylene bridge connecting the 2′ oxygen and 4′ carbon. Thereby, the ribose is 'locked' in the C3′-endo confirmation, which enhances base stacking and backbone pre-organization in A-form duplexes and protects from nuclease degradation [16]. Therefore, the most prominent anti-miR drug candidate is the LNA-PS-modified antisense oligonucleotide Miravirsen. The 15-mer Miravirsen was developed by Santaris Pharma A/S (acquired by F. Hoffmann-La Roche AG in 2014 for US $450 million), and tested successfully in Phase II clinical trials for the treatment of hepatitis C virus (HCV) infection [17]. Miravirsen's target is the human liver-expressed miRNA-122 (miR-122). miR-122 acts as an important host factor for HCV interacting with the 5′ untranslated region (5′UTR) of the virus RNA by binding to two miR-122 sites in complex with the Argonaute protein (Fig. 3) [18]. The binding of the HCV genome to the miR-122-Argonaute complex protects the viral RNA from nucleolytic degradation [19, 20]. Miravirsen blocks

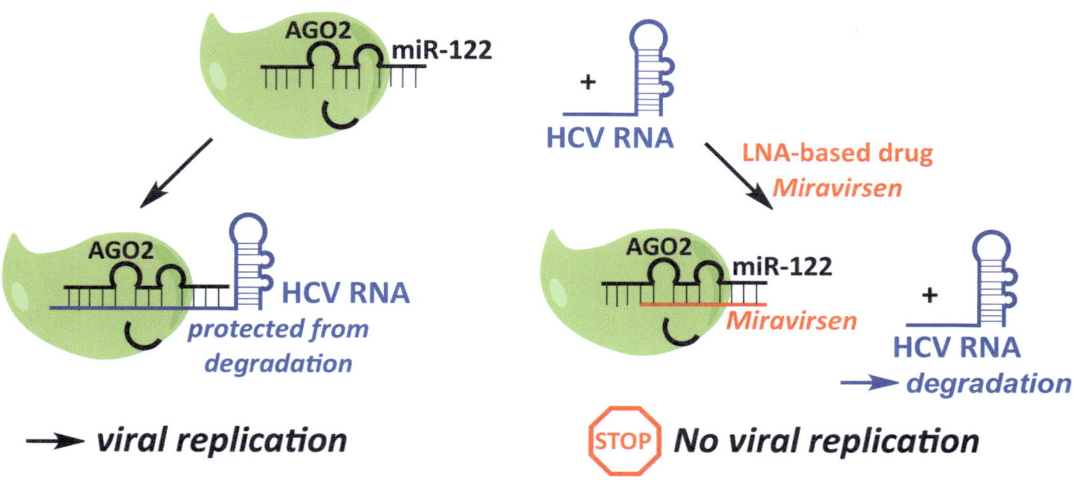


**Fig. 3** Mechanism of the LNA-PS-modified oligonucleotide Miravirsen. Hepatitis C virus is either protected by AGO2 in the absence of Miravirsen (*left*) or allowed to degrade in its presence (*right*). Figure from [7] with permission

the miR-122-AGO complex, thereby, inhibiting the essential interaction with HCV RNA for viral replication [21]. Nevertheless, Miravirsen is an exception in miRNA drug discovery. Due to its phosphorothioate modification Miravirsen accumulates in the liver after injection, where its target miR-122 is exclusively expressed [22]. From there, the development of anti-miRs targeting miRNAs outside of the liver is still a challenge.

In conclusion, different chemical modifications on the ribose ring have been developed and are widely used in different combinations in respect to yield an anti-miR with necessary pharmacodynamic and pharmacokinetic parameters for therapeutic use. Until today, only the DNA/LNA-PS-modified anti-miR Miravirsen has reached the stage of a clinical phase III trial that—ironically—works as an exception. However, this raises the question whether classical antisense agents are generally suitable for clinical application. Probably, non-nucleotide modifiers may be promising for the development of more effective entities in miRNA drug discovery. One such example is *N,N*-diethyl-4-(4-nitronaphthalen-1-ylazo)-phenylamine (ZEN): Behlke and co-workers from Integrated DNA Technologies, Inc. developed the ZEN monomer. They incorporated the ZEN monomer at both ends of a 2′-OMe-modified anti-miR demonstrating that ZEN modification increases potency and specificity compared to the un-modified oligonucleotide while the modifications also showed low toxicity in cell culture [23].

#### 3.1.2 Advanced Delivery Strategies

The introduction of chemical modifications in anti-miR oligonucleotides improved effectively their resistance against serum nucleases. However, due to their negatively charged backbone efficient delivery of antisense agents in vivo is still a challenge [7, 8]. Chemically modified anti-miR oligonucleotides are usually administered in high doses to show any effect and, consequently, often taken up directly by the liver and the kidney, so that they rapidly excreted in urine [8]. Therefore, three strategies to enhance anti-miRs in vivo delivery have been widely investigated: the use of covalent conjugation with up-take enhancers, liposomes, and nanoparticles.

In 2004, Krützfeld et al. reported the use of 2′-OMe/PS-modified ribonucleic acids conjugated with a cholesterol tag at their 3′-end, so-called antagonistic miRNAs (antagomiRs), to improve their cellular up-take [24]. Although the cholesterol tag enhances cell-permeability, antagomiRs delivery is still insufficient for therapeutic use as their doses required for in vivo administration is very high with 80 mg/kg [24, 25].

More successful is the conjugation of an anti-miR oligonucleotide with a trivalent *N*-acetylgalactosamine (GalNAc) carbohydrate tag. The trivalent GalNAc tag shows high binding affinity to the asialoglycoprotein receptor (ASGPR). Originally, ASGPR is responsible for the efficient up-take of glycoproteins from the serum via clathrin-mediated endocytosis. This mechanism has been adapted for effective delivery of conjugated anti-miRs with remarkable in vivo activity with less than 0.05 mg/kg median effective dose ($ED_{50}$) [26]. The ASGP receptor is well conserved across species. From there, the GalNAc delivery strategy can also be applied apart from human medicine.

An example for successful delivery of antisense agents is MRX34, a liposomal nanoparticle loaded with synthetic miRNA-34 mimics, developed by Mirnarx Therapeutics, Inc. [27, 28]. Human miRNA-34a is a downregulated tumor suppressor in various cancers regulating more than 20 oncogenes, including the epidermal growth factor receptor (EGFR) pathway. It was shown that addition of artificial miRNA-34a to cancer cells suppresses oncogenes and, from there, displays a possible therapy. MRX34 has recently entered Phase II clinical trials. Andreas Bader and coworkers reported recently that MRX34 was tested against cancer cells in combination with the EGFR tyrosine kinase inhibitor (EGFR-TKI) Erlotinib, giving evidence that several cancers previously not suited for Erlotinib may prove sensitive to the drug when used in combination with MRX34 [28].

In conclusion, MRX34 represents two trends in miRNA drug discovery. On one hand, it is administered by an advanced formulation (liposomal nanoparticles) to increase the delivery of oligonucleotides into the cell. On other hand, MRX34 is tested in combination with reported drugs to identify synergistic effects.

### 3.1.3 Challenges of Antisense Agents in miRNA Drug Discovery

The main challenge of antisense agents in miRNA drug discovery is still the delivery from the injection site via blood stream and tissue into the cell. Admittedly, some tissues such as liver and kidney are much easier to access for antisense agents than other. That explains the success of Miravirsen [17] and MRX34 [27] whose both targets are located in the liver. However, even when anti-miRs reach their target tissue from the injection site, the most limiting step is the cellular up-take and internal release of the anti-miR into the cytosol. For instance, Gilleron et al. reported recently an assay to track quantitatively the up-take and intracellular release of liposomal nanoparticles encapsulated siRNA based on fluorescence and electron microscopy. Herein, it was shown that the nanoparticles entered the cell via clathrin-mediated endocytosis and macropinocytosis whereas only 1–2% of the nanoparticles reached the cytosol after escaping from the endosomes [29]. This result indicates that, firstly, hitherto existing up-take strategies such as liposomal nanoparticles are still insufficient for the delivery of anti-miRs into the cytosol and, secondly, the clinically tested anti-miRs (Miravirsen, MRX34, etc.) have to be administered in high doses to initiate an effect. And administration of high doses always bears the risk of inducing off-target effects.

There are two types of anti-miRs' off-target effect: hybridization-associated and hybridization-independent. The hybridization-associated off-target effects rely on the promiscuous binding behavior of an anti-miR to all family members of the miRNA target [30]. The reason for this is that the target miRNA is bound to the Argonaute 2 protein as part of miRISC in the cell and only the nucleotides at miRNA's 5′-end, the so-called seed region, are solvent-exposed. So, anti-miR's binding to its target miRNA occurs in a first, rate-depending step to its seed region and only in a second, fast step to the whole sequence [31]. As the seed region is mostly the same in all family members, targeting of one specific family member with one anti-miR in vivo is very difficult. The only solution at the moment for antisense agents in miRNA drug discovery seems a careful selection of a miRNA target with a small number of family members or the deliberate inhibition of a full miRNA family.

In contrast, the hybridization independent off-target effects are associated with immune stimulation and in vivo toxicity. Anti-miRs, especially when administered in high doses, are recognized by the innate immune system. Cells of the innate immune system express Toll-like receptors (TLRs), a type of pattern recognition receptor (PRR), those recognize molecules from pathogens and, therefore, play a central role in microbial defense. Several TLRs (TLR3, TLR7, TLR8, and TLR9) have been identified that induce interferon alpha (IFN-$\alpha$) response after binding a short, both single- or double-stranded nucleic acid [32]. Because of this, the interaction of a potential anti-miR drug is routinely investigated in vitro and in vivo in hope to avoid receptor activation. Herein, an interesting finding was that for the activation of a TLR only the nine nucleotides at the 3′-end of the oligonucleotide, those directly correspondent with miRNA's seed region, are crucial [33]. Another sequence-independent off-target effect is in vivo toxicity. This is often recognized by inhibition of coagulation, activation of the complement cascade and hepatotoxicity. Herein, it was shown that PS-modified anti-miRs inhibit coagulation and transiently prolong clotting times in monkeys, probably due to their ability to bind blood plasma proteins [34]. In case of LNA-modified oligonucleotides for instance, hepatotoxicity is often observed indicated by organ and body weight loss in preclinical animal tests [35].

In conclusion, antisense miRNA modifiers only work under certain circumstances such as liposomal nanoparticles, in high doses with the danger of off-target effects, in combination with other drugs, or in case of Miravirsen as an exception. However, their general application is hampered due to their poor delivery and up-take properties as well their off-target effects, likely because of their molecular size of more than 6000 Da and their negatively charged backbone. In addition, antisense oligonucleotides have to be applied by injection, thereby making the treatment less convenient. In contrast to that, the success of protein-targeting small-molecule drugs relies mostly on their oral application and their ability to reach in-cell targets by simple diffusion [4, 5]. The question may therefore be asked, why the concept of protein-based drug discovery cannot be adopted to target miRNAs with small molecules?

### 3.2 Small-Molecule Modulators in miRNA Drug Discovery

Small molecules are low-molecular-weight (<1000 Da) organic compounds. Due to their mostly hydrophobic structure they can bind to macromolecules and, thereby, they can modulate the macromolecule's function. Most drugs are small molecules. Their success in drug discovery relies on their ability to cross easily cell membranes and reach their target macromolecule by simple diffusion. Additionally, small molecules are resistant against degradation in the blood stream and, from there, they show a high bioavailability. Adopting this concept to miRNAs may solve the problem of poor cell-permeability and pharmacokinetics. So, why small molecules are not the standard in miRNA drug discovery?

Binding of a small molecule to a macromolecule requires a binding site that can accommodate a small-molecule ligand. Therefore, most small-molecule drugs bind to enzymes, receptors, and transporters that display a defined binding pockets for their native binders, e.g. metabolic substrates, hormones, transmitters, etc. Efforts have been made to set up protocols, e.g. *Lipinski's Rule of Five* (MW < 500 Da, H donors ≤ 5, H acceptors ≤ 10, Log$P$ < 5), how to design efficiently a small-molecule drug [4]. Nonetheless, the concept of small molecule drugs for protein drug targets cannot applied to miRNA drug targets as a single-stranded, 23 nucleotides long miRNA does not display a rigid structure with a defined binding site for a small-molecule ligand. According to this, there is still no report of a small-molecule ligand according to the *Lipinski's Rule of Five* binding to a single-stranded miRNA selectively. Even though, several drug-like compound libraries were screened successfully against different miRNAs in cellular assays. Further investigations of in these screens identified small molecule ligands showed that miRNAs' function can be targeted by small-molecule ligands; however, these ligands do not bind directly to target miRNA.

#### *3.2.1 Small-Molecule miRNA Modulators Identified in Cellular Screens*

Alexander Deiters and co-workers were among the first who developed a cellular assay based on luciferase expression for the screening of small-molecule modulators targeting miRNA functions [36, 37]. miRNA activity was monitored by introducing a complementary sequence of the target miRNA downstream of the luciferase reporter gene (Fig. 4). Herein, the luciferase activity was downregulated when the miRNA of interest bound to the miRNA binding sequence in the 3' untranslated region (3'UTR) of the transcribed reporter construct. Finally, several small-molecule libraries were screened with this cellular assay against different miRNAs, yielding several selective small-molecule inhibitors of miRNA-21 (an anti-apoptopic factor), miRNA-34a (cancer target), and miRNA-122 (prevents HCV infection) as well as a selective activator of miRNA-122 (Fig. 4). Nonetheless, none of these compounds were found to bind directly to their target miRNA as

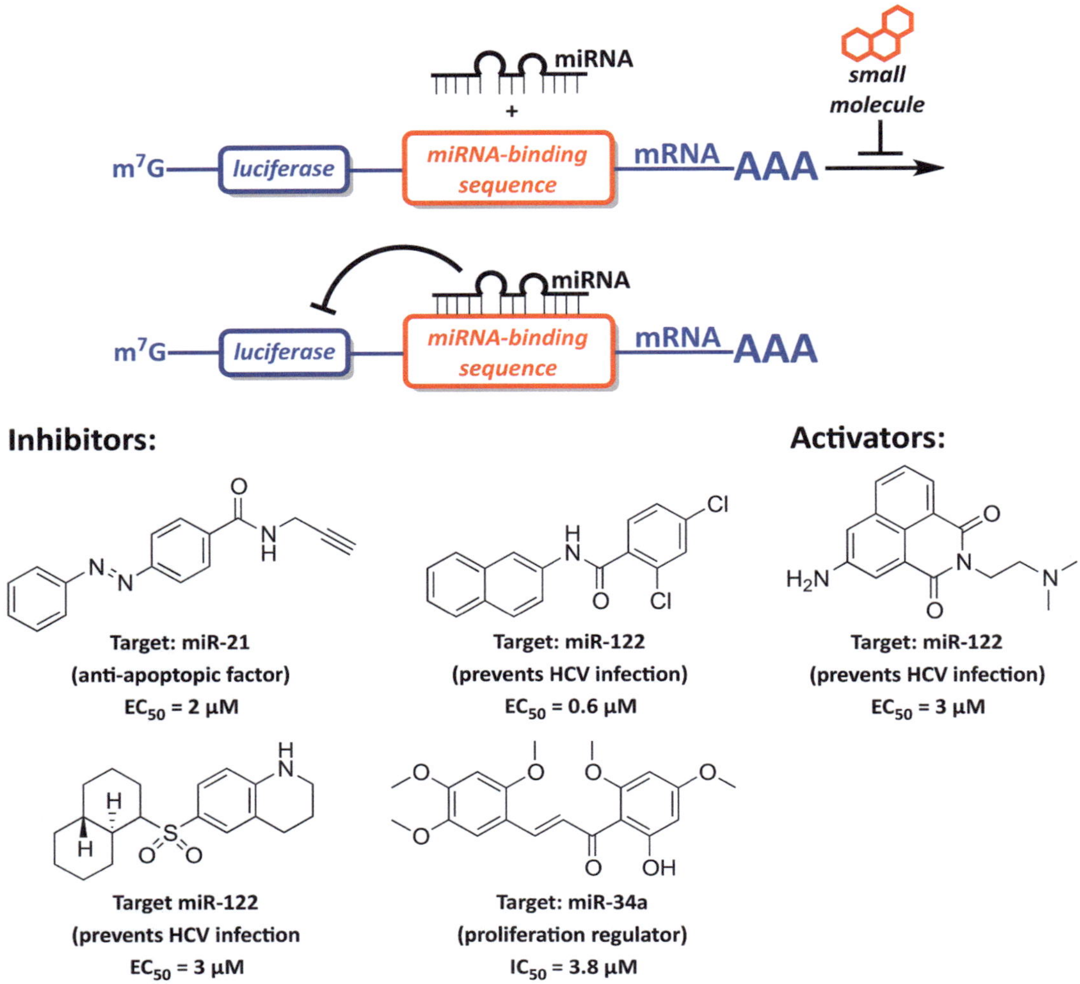


**Fig. 4** Cellular screening assays based on luciferase expression for identification of miRNA small-molecule modulators. Target miRNA downregulates luciferase activity when paired with their specific binding sequence. Figure from [7] with permission

further investigations in in-vitro assays showed [36, 37]. Presumably, the here identified hits bind to somewhere in the complex machinery of the miRNA pathway. Target identification experiments were conducted, however, failed to determine these binding partners.

Nevertheless, Deiters' work is an important milestone in small-molecule miRNA drug discovery as it was shown that a miRNA can be modulated selectively by a small molecule, albeit only indirectly via binding to a protein (most likely) or another macromolecule involved in RNAi pathway. In conclusion, it remains the question what other macromolecules exist that can be targeted by a small molecule modulating only one miRNA function specifically?

### 3.2.2 Small-Molecule Enhancers of DICER-Mediated miRNA Processing

In parallel to Deiters' group, Jin and co-workers developed a *g*reen *f*luorescence *p*rotein (GFP) expression cellular assay and screened a collection of 2000 approved drugs. They identified a small-molecule drug named Enoxacin. Enoxacin induced siRNA-mediated mRNA degradation via general upregulation of miRNA population [38]. Enoxacin is an approved antibiotic drug based on fluoroquinolone scaffold that inhibits bacterial DNA topoisomerase. It was demonstrated that in human tumors miRNA expression is downregulated indicating that miRNA impairment likely contributes to cancer development [39]. Hence, small-molecule inducers of general upregulation of miRNA population may have enormous potential in cancer therapy. From there, it is crucial to elucidate Enoxacin's molecular mechanism. Esteller and co-workers showed that Enoxacin induces DICER-mediated miRNA maturation by binding to TRBP with a $K_D$ of 13 μM (Fig. 5, left) [40]. While Enoxacin is routinely used in antibiotic therapy, its binding affinity to TRBP is too weak that it has no clinical effect. Nonetheless, TRBP is a high-potential drug target for future cancer therapy. This is supported by Maiti and co-workers' findings that quinazoline-based small molecules enhance upregulation of miRNA population (likely through the same mechanism as Enoxacin does) validating this effect is not exclusively dependent on fluoroquinolone scaffold [40].

In summary, miRNA function can be modulated indirectly via targeting TRBP by a small-molecule ligand and represents a promising approach for cancer therapy. However, there are two bottleneck of this approach. Firstly, the identified compounds are still not active enough for the clinical use and it is questionable whether such highly potent can be developed. Secondly, targeting TRBP does not allow the selective modulation of one miRNA of interest. Therefore, targeting TRBP does not fulfill all demands in miRNA drug discovery.

### 3.2.3 Small-Molecule Inhibitors of DICER-Mediated miRNA Processing

Due to miRNAs' short sequence they do not form a complex structure that can accommodate a small-molecule ligand selectively as reported for protein drug targets. From there, the development of a small molecule targeting a miRNA of interest selectively is still a challenge. In contrast to miRNAs, the precursor microRNAs (pre-miRNAs) display a more complex structure increasing the ability to accommodate a small-molecule ligand, referred to as ligandability, providing a higher chance of finding a small molecule binding to them than to miRNA [41].

The groups of Christoph Arenz and Souvik Maiti were the first who focused on pre-miRNA in miRNA drug discovery. They reported independently that aminoglycoside antibiotics such as kanamycin and streptomycin generally block DICER-mediated miRNA maturation by nonspecific binding to the double-stranded DICER substrate pre-miRNA (Fig. 5, right) [42, 43]. Again,

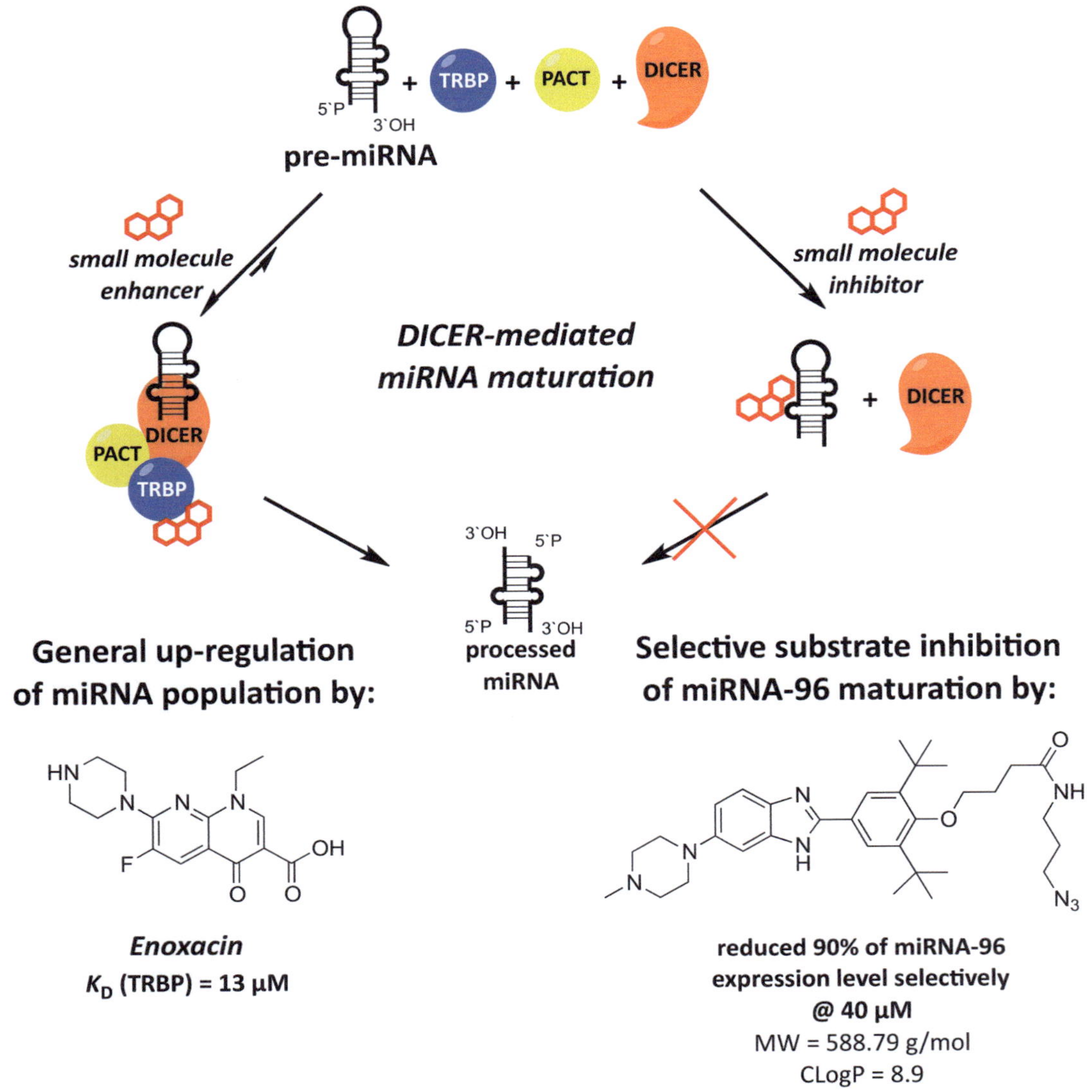


**Fig. 5** Enhancement (*left*) or inhibition (*right*) of DICER-mediated miRNA maturation induced by small molecules. Figure from [7] with permission

inhibition of one specific miRNA selectively was not possible. However, the double-stranded pre-miRNA forms a more stabile secondary structure than miRNA and, from there, provides a good starting point for the rational design of small-molecule ligands. Several approaches have been reported to target pre-miRNA with small molecules specifically. For example, Disney and co-workers predicted secondary structure s of reported pre-miRNAs and compared them to a database of RNA motif small-molecule interactions [44]. They identified a small molecule that binds selectively to pre-miRNA-96, thereby inhibiting the maturation of miRNA-96 (Fig. 5, right). Further investigation showed that this inhibitor selectively reduced 90% of miRNA-96 expression level at a concentration of 40 μM in cellular assays. In conclusion, the more complex pre-miRNA offers a way to target specifically a single miRNA of interest with a small-molecule ligand. However, comparison of identified small-molecule pre-miRNA ligands indicates that these ligands obviously tend to be larger and more lipophilic than members of compound libraries according to the *Lipinski's Rule of Five* [4]. For instance, the identified pre-miRNA-96 ligand by Disney et al. had a higher molecular weight of 588.79 Da and a more lipophilic CLogP of 8.9 than mandatory according to the *Lipinski`s Rule of Five* for protein small molecule ligands. According to this, several high-throughput screening campaigns of drug-like compound libraries against pre-miRNAs yielded insufficient results in regard of potency and selectivity [45, 46]. The question arises whether more lipophilic and larger compounds are suitable for clinical use or do they fail in clinical testing due to their likely inappropriate chemical structure. Summarized, targeting pre-miRNA with its more complex structure has enormous potential for the design of selective miRNA small-molecule ligands. However, it is still the question, whether potent compounds binding to miRNA will work in clinics. The question whether there are no better protein targets in miRNA pathway remains.

### 3.3 Argonaute 2 Protein in miRNA Dug Discovery

miRNA's function is executed via the protein Argonaute 2 (AGO2). miRNA guides the AGO2 protein to the target mRNA by sequence-specific complementarity [2, 3]. Then, AGO2 protein itself recruits several other proteins that form the microRNA-induced silencing complex (miRISC). Recently, the first crystal structures of human Argonaute 2 (hAGO2) protein have been reported [47, 48]. The 859 amino acids long hAGO2 shapes four globular domains: N-terminal, PAZ, MID, and a C-terminal PIWI domain. miRNA binds with its 5′ end to the MID domain. The nucleotides 2–10 track along the RNA binding grove, and nucleotides 17–20 interferes with the PAZ domain. The PIWI domain forms a ribonuclease H-like active site that is responsible for the cleavage of target mRNA specifically after nucleotide 10 at its 3′ end.

The Argonaute 2 protein plays a crucial role in miRNA and, as it is a protein, displays a key target of small molecules in miRNA drug discovery. Several approaches and strategies have been developed to identify small molecules modulating miRNA function via targeting AGO2 protein:

#### 3.3.1 Inhibitors of miRNA Binding to AGO2 (miRISC Loading Inhibitors)

The most prominent small-molecule ligands targeting AGO2 are inhibitors that block the binding of miRNA to AGO2, the so-called miRISC loading inhibitors (Fig. 6a) [49, 50]. However, their therapeutic potential is limited due to the fact the general blockage of AGO2 loading does not allow the modulation of one specific miRNA. A further application of them in clinics is

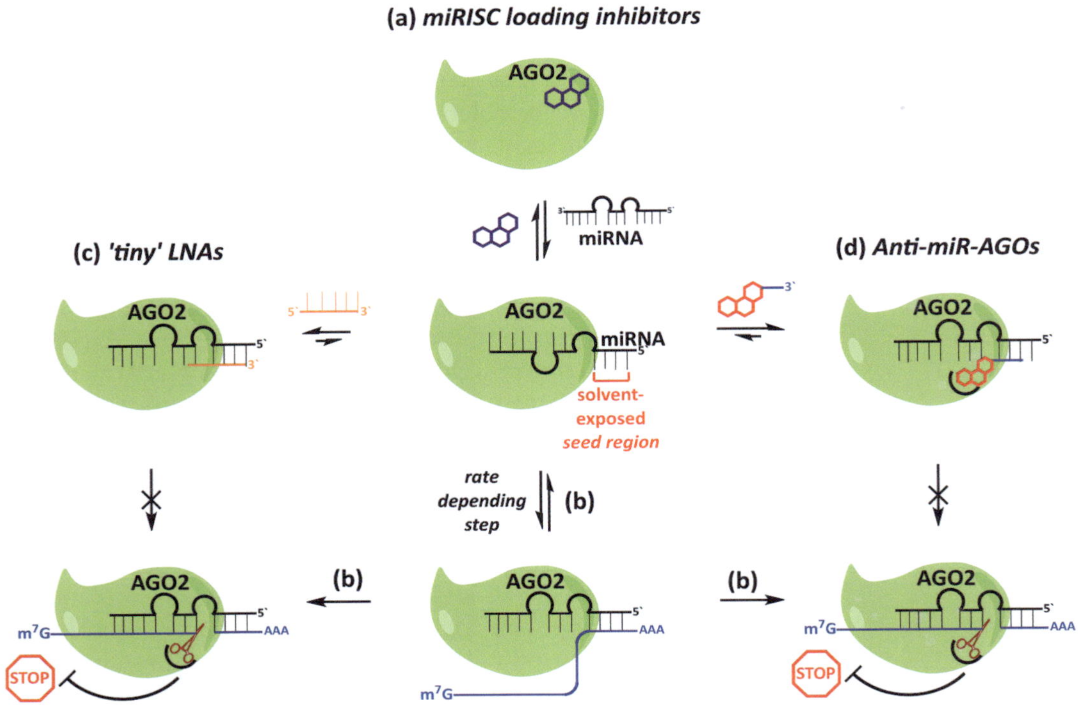


**Fig. 6** Targeting Argonaute 2 protein to modulate miRNAs' function. (**a**) Small-molecule inhibitor of RISC loading (*violet*) blocks generally every miRNA. (**b**) Binding of substrate mRNA occurs in two steps: Firstly, mRNA binds a rate-dependent step to miRNA's 5′-end (seed region). Then, full binding to the miRNA/AGO2 complex occurs. Next, the target mRNA is cleaved by AGO2. (**c**) According to that, short, octamer LNAs (*orange*), so-called 'tiny LNAs', only by blocking miRNA's seed region, inhibit miRNA totally. (**d**) Analogously, an anti-miR-AGO blocks miRNA's seed region (*blue* part of the inhibitor) and then binds additionally in AGO2's active site (*red* part of the inhibitor), thus inhibiting the silencing of target mRNA more effectively. Figure from [7] with permission

questionable. Nonetheless, these compounds have more significance as suitable tools for pathway studies. For instance, Del Rio et al. reported recently that inhibition of miRISC loading showed similar effects to AGO2 *s*mall *h*airpin *RNA* (shRNA)-mediated (a tool to silence gene expression via RNAi) downregulation [50].

### *3.3.2 Antagonists of the miRNA-Argonaute 2 Protein Complex: Anti-miR-AGOs*

Recently, several crystal structures of bacterial and human Argonaute proteins with bound guide strands and RNA substrate have been reported [51]. This together with biochemical investigations gave insights into the molecular mechanism of the gene silencing process [52–54]. The most important finding: The binding of substrate mRNA to the complex of guide miRNA and AGO2 occurs in two steps. Firstly, substrate mRNA binds in a slow, rate-dependent step to the solvent-exposed first eight nucleotides of miRNA's 5′-end, also referred to as 'seed region'. Next, the full binding of substrate mRNA to the miRNA/AGO2 complex happens in fast step (Fig. 6b). Thus, only the blockage of the substrate binding to miRNA's seed region should inhibit the gene silencing.

Indeed, as one of the first Kauppinen and co-workers from Santaris Pharma A/S (now F. Hoffmann-La Roche AG) demonstrated that short, octamer LNAs, so-called 'tiny LNAs', blocking only miRNA's seed region, inhibit miRNA function totally (Fig. 6c) [55]. According to these findings, a new inhibitor class, the *ant*agonists of the *miR*NA-*Argo*naute 2 protein complex (anti-miR-AGOs), were designed [56, 57]: Anti-miR-AGOs consist of a short oligonucleotide sequence and a small-molecule moiety. Analogously to 'tiny LNAs', anti-miR-AGOs bind with their oligonucleotide sequence to the solvent-exposed miRNA's seed region. Next, as anti-miR-AGOs bear a small-molecule moiety at their 3′ end, this small-molecule moiety binds to the active site of AGO2, such as a small-molecule enzyme inhibitor does (Fig. 6c). Finally, anti-miR-AGOs bind to two sites (miRNA's seed region and AGO's active site) benefiting from cooperative binding effects [58–60]. Although anti-miR-AGOs' nucleotide sequence is short (<10 nucleotides), their binding to target mRNA is selectively, as only approximately 2000 miRNAs exist (www.mirbase.org), thus, a hexamer oligonucleotide sequence potentially results in 4096 permutations (four different bases per position). In conclusion, adopting the concept of small molecule to target the AGO2 protein's active site, combined with a short but specific oligonucleotide sequence addressing the miRNA of interest, opens the chance for the development of more hydrophobic molecules with lower molecular weight than reported oligonucleotides inhibitors. Therefore, anti-miR-AGOs may promise better pharmacokinetic properties, providing a chance of tackling delivery issues compared with reported oligonucleotide-based inhibitors, and hopefully enabling them for therapeutic use.

## 4 Conclusion

Until today, several approaches have been developed to modulate miRNAs' function in the hope of potential therapeutic use. Due to the simple structure of miRNA it is a challenge to develop potent drug molecules with appropriate pharmacokinetic properties. Herein, three general strategies have been established to overcome these challenges: Firstly, due to their poor cell permeability, antisense agents targeting miRNA are applied in advanced formulations, or are chemically optimized to increase their delivery. Secondly, efforts were made to develop small-molecule miRNA modulators to overcome antisense agents' limitations. Especially, DICER-mediated miRNA maturation is a target for small molecules. General enhancers of miRNA maturation, as well specific substrate inhibitors, were identified, thereby demonstrating the potential of adopting the concept of small molecules to target miRNA functions. Thirdly, as miRNA function is executed by the

Argonaute 2 protein, new chemical entities, addressing this protein (or its complex with target miRNA of interest) with likely better pharmacokinetic parameters than reported oligonucleotides, may open new perspectives in miRNA drug discovery. In conclusion, miRNAs can be targeted for clinical use. However, it is still a challenge to develop drug molecules with appropriate pharmacokinetic properties as established protocols from protein drug discovery such as *Lipinski's Rule of Five* cannot be directly adopted. Therefore, new concepts differing from established techniques in drug discovery need to be developed. Nevertheless, it is still my firm belief that successful application of these different approaches targeting miRNAs will yield a new generation of drugs enabling the cure of diseases, which presently seem un-curable.

## Acknowledgement

The author thanks Dr. Rajavel Srinivasan for critical proofreading of the manuscript.

### References

1. Bartel DP (2004) MicroRNAs: genomics, biogenesis, mechanism, and function. Cell 116:281–297
2. Dykxhoorn DM, Novina CD, Sharp PA (2003) Killing the messenger: short RNAs that silence gene expression. Nat Rev Mol Cell Biol 4:457–467
3. Fabian MR, Sonenberg N (2012) The mechanisms of miRNA-mediated gene silencing: a look under the hood of miRISC. Nat Struct Mol Biol 19:586–593
4. Overington JP et al (2006) How many drug targets are there? Nat Rev Drug Discov 5:993–996
5. Hopkins AL, Groom CR (2002) The druggable genome. Nat Rev Drug Discov 1:727–730
6. Cheng AC et al (2007) Structure-based maximal affinity model predicts small-molecule druggability. Nature Biotech 25:71–75
7. Schmidt MF (2014) Drug target miRNA: chances and challenges. Trends Biotechnol 32:578–585
8. Li Z, Rana TM (2014) Therapeutic targeting of microRNAs: current status and future challenges. Nat Rev Drug Discov 13:622–638
9. Hutvagner G, Simard MJ, Mello CC, Zamore PD (2004) Sequence-specific inhibition of small RNA function. PLoS Biol 2, E98
10. Meister G, Landthaler M, Dorsett Y, Tuschl T (2004) Sequence-specific inhibition of microRNA- and siRNA-induced RNA silencing. RNA 10:544–550
11. Geary RS (2009) Antisense oligonucleotide pharmacokinetics and metabolism. Expert Opin Drug Metab Toxicol 5:381–391
12. Lennox KA, Behlke MA (2011) Chemical modification and design of anti-miRNA oligonucleotides. Gene Ther 18:1111–1120
13. Esau CC (2008) Inhibition of microRNA with antisense oligonucleotides. Methods 44:55–60
14. Kawasaki AM et al (1993) Uniformly modified 2′-deoxy-2′-fluoro phosphorothioate oligonucleotides as nuclease-resistant antisense compounds with high affinity and specificity for RNA targets. J Med Chem 36:831–841
15. Rigo F et al (2012) Synthetic oligonucleotides recruit ILF2/3 to RNA transcripts to modulate splicing. Nature Chem Biol 8:5974–5982
16. Koshkin AA et al (1998) LNA (locked nucleic acid): synthesis of the adenine, cytosine, guanine, 5-methyl cytosine, thymine, and uracil nicyclonucleoside monomers, oligomers, and unprecedented nucleic acid recognition. Tetrahedron 54:3607–3630
17. Janssen HL et al (2013) Treatment of HCV infection by targeting microRNA. N Engl J Med 368:1685–1694
18. Jopling CL et al (2005) Modulation of hepatitis C virus RNA abundance by a liver-specific microRNA. Science 309:1577–1581
19. Lanford RE et al (2010) Therapeutic silencing of microRNA-122 in primates with chronic hepatitis C virus infection. Science 327:198–201

20. Machlin ES et al (2011) Masking the 5′ terminal nucleotides of the hepatitis C virus genome by an unconventional microRNA-target RNA complex. Proc Natl Acad Sci USA 108:3193–3198
21. Shimakami TD et al (2012) Base pairing between hepatitis C virus RNA and microRNA 122 3′ of its seed sequence is essential for genome stabilization and production of infectious virus. J Virol 86:7372–7383
22. Lindow M, Kauppinen S (2012) Discovering the first microRNA-targeted drug. J Cell Biol 199:407–412
23. Lennox KA, Owczarzy R, Thomas DM, Walder JA, Behlke MA (2013) Improved performance of anti-miRNA oligonucleotide using a novel non-nucleotide modifier. Mol Ther Nucleic Acids 2, e117
24. Krützfeld J, Rajewsky N, Braich R, Rajeev KG, Tuschl T, Manoharan M, Stoffel M (2005) Silencing of microRNAs in vivo with antagomirs. Nature 438:685–689
25. Elmen J et al (2008) LNA-mediated microRNA silencing in non-human primates. Nature 452:896–899
26. Akinc A et al (2010) Targeted delivery of RNAi therapeutics with endogenous and exogenous ligand-based mechanism. Mol Ther 18:1357–1364
27. Bader AG (2012) miR-34 – a microRNA replacement therapy is headed to the clinic. Front Gene 3:120
28. Zhao J et al (2013) In-depth analysis shows synergy between erlotinib and miR-34a. PLoS ONE 9, e89105
29. Gilleron J et al (2013) Image-based analysis of lipid nanoparticle-mediated siRNA delivery, intracellular trafficking and endosomal escape. Nature Biotech 31:638–646
30. Li Z, Yang CS, Nakashima K, Rana TM (2011) Small RNA-mediated regulation of iPS cell generation. EMBO J 30:823–834
31. Bartel DP (2009) MicroRNAs: target recognition and regulatory functions. Cell 136:215–233
32. Sarvestani ST et al (2015) Sequence-dependent off-target inhibition of TLR7/8 sensing by synthetic microRNA inhibitors. Nucleic Acids Res 43:1177–1188
33. Hornung V et al (2005) Sequence-specific potent induction of IFN-α by short interfering RNA in plasmacytoid dendritic cells through TLR7. Nature Med 11:263–270
34. Bennett CF, Swayze EE (2010) RNA targeting therapeutics: molecular mechanisms of antisense oligonucleotides as a therapeutic platform. Annu Rev Pharmacol Toxicol 50:259–293
35. Swayze EE et al (2007) Antisense oligonucleotides containing locked nucleic acid improve potency but cause significant hepatotoxicity in animals. Nucleic Acids Res 35:687–700
36. Gumireddy K et al (2008) Small-molecule inhibitors of microRNA miR-21 function. Angew Chem Int Ed 47:7482–7484
37. Young DD et al (2010) Small molecule modifiers of microRNA miR-122 function for the treatment of hepatitis C virus infection and hepatocellular carcinoma. J Am Chem Soc 132:7976–7981
38. Shan G et al (2010) A small molecule enhances RNA interference and promotes microRNA processing. Nat Biotechnol 26:933–940
39. Lu J et al (2005) MicroRNA expression profiles classify human cancers. Nature 435:834–838
40. Melo S et al (2011) Small molecule enoxacin is a cancer-specific growth inhibitor that acts by enhancing TAR RNA-binding protein 2-mediated microRNA processing. Proc Natl Acad Sci USA 108:4394–4399
41. Nahar S et al (2014) Anticancer therapeutic potential of quinazoline based small molecules via upregulation of miRNAs. Chem Comm 50:4639–4642
42. Davies BP, Arenz C (2006) A homogenous assay for microRNA maturation. Angew Chem Int Ed 45:5550–5552
43. Bose D et al (2012) The tuberculosis drug streptomycin as a potential cancer therapeutic: inhibition of miR-21 function by directly targeting its precursor. Angew Chem Int Ed 51:1019–1023
44. Velagapudi SP et al (2014) Sequence-based design of bioactive small molecules that target precursor microRNAs. Nat Chem Biol 10:291–297
45. Bose D et al (2013) A molecular-beacon screen for small molecule inhibitors of miRNA maturation. ACS Chem Biol 8:930–938
46. Neubacher S et al (2011) A rapid assay for miRNA maturation by using unmodified pre-miRNA. ChemBioChem 12:2302–2305
47. Schirle NT, MacRae IJ (2012) The crystal structure of human Argonaute 2. Science 336:1037–1040
48. Elkayam E et al (2012) The structure of human Argonaute-2 in complex with miR20a. Cell 150:100–110
49. Tan GS et al (2012) Small molecule inhibition of RISC loading. ACS Chem Biol 7:403–410
50. Masciarelli S et al (2014) A small-molecule targeting the microRNA binding domain of Argonaute 2 improves the retinoic acid differentiation response of the acute promyelocytic

leukemia cell line NB4. ACS Chem Biol 9:1674–1679
51. Wang Y et al (2009) Nucleation, propagation, and cleavage of target RNAs in Ago silencing complexes. Nature 461:754–761
52. Kole R, Krainer AR, Altman S (2012) RNA therapeutics: beyond RNA interference and antisense oligonucleotides. Nat Rev Drug Discov 11:125–140
53. Chi SW et al (2012) An alternative mode of microRNA target recognition. Nat Struct Mol Biol 19:321–327
54. Kumar S et al (2014) Understanding the effect of LNA and 2′-O methyl modification on the hybridization thermodynamics of miRNA-mRNA pair in the presence and absence of AfPiwi protein. Biochemistry 53:1607–1615
55. Obad S et al (2011) Silencing of microRNA families by seed-targeting tiny LNAs. Nat Genet 43:371–378
56. Schmidt MF, Korb O, Abell C (2013) MicroRNA-specific Argonaute 2 protein inhibitors. ACS Chem Biol 8:2122–2126
57. Matsuyama Y et al (2013) Functional regulation of RNA-induced silencing complex by photoreactive oligonucleotides. Bioorg Med Chem 22:1003–1007
58. Schmidt MF, Rademann J (2009) Dynamic template-assisted strategies in fragment-based drug discovery. Trends Biotechnol 27:512–521
59. Schmidt MF et al (2008) Sensitized detection of inhibitory fragments and iterative development of non-peptidic protease inhibitors by dynamic ligation screening. Angew Chem Int Ed 47:3275–3278
60. Schmidt MF et al (2009) Selective identification of cooperatively binding fragments in a high-throughput ligation assay enables development of a picomolar caspase-3 inhibitor. Angew Chem Int Ed 48:6346–6349

# Part II

## Protocols

# Chapter 2

# Functional Analysis of miRNAs Using the DIANA Tools Online Suite

**Ioannis S. Vlachos and Artemis G. Hatzigeorgiou**

## Abstract

microRNAs (miRNAs) are central regulators of gene expression. They are actively studied for their involvement in numerous physiological and pathological conditions but also as diagnostic biomarkers or promising therapeutic targets. The increased complexity of the miRNA interactomes hinders straightforward interpretation of miRNA expression differences between states and conditions. To this end, functional analysis web servers process and combine experimental and in silico data, enabling researchers to uncover targeted pathways and transcriptional mechanisms that are hidden within numerous interactions and vast expression datasets. DIANA-tools (www.microrna.gr) is a web server hosting state-of-the-art utilities and databases for miRNA functional investigation. Available utilities cover a wide scope of different needs and research scenarios, rendering DIANA website a one-stop-shop for miRNA analyses. The most commonly utilized databases and algorithms include DIANA-microT-CDS, DIANA-TarBase v7.0, DIANA-lncBase v2.0, DIANA-miRGen v3.0, DIANA-miRPath v3.0, and DIANA-mirExTra v2.0.

In the presented protocol, we will utilize different online tools in order to explore miRNA functions and to identify probable targets of interest for downstream analyses and wet lab experiments. The combined use of different applications from the DIANA suite can shed light to numerous different aspects of miRNA regulation and regulatory function, without the necessity for extensive bioinformatics expertise or computational infrastructure.

**Key words** microRNA, miRNA, Transcription factor, RNA-Seq, Small RNA-Seq, miRNA-Seq, Pathways, Gene ontology, Transcription start site, CLIP-Seq

## 1 Introduction

microRNAs (miRNAs) are central regulators of gene expression. They are actively studied for their involvement in numerous physiological and pathological conditions but also as diagnostic biomarkers or promising therapeutic targets [1]. From very early on, progress in our understanding of miRNA biogenesis and function went hand in hand with advances of relevant in silico tools and experimental methodologies.

Currently available in silico tools and databases cover an extensive array of services and applications, including target prediction,

Marco F. Schmidt (ed.), *Drug Target miRNA: Methods and Protocols*, Methods in Molecular Biology, vol. 1517,
DOI 10.1007/978-1-4939-6563-2_2, © Springer Science+Business Media New York 2017

functional investigation, as well as repositories of expression, sequences, and experimental findings [1]. miRNA target prediction algorithms were the first implementations that enabled researchers to select probable candidates for wet lab validation or for the investigation of miRNA involvement in biological mechanisms. Current implementations use sophisticated models, machine learning, and biophysical properties in order to identify miRNA:mRNA or miRNA:lncRNA interactions. Despite the progress in the field, even the most advanced implementations do not still exhibit perfect predictive accuracy [2]. Therefore, databases of experimentally validated targets have become essential tools for mapping the complex miRNA interactome, where a single miRNA can target dozens or even hundreds of mRNAs [3]. We now know that multiple miRNAs collaborate by sharing targets or by targeting different genes participating to the same pathways or functions. The increased complexity of the combined miRNA actions hinders straightforward interpretation of miRNA expression differences between states and conditions. To this end, functional analysis web servers analyze and combine experimental and in silico data, enabling researchers to uncover targeted pathways and transcriptional mechanisms that are hidden within the vast interactome and expression datasets.

DIANA-tools (www.microrna.gr) is a web server hosting state-of-the-art tools and databases for miRNA research and functional investigation [4]. Available utilities cover a very large scope of different needs and research scenarios, rendering DIANA website a one-stop-shop for miRNA analyses. The most commonly utilized databases and algorithms, include DIANA-microT-CDS [4], DIANA-TarBase v7.0 [3], DIANA-lncBase v2.0 [5], DIANA-miRGen v3.0 [6], DIANA-miRPath v3.0 [7], and DIANA-mirExTra v2.0. A brief introduction to each tool is presented below:

*DIANA-microT* was one of the first implemented algorithms for miRNA:mRNA target identification [8]. DIANA-microT-CDS (http://www.microrna.gr/microT-CDS/) is its fifth version [4] and enables the accurate detection of miRNA targets in mRNA 3′UTR and CDS sequences. It supports 4 species: *Homo sapiens*, *Mus musculus*, *Drosophila melanogaster*, and *Caenorhabditis elegans*.

*DIANA-TarBase* is the largest manually curated repository of experimentally validated miRNA:mRNA interactions. DIANA-TarBase v7.0 (www.microrna.gr/tarbase) comprises more than 600,000 experimentally supported miRNA:gene interactions spanning 24 species and 356 different cell types [3]. The interactions are derived from thousands of manually curated publications, specific experiments as well as in-house analyzed high-throughput methodologies, including CLIP-Seq, CLASH, RNA-Seq, Degradome-Seq, microarrays, biotin pull-down, miTRAP, IMPACT-Seq, and 3′LIFE.

*DIANA-LncBase* is the first database of miRNA:lncRNA interactions. Its second version, DIANA-LncBase v2.0 [5], hosts in silico-predicted and experimentally supported interactions as well as extensive lncRNA expression data for human and mouse. The experimentally supported interactions have been derived from manually curated publications and the analysis of >150 AGO-CLIP-Seq datasets.

*DIANA-miRGen* is a database of miRNA transription regulation [6]. DIANA-miRGen v3.0 comprises accurate cell-line-specific miRNA transcription start sites (TSS) and genome-wide maps of transcription factor (TF) binding sites derived from the in silico/experimental microTSS [9] framework and the analysis of more than seven billion next generation sequencing (NGS) reads.

*DIANA-miRPath* is a web server dedicated to the assessment of miRNA regulatory roles and combined miRNA function [7]. DIANA-miRPath v3.0 enables the functional annotation of one or more miRNAs and the identification of miRNA-controlled pathways. It utilizes sophisticated statistics including meta-analysis methodologies and empirical distributions in order to translate large experimentally validated and in silico predicted miRNA interactomes to functional information. Experimentally supported information is derived from TarBase v7.0, while predictions are calculated using microT-CDS and/or TargetScan v6.2 [10]. It fully supports seven species: *Homo sapiens*, *Mus musculus*, *Rattus norvegicus*, *Drosophila melanogaster*, *Caenorhabditis elegans*, *Gallus gallus*, and *Danio rerio*.

*DIANA-mirExTra v2.0* is a web server that can analyze miRNA and mRNA NGS expression datasets, in order to uncover miRNAs and TFs playing central regulatory roles between two investigated states or conditions. Users can upload and analyze their NGS miRNA/mRNA expression datasets or combine them with the extensive mirExTra expression database. DIANA-mirExTra v2.0 can identify miRNAs controlling mRNAs, TFs regulating mRNAs and TFs regulating miRNAs between two conditions. It supports 4 species: *Homo sapiens*, *Mus musculus*, *Drosophila melanogaster*, and *Caenorhabditis elegans*.

In the presented protocol, we will utilize different DIANA online tools in order to uncover miRNA functions and to identify probable targets of interest for downstream analyses and wet lab experiments. Certainly, all tools are completely autonomous and can be utilized separately. However, most research scenarios can benefit from information provided from different algorithms and databases. The combined use of DIANA-tools can shed light to numerous different aspects of miRNA regulation and regulatory function, without the necessity for extensive bioinformatics expertise or computational infrastructure.

## 2 Materials

All DIANA web servers, tools, and databases are free to use without requiring login or registration. Users should have access to a personal computer, work station, or server (Windows, Linux, Unix, or Mac OS) with an installed web browser (e.g. Mozilla, Chrome, Safari, Opera) and an internet connection. DIANA-tools can also be accessed from most web browser-enabled smartphones or tablets. DIANA web servers also offer files for download in order to be stored or used subsequent analyses. These files are provided in image (.jpg or .png), text, spreadsheet (.xls or .csv) and compressed (.zip) files. Therefore, applications for image viewing, text editing, spread sheet file processing (e.g. MS Office, OpenOffice, or LibreOffice) and file decompression should be installed. This analysis will utilize solely online stored files and data. However, all tools also support user data import. The relevant formats and examples will be provided in each specific step in the Subheading 3, while tips for optimal setup are presented in Subheading 4. Most DIANA applications also support user accounts, which can further extend existing functionalities (*see* **Note** 1).

## 3 Methods

The latest human miRBase (v21) annotation comprises around 2.5K human miRNAs [11], while each of those miRNAs can target numerous different mRNAs. Wet lab studies require resources, time, and cost. Selection of the best candidate miRNAs for further investigation can be often crucial to the project's outcome. Plausible miRNAs for study can be identified through literature searches (known miRNAs), from their targets (bottom-up search), their function or pathways they control (functional analyses and reverse search), as well as based on whether they significantly alter their expression between conditions (differential expression analysis) or whether they control most of the mRNAs that alter their expression between states (functional differential expression analysis). This protocol utilizes all these techniques to select miRNAs for downstream studies as possible therapeutic targets, key regulators, or biomarkers. These fundamental techniques can be mixed and matched in order to support a wide scope of research topics.

### 3.1 Selecting Candidate miRNAs for Downstream Studies from NGS Differential Expression Analyses

miRNAs significantly altering their expression between two groups, states or conditions (e.g. healthy vs patient, tumor vs normal tissue, treated vs untreated cells, etc.) can affect targeted gene expression and contribute to the observed phenotypic differences. High-throughput methodologies such as microarrays or NGS are often utilized for a hypothesis-free identification of such miRNAs. Small-RNA-Seq is an advantageous method, since the expression of all known miRNAs can be assessed in the examined samples (*see* **Note 2**). Following sequencing, pre-processing and alignment, small-RNA-Seq experiments result in long lists of miRNA identifiers associated with read counts as measures of expression. The comparison of the estimated expression levels between two states is often referenced as "differential expression analysis". This section shows how to perform such analyses online using DIANA-mirExTra v2.0.

1. Using a web browser navigate to http://www.microrna.gr/mirextrav2.
2. Select "Differential Expression Analysis" from the main menu. In the differential expression analysis (DE) web page of mirExTra (Fig. 1), users can perform miRNA or gene DE by uploading their own expression datasets or using pre-analyzed NGS data from the mirExTra database. Imported data can be derived from user-performed experiments or from datasets available in public repositories such as Gene Expression Omnibus (GEO) [12], UCSC [13] and ENCODE [14]. mirExTra can directly import NGS expression datasheets by pressing the "Your miRNAs (or genes) expr. File" button. The compatible file format is explained in the help section of the web server, which is accessible through the "Help (?)" button. In this protocol, we will utilize expression data from the extensive mirExTra database. Select "Use stored" in the miRNA expression file menu.
3. In the pop-up miRNA expression database window, select: Species: "Human", Group A: "Fetal Lung Fibroblasts" [Fetal Lung Fibroblasts (Lung,Embryonic/Fetal,Stem/Progenitor, Ag04450)].
   Group B: "Embryonic Stem Cells" [Embryonic Stem Cells (Embryo,Embryonic/Fetal,Stem/Progenitor,H1hESC)].

Of course, users can substitute any of the selected groups in this example with any groups relevant to their field of study. Press "Go!" and the web page automatically returns to the DE settings pane.

4. Subsequently, setup the DE settings: Species: "Human", Statistical Method: "DESeq", miRNA FDR threshold: 0.05, Gene FDR Threshold: 0.05, Create comparison graphs: ticked, Create group homogeneity graphs: ticked and Results format: xls (Fig. 1). With these settings, we have asked mirExTra to perform the miRNA DE analysis using DESeq algorithm [15], we have selected the necessary thresholds for calling statistically significant results and the output file format. We have also requested all relevant graphs to be produced, which help in understanding the possible differences between the two sample groups (comparison graphs) or to check for consistency between replicates (homogeneity graphs) (*see* **Note 3**). mirExTra also supports other state of the art algorithms, such as limma [16] and edgeR [17], which can be used by changing the relevant selection in the dropdown list.

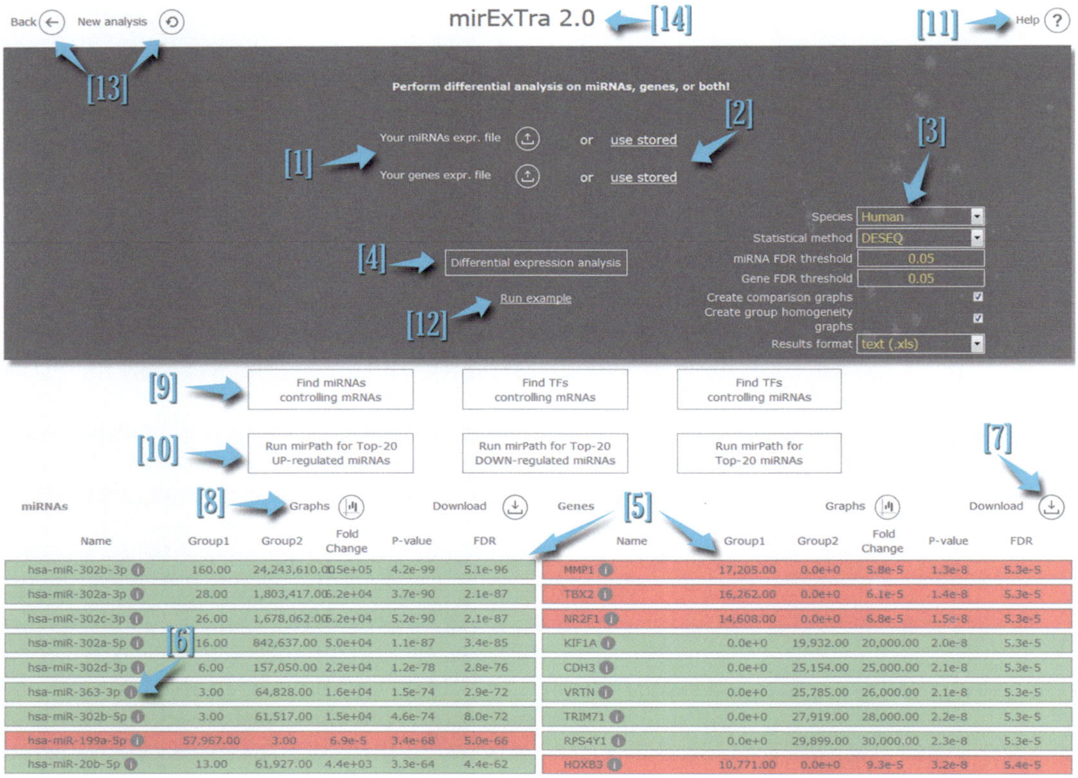


**Fig. 1** DIANA-mirExTra v2.0 Differential Expression Module following a parallel miRNA and mRNA expression analysis. In this module users can directly upload miRNA/mRNA expression files (*1*) or use the mirExTra expression database (*2*). From the options panel (*3*) users can set up the analysis and select the employed algorithm, produced graphs and utilized thresholds. The procedure starts by pressing the relevant button (*4*). The results panel is divided into two sub-panes for miRNAs and mRNAs, respectively (*5*). Meta-data and links for each molecule are available from the accompanying information button (*6*). All results can be downloaded for later use (*7*). Requested graphs are shown by pressing the "Graphs" button (*8*). The regulator identification (miRNAs or TFs) modules can be directly invoked following a parallel miRNA and mRNA differential expression analysis (*9*). Top results can be exported to miRPath for further functional investigation (*10*). Help (*11*), Example run (*12*), Back/Reset (*13*), and Home (*14*) buttons assist user navigation

5. Select "Differential expression analysis" in order to start the procedure. In analyses that are estimated to require more than 1 min to complete, the web server provides a unique link, enabling users to return to the results at a later point in time.
6. Results for miRNA DE analysis are presented on the lower right part of the web page. Significantly up- and downregulated miRNAs are marked with green and red, respectively.
7. Press the "Graphs" button to examine the created graphs. All graphs can be saved for later use from the web browser.
8. To save the results file, select the "Download" button above the results pane.

9. Candidate miRNAs for further analysis are located in the top positions of the list. Since many of those miRNAs can exhibit significant deregulation between the two conditions, further information is often required to reduce the number of possible candidates. Such information includes: miRNA targets (predicted and validated), metadata, and functional information. Press the information button "(i)" next to the miRNA names, in order to open the miRNA information pane. This pane leads to miRNA metadata, including its name, sequence, and identifiers; while providing links to external databases, as well as DIANA-tools in order to further examine the candidate microRNA. Specifically, the available links include:
   (a) "microT-CDS": to examine predicted targets of the selected miRNA.
   (b) "TarBase v.7": for experimentally validated targets.
   (c) "LncBase Experimental": to access experimentally supported targets of this miRNA on lncRNAs.
   (d) "LncBase Predicted": for predicted targets on lncRNAs.
   (e) "miRPath v.3": to analyze the function of this miRNA and its effects on molecular pathways.
10. Keep the web page in a separate tab, in order to continue this analysis in Subheading 3.4.

### 3.2 Examining miRNA Targets in mRNA 3′ UTR and CDS Regions In Silico with DIANA-microT-CDS

We will further examine the top result of the analysis conducted in 3.1 (hsa-miR-302b-3p) and identify its predicted targets in 3′UTR and CDS sequences. This analysis can be performed for any other miRNA.

1. In the web page of the DE results (Subheading 3.1, **step 10**), press the "(i)" information button next to the miRNA name (hsa-miR-302b-3p) and then select "microT-CDS" or visit directly the microT-CDS web page (http://www.microrna.gr/microT-CDS) and enter "hsa-miR-302b-3p" in the search box (Fig. 2).
2. All in silico predicted targets for this miRNA are presented in the results pane, which shows the Gene target ID, its name, prediction score, and whether this interaction is predicted from other algorithms.
3. Further information regarding the interaction can be derived from the black arrow pointing downwards on the right side of the results pane. The pane includes the following information:
   (a) Gene details and metadata: accessible from the "(i)" information button. The metadata include a list of tissues and cell types where this gene is expressed, links to Ensembl [18] database and to DIANA-tools.
   (b) miRNA details and metadata: accessible from the relevant "(i)" information button. The metadata include the

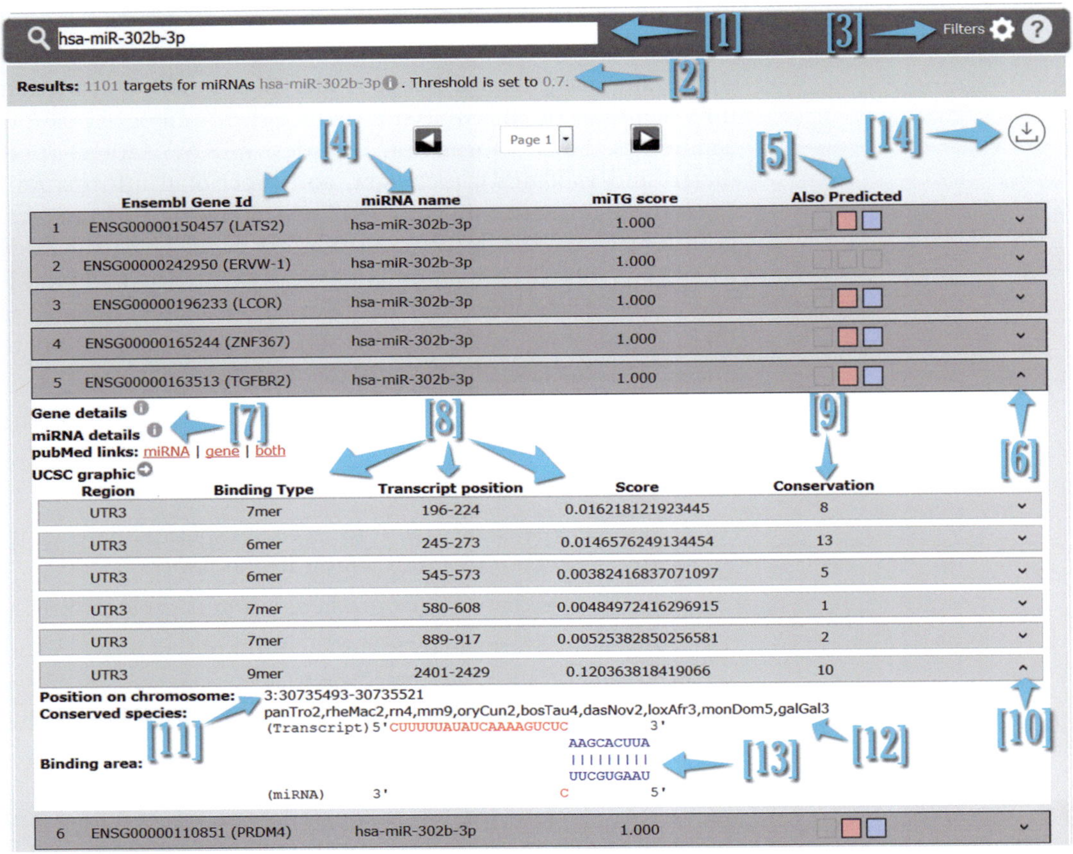


**Fig. 2** DIANA-microT-CDS interface. Following a query for a miRNA in microT-CDS (*1*), the result summary is presented below the relevant edit box (*2*). Results can be further filtered by selecting the gear button (*3*). The identified interactions populate the results pane (*4*). Colors are used to mark interactions also predicted by other algorithms (*5*). The MRE panel can be expanded for each interaction (*6*). This panel provides access to tools and metadata for the interacting miRNA and mRNA (*7*), as well as extensive information regarding the identified binding sites (*8*). Each binding site can be further expanded (*10*). The sub-panel shows the MRE genomic location (*11*), conserved species (*12*), and the miRNA:mRNA duplex conformation (*13*). All results can be saved and downloaded (*14*)

miRNA name, sequence, links to miRBase database and a tag cloud of terms related to this miRNA from available publications.

(c) PubMed links: queries for PubMed articles mentioning the miRNA, the target gene or both.

(d) UCSC graphic: leads to a pop up window showing the genomic region of the target gene and its binding site in UCSC genome browser.

(e) The individual microRNA binding elements (MREs) or binding sites: each MRE is characterized by each region (UTR3 or CDS), its binding type (6mer, 7mer, 8mer,

9mer), transcript position, MRE prediction score, and conservation index (number of species where this MRE is found conserved) (see Note 4).

(f) Further MRE information: accessed from expanding each MRE section, providing its genomic location, the species where the MRE is conserved and the binding conformation graphic (see Note **4**).

4. Each miRNA can have hundreds of predicted targets. DIANA-microT-CDS offers the option to filter results based on their interaction score. The option is revealed after selecting the gear button on the top right of the pane. One is the maximum score and lower values signify smaller probabilities of functional impact. Depending on the type of the study (highly specific or investigative) different thresholds can be utilized (*see* **Note 5**).
5. Download all results for later use or inclusion to local pipelines by pressing the download button on the right of the navigation panel.

### 3.3 Meta-Analyzing Thousands of miRNA Experiments in DIANA-TarBase

Even the most sophisticated miRNA target prediction algorithms still cannot achieve perfect predictive accuracy. DIANA-TarBase v7.0 hosts hundreds of thousands of experimentally supported miRNA:gene interactions. We will use DIANA-TarBase v7.0 to examine also if the selected miRNA (hsa-miR-302b-3p) has also experimentally validated interactions with genes of interest. This analysis can be also repeated for any other miRNA.

1. In the web page of the DE results (Subheading 3.1, **step 10**), press the "(i)" information button next to the miRNA name (hsa-miR-302b-3p) and then select "TarBase v.7" or visit TarBase web page (http://www.microrna.gr/tarbase) and enter "hsa-miR-302b-3p" in the search box (Fig. 3).
2. The results pane shows the gene target's name, the targeting miRNA, the experimental methods that support the interaction, and a prediction score if an interaction is also predicted by microT-CDS. All positive results are marked with green in the methods section, negative are shown in red, while experiments showing conflicting results use both colors (*see* **Note 6**).
3. Further information regarding each interaction can be accessed by pressing the downwards pointing arrow. The revealed pane shows the supporting studies, methods used in each publication, as well as the tissue, cell line, and experimental conditions for each experiment (*see* **Note 2**). When binding site coordinates are available, these are also presented in the relevant pane. For reporter gene assays, the primers utilized for cloning can be accessed by pressing the "(i)" button between the "Location" and "Method" columns. In the revealed pop-up window, a link is also provided that leads to Ensembl Genome browser showing the exact binding site location.

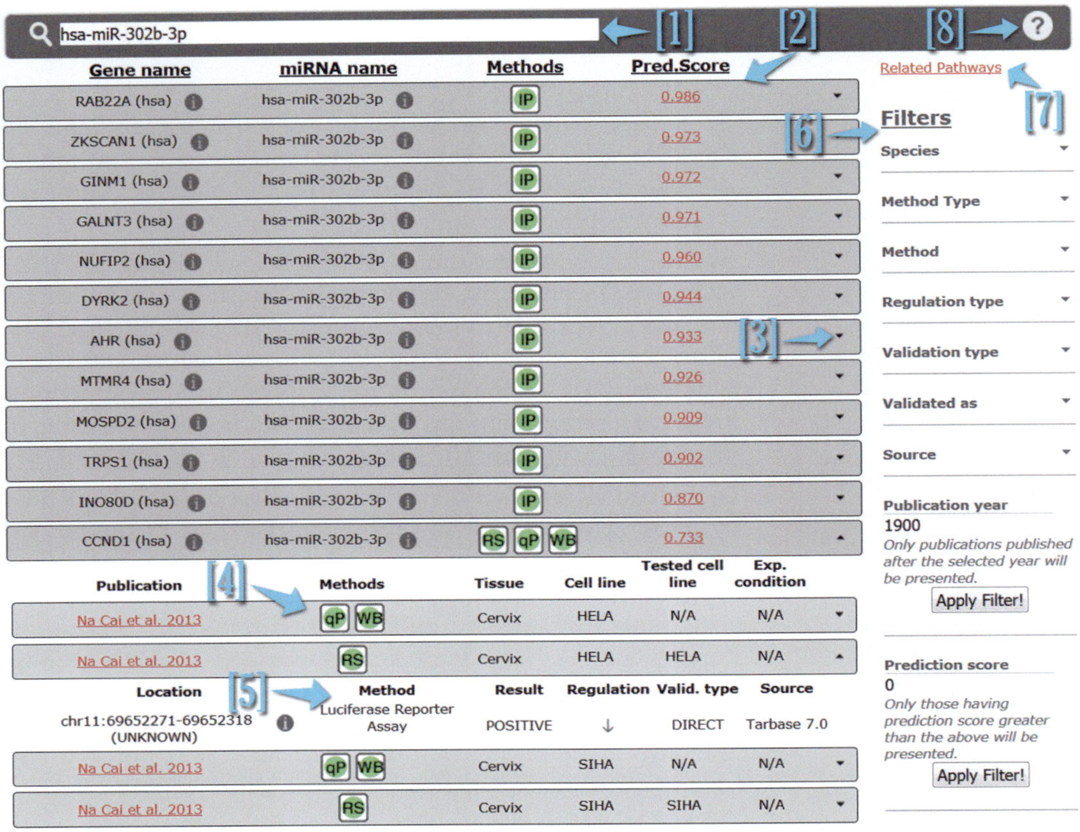


**Fig. 3** The interface of DIANA-TarBase v7.0. miRNA and gene names can be inserted into the query edit box (*1*). All results are presented below (*2*). Each interaction can be further expanded to provide more detailed information (*3*), including the supporting publication, and the experimental methods (*4*). By further expanding an experiment, we have access to the binding site location, the employed method (*5*), as well as the outcome of the interaction. All results can be filtered with multiple parameters (*6*). The investigated miRNA can be forwarded to miRPath for functional examination (*7*). Detailed use information can be found in the help section (*8*)

4. The column on the right offers advanced filtering options. All results can be filtered based on numerous features, including species, method type, method, regulation type, validation type, and publication year (*see* **Note 7**). For instance, in order to select all the entries that have been also validated by reporter gene assays, press "Method" on the filter pane and check the "Luciferase Reporter Assay" check box. All entries that have been validated with this technique are shown in the results pane. In order to remove the filter, press the "X" button next to "Remove all" in the Filters box.
5. By combining predicted interactions from DIANA-microT-CDS with high-quality experimentally supported interactions from DIANA-TarBase v7.0, we can chart the interactome of the investigated miRNAs and find important targets that have already been validated or candidates for wet lab assessment.

### 3.4 Identifying miRNAs with Regulatory Roles Through Combined Analyses of Small-RNA-Seq and RNA-Seq Expression Data with DIANA-mirExTra v2.0

Often, the deregulated miRNAs identified in Subheading 3.1 are many and those exhibiting the most potent regulatory roles have to be selected for downstream investigations. DIANA-mirExTra v2.0 can combine mRNA and miRNA expression data, in order to identify miRNAs having the most significant impact on mRNA expression between two conditions (*see* **Note 2**). This is a powerful analysis and can be performed on user-provided data, mirExTra expression database datasets, or their combinations.

1. In the web page of the DE results (Subheading 3.1, **step 10**) select genes - > "used stored" and select Group A: "Fetal Lung Fibroblasts" [Fetal Lung Fibroblasts (Lung,Embryonic/Fetal,Stem/Progenitor,IMR90)] and Group B: "Embryonic Stem Cells" [Embryonic Stem Cells (Embryo,Embryonic/Fetal,Stem/Progenitor,H1hESC)].

   Alternatively, navigate to http://www.microrna.gr/mirextrav2 and select: miRNAs → "use stored" and Group A: "Fetal Lung Fibroblasts" [Fetal Lung Fibroblasts (Lung,Embryonic/Fetal,Stem/Progenitor,Ag04450)], Group B: "Embryonic Stem Cells" [Embryonic Stem Cells (Embryo,Embryonic/Fetal,Stem/Progenitor,H1hESC)]. Subsequently, select genes → "used stored" and select Group A: "Fetal Lung Fibroblasts" [Fetal Lung Fibroblasts (Lung,Embryonic/Fetal,Stem/Progenitor,IMR90)] and Group B: "Embryonic Stem Cells" [Embryonic Stem Cells (Embryo,Embryonic/Fetal,Stem/Progenitor,H1hESC)].

2. We will use the same settings for DE analysis as in Subheading 3.1, **step 3** (Species: "Human", Statistical Method: DESeq, miRNA FDR threshold: 0.05, Gene FDR Threshold: 0.05, Create comparison graphs: ticked, Create group homogeneity graphs: ticked and Results format: xls) but this time mirExTra will analyze mRNA and miRNA expression datasets in parallel, since both have been selected.
3. Press "Differential expression analysis" to commence the procedure. The results will be presented in the main panel below, with miRNA and mRNA DE in the left and right sub panes, respectively (Fig. 1) (*see* **Note 8**).
4. When both miRNA and mRNA expression datasets have been concurrently analyzed, mirExTra enables the "Find miRNAs and TFs with crucial roles" module (*see* **Note 9**). This module permits users to identify the most important regulators (miRNAs and TFs) that control mRNA or miRNA expression changes between two conditions. These modules can be also directly accessed by selecting "Find miRNAs and TFs with crucial roles" in the mirExTra home page. In that case, users must upload DE datasets for mRNAs (for TF:mRNA investigations) or DE miRNA and DE mRNA datasets for TF:miRNA and

miRNA:mRNA combined analyses. The format of these files is explained in mirExTra help section in detail. The module can also be populated with data generated from a mirExTra DE analysis, without the necessity of importing data files. In this case study, we have just generated these datasets by performing a parallel DE analysis of miRNAs and mRNAs, enabling the functionality of the relevant modules. Press the "Find miRNAs controlling mRNAs" button.

5. In the "Find miRNAs with central roles by combining mRNA and miRNA expression" module, we can utilize predicted (microT-CDS) or experimentally supported (TarBase v7.0) miRNA interactions, in order to identify which differentially expressed miRNAs had a significant functional impact on mRNA expression between the two studied conditions. We usually perform both analyses and compare the result sets, since they depend on different rules and interaction datasets. Experimentally supported targets have higher specificity, while predicted interactions tend to be more sensitive. However, the specificity level of predictions can be adjusted in mirExTra from the microT-CDS score threshold option, with higher values increasing specificity but reducing sensitivity (*see* **Note 5**). The threshold type is a means to select which miRNAs or mRNAs will be considered as differentially expressed between the two conditions. This module offers more options than the relevant DE module, since users can select to set thresholds based on fold change, *p*-values, and FDR levels or arbitrarily select those subsets in user imported files (*see* **Note 10**). For this case study, select: species: "Human", Interactions based on: microT-CDS, microT-CDS score threshold: 0.7, "Threshold type: FDR, miRNAs threshold value 0.05, Genes threshold value: 0.05. Press "Find miRNAs" to commence the analysis (Fig. 4).
6. The results are presented below in two different sub-panes. Upregulated and downregulated miRNAs are presented separately in the left and right panel, respectively. Each miRNA name is accompanied with the relevant *p*-value, showing the functional analysis significance level. miRNAs having more targets in the oppositely differentially expressed mRNAs (upregulated miRNAs having many downregulated mRNA targets and vice versa) will exhibit the lowest *p*-values. The top results in this analysis are often the best candidate molecules for downstream investigation.
7. All results can be downloaded for later use by pressing the individual "Download" buttons above the up- and downregulated miRNA columns or the "Download all" button on the right. The result files offer extensive metadata and information regarding the examined miRNAs.

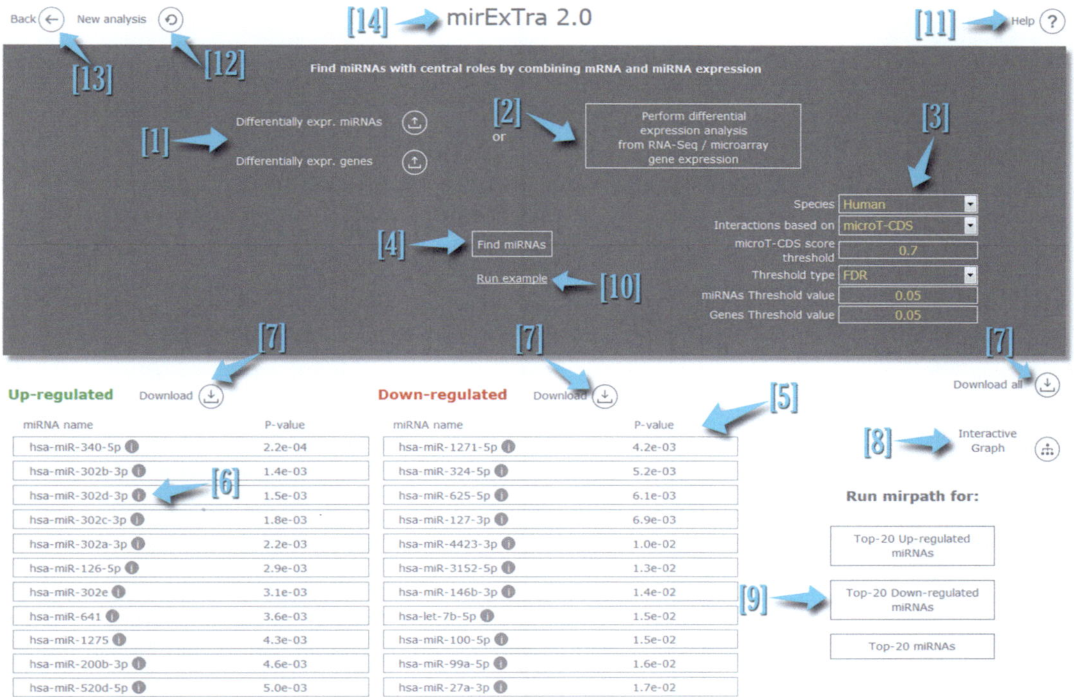


**Fig. 4** DIANA-mirExTra v2.0 "Find miRNAs with central roles" module. Users can directly upload differentially expressed genes and miRNAs (*1*) or perform the analysis within mirExTra v2.0 (*2*). The investigation can be fine-tuned from the options menu (*3*) and initiated from the relevant button (*4*). All results are presented below (*5*). Further information for each miRNA, metadata, and tools can be accessed with the information button (*6*). All results can be downloaded (*7*). The interactive network graphs are presented in a separate web page (*8*), while top results can be forwarded to miRPath v3.0 for functional investigation (*9*). Example (*10*), Help (*11*), Reset (*12*), Back (*13*), and Home (*14*) buttons assist user interaction with the module

8. An interactive network graph can be accessed by pressing the "Interactive Graph" button. The graph depicts the top up- and downregulated miRNAs along with their targets. Up- and downregulated miRNAs and mRNAs are presented in different colors, enabling the assessment of the role of each regulator within the network (*see* **Note 11**).
9. As in all DIANA-tools (microT-CDS, TarBase, lncBase, and miRGen), each individual miRNA can be sent to DIANA-miRPath v3.0 for functional analysis. DIANA-mirExTra offers also the option to send the top up- or downregulated miRNAs directly to miRPath for combined miRNA functional analyses.
10. Select Run mirpath for "Top-20 Upregulated miRNAs", in order to proceed to the miRPath functional analysis presented in Subheading 3.5.

### 3.5 Investigating miRNA Function and Identifying miRNA-Controlled Pathways with DIANA-miRPath v3.0

miRNA functional investigation is a versatile process enabling the examination of miRNA activities and the identification of targeted pathways of one or more microRNAs. miRNAs selected from bibliography or by relevant analyses such as those performed in Subheadings 3.1, 3.2, 3.3, and 3.4 can often have hundreds of mRNA targets, hindering the translation of their function to biological insight. Furthermore, miRNAs can often exhibit complementary actions by co-targeting molecular pathways and regulating extensive biological mechanisms. Therefore, tools for the assessment and direct comparison of miRNA function are essential for identifying the most relevant molecules. DIANA-miRPath v3.0 is an extensive suite capable of performing sophisticated statistics in order to uncover miRNA functional impact and to identify targeted pathways. All analyses can be performed using in silico predicted interactions from DIANA-microT-CDS and TargetScan 6.2 or experimentally supported data from DIANA-TarBase v7.0.

1. Select Run mirpath for "Top-20 Upregulated miRNAs" in Subheading 3.4, **step 10** or directly navigate to http://www.microrna.gr/miRPathv3/ and manually select the 20 investigated miRNAs from the main menu (Fig. 5). The miRNAs used in this example are: hsa-miR-126-5p, hsa-miR-1275, hsa-miR-1322, hsa-miR-200b-3p, hsa-miR-302a-3p, hsa-miR-302b-3p, hsa-miR-302c-3p, hsa-miR-302d-3p, hsa-miR-302e, hsa-miR-3145-3p, hsa-miR-488-3p, hsa-miR-518a-5p, hsa-miR-520d-5p, hsa-miR-520e, hsa-miR-524-5p, hsa-miR-527, hsa-miR-548n, hsa-miR-641, and hsa-miR-96-5p (alphanumeric order).
2. Results in DIANA-miRPath v3.0 are calculated in real time without having to press a relevant button. They are presented below in the dedicated panel (Fig. 6). The default analysis uses predicted interactions from DIANA-microT-CDS with a medium-strict threshold (0.8). This threshold can be changed for more sensitivity (lower values) or increased specificity (higher values) (*see* **Note 5**). However, all analyses for human and mouse can be performed using experimentally supported interactions. This can be set individually for each miRNA from the panel right next to its identifier. The number of interactions available for each miRNA is presented at the end of the table row and can be directly examined by pressing "see genes".
3. Press "see genes" for any miRNA in the list, in order to examine the relevant table. The new tab that opens shows the targeted gene names, their IDs (with a direct link to Ensembl), the predicted interaction score, if this entry is also experimentally supported in TarBase v7.0, and if there is a pathogenic SNP in the predicted binding site. The "see interactions" link will open the relevant page from microT-CDS.

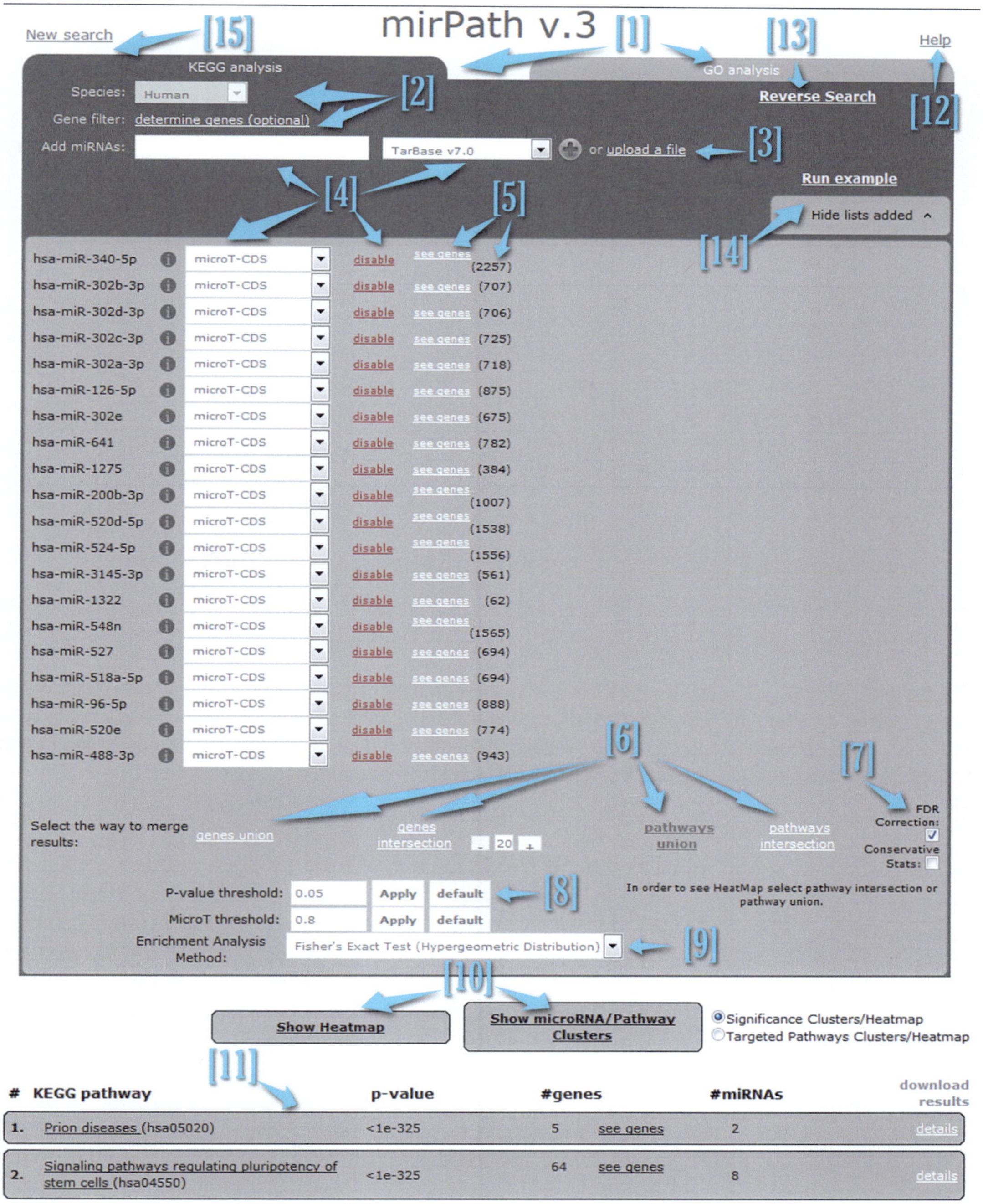


**Fig. 5** The options menu of DIANA-miRPath v3.0. Users can initially choose between pathway or functional analysis (*1*). Subsequently, the species and (optionally) expressed mRNAs can be inserted (*2*). Users can upload the miRNA names and options for the analysis (*3*) or select each miRNA individually (*4*). The identified interactions can be accessed through the accompanying link (*5*). miRPath v3.0 offers numerous options: users can select the analysis mode (*6*), use of FDR or conservative statistics (*7*), thresholds (*8*), or to employ empirical or hypergeometric distributions (*9*). Advanced visualizations are created in high resolution (*10*). All results are presented in the panel below (*11*). Detailed help is provided for all functions (*12*). The Reverse Search module can be accessed from the relevant link (*13*). The example (*14*) and reset buttons (*15*) assist users to familiarize with the interface

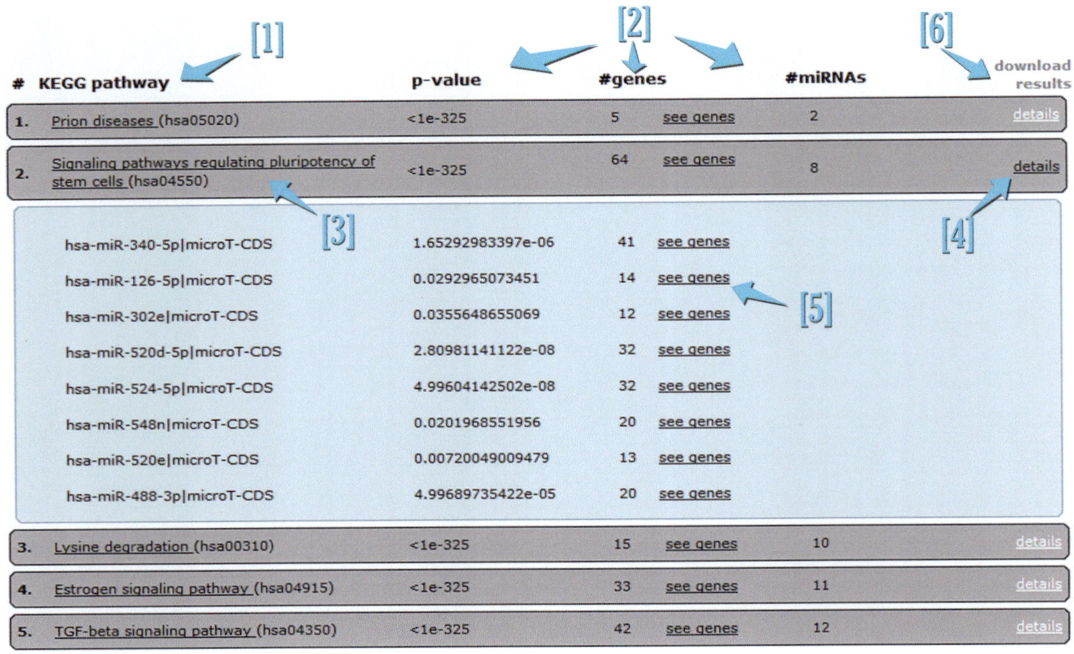


**Fig. 6** DIANA-miRPath v3.0 results panel. The panel shows the name of the targeted pathways (*1*), as well as the number of targeting miRNAs, targeted genes, and the enrichment *p*-value (*2*). Each pathway name is an active link to the pathway graph (*3*). The details button (*4*) offers further information for each targeting miRNA and the genes it controls (*5*). All results can be downloaded for future reference (*6*)

4. The default miRPath analysis mode is "genes union", where all targets of all selected miRNAs are combined into one union set. However, when analyzing concurrently numerous miRNAs this analysis is not always optimal, since it results into sets of thousands of genes. miRPath offers other modes of analysis, such as genes (soft) intersection, where genes targeted by more than one miRNAs (the exact number of targeting miRNAs is set by the user from the relevant dial), and pathways union and intersection. The latter utilize meta-analysis statistics to identify pathways targeted by more than one miRNAs. Press "pathways union" to enable this analysis.
5. There are also other options that can be used to customize an analysis to user-specific needs: users can set different thresholds (e.g. statistical significance level for pathways or microT-CDS score thresholds), whether to use FDR correction, more conservative statistics, empirical distributions instead of Fisher's exact test and more. Depending on the analysis aim (sensitive/investigative or specific) these options can change the utilized miRNA interactome and statistics machinery employed by miRPath v3.0, in order to uncover different aspects of miRNA function.

6. In the results pane we see the targeted pathways, the relevant *p*-values, the number of targeted genes, and targeting miRNAs (Fig. 6). There are many pathways that seem quite relevant to our analysis, including “Signaling pathways regulating pluripotency of stem cells” and “TGF-beta signaling pathway” among others. Press “details” next to one of those pathways, in order to further examine which miRNAs are exactly targeting them.
7. The revealed pane presents the miRNAs, their interactome sources, the *p*-value for the targeting enrichment and the number of targeted genes in this pathway from each miRNA. By selecting “see genes”, we can examine exactly which genes are targeted from each miRNA.
8. Press the name of the pathway “Signaling pathways regulating pluripotency of stem cells” in order to see the targeted genes in a relevant graph (Fig. 7). The graph shows the targeted genes and their positions within the KEGG [19] pathway. Genes marked with yellow and orange are targeted by one or

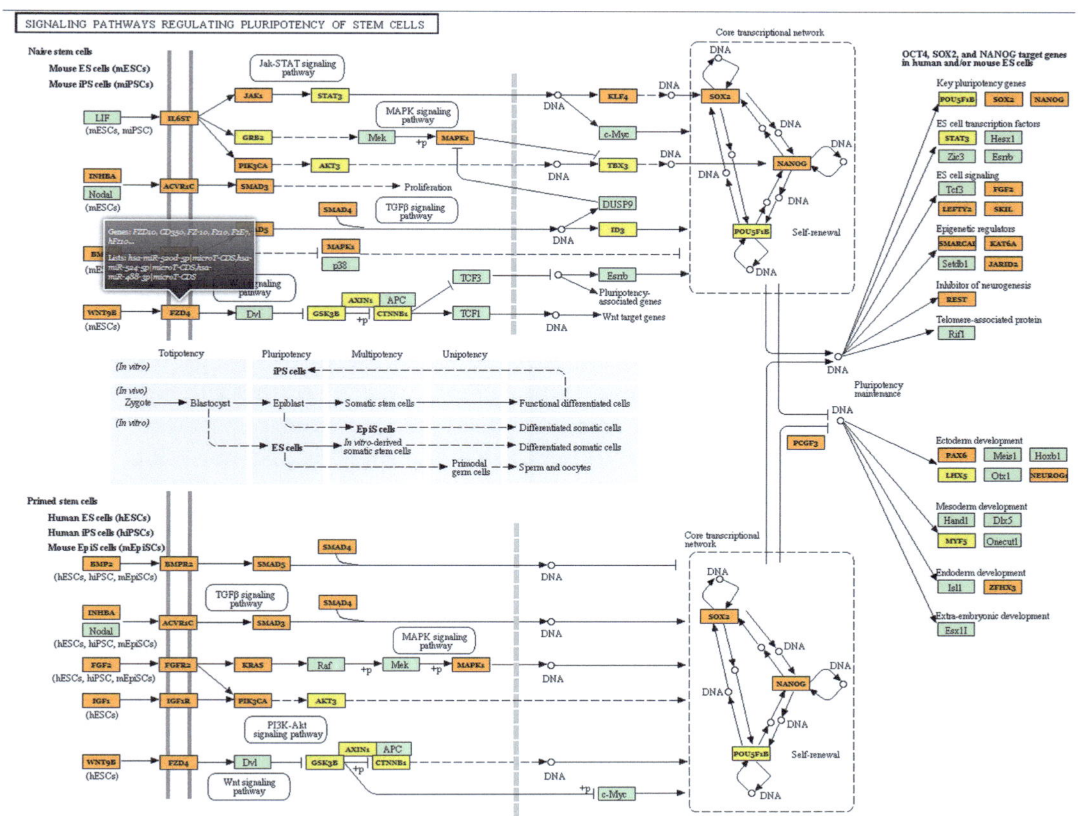


**Fig 7** A pathway graph showing targeted genes by one (*yellow*) or more microRNAs (*orange*). Targeting miRNA names are revealed by hovering the mouse cursor over a targeted gene. The position of each gene can provide important insight on the function of the targeting miRNA

more miRNAs, respectively. By hovering the mouse pointer above a targeted gene (mouseover), we can see exactly which miRNAs are doing the targeting.

9. By selecting the "pathways union" type of analysis, we unlock the advanced visualization modules of DIANA-miRPath v3.0. Using these modules we can create sophisticated graphs, such as miRNA or pathway hierarchical clustering dendrograms or pathway vs miRNA heat maps (Fig. 8). Importantly, miRNAs are clustered based on their impact on pathways and pathways based on the miRNAs that target them, providing crucial functional insight on both. By using these features we can see which subgroups of miRNAs are present in our list and which are their common or different functions. Furthermore, if we have a miRNA or miRNAs of interest, we can discover which miRNAs exhibit similar functionalities or which pathways are also targeted by our miRNA(s). Press the "Show microRNA/Pathway clusters" to create the relevant graph.

10. In the miRNA cluster graph, we can see that there are two or three major miRNA clusters by taking into account the first or second level of refinement (Fig. 9). We can see that the miRNAs belonging to the miR-302 family are clustered together by exhibiting similar function.

11. Press "Show Heatmap" button to access the miRNA vs pathways heat map graph. This graph and the clustering analysis of Subheading 3.5, **step 9** can be implemented using the *p*-values for each interaction or using a binary setup (targeted or not targeted). This can be changed by selecting "Significance Clusters/Heatmap" (*p*-value/default setting) or "Targeted Pathways Clusters/Heatmap" (binary setting). After selecting "Show Heatmap", the graph is created in high resolution and in real time. In this graph, we can see that the miRNAs of the mir-302 family indeed target similar pathways (Fig. 8). However, other miRNAs, such as hsa-mir-520e, hsa-miR-524-5p, and hsa-miR-340, have a high functional overlap with mir-302 family. This is a very powerful graph that can significantly assist us to decide which miRNAs and pathways we can select for further experimentation. For instance, we can identify which miRNAs target a specific pathway of interest (e.g. "Signaling pathways regulating pluripotency of stem cells") and also which miRNAs have relevant or not targeting profiles to our research. We can subsequently repeat our investigation with miRPath following selection of specific miRNA subgroups, in order to drill down further to more detailed information.

12. DIANA-miRPath v3.0 can also support gene ontology (GO) [20] analyses. This mode enables the identification of individual or common miRNA functions. To perform the analysis, select the "GO analysis" tab. The results are also calculated in real time.

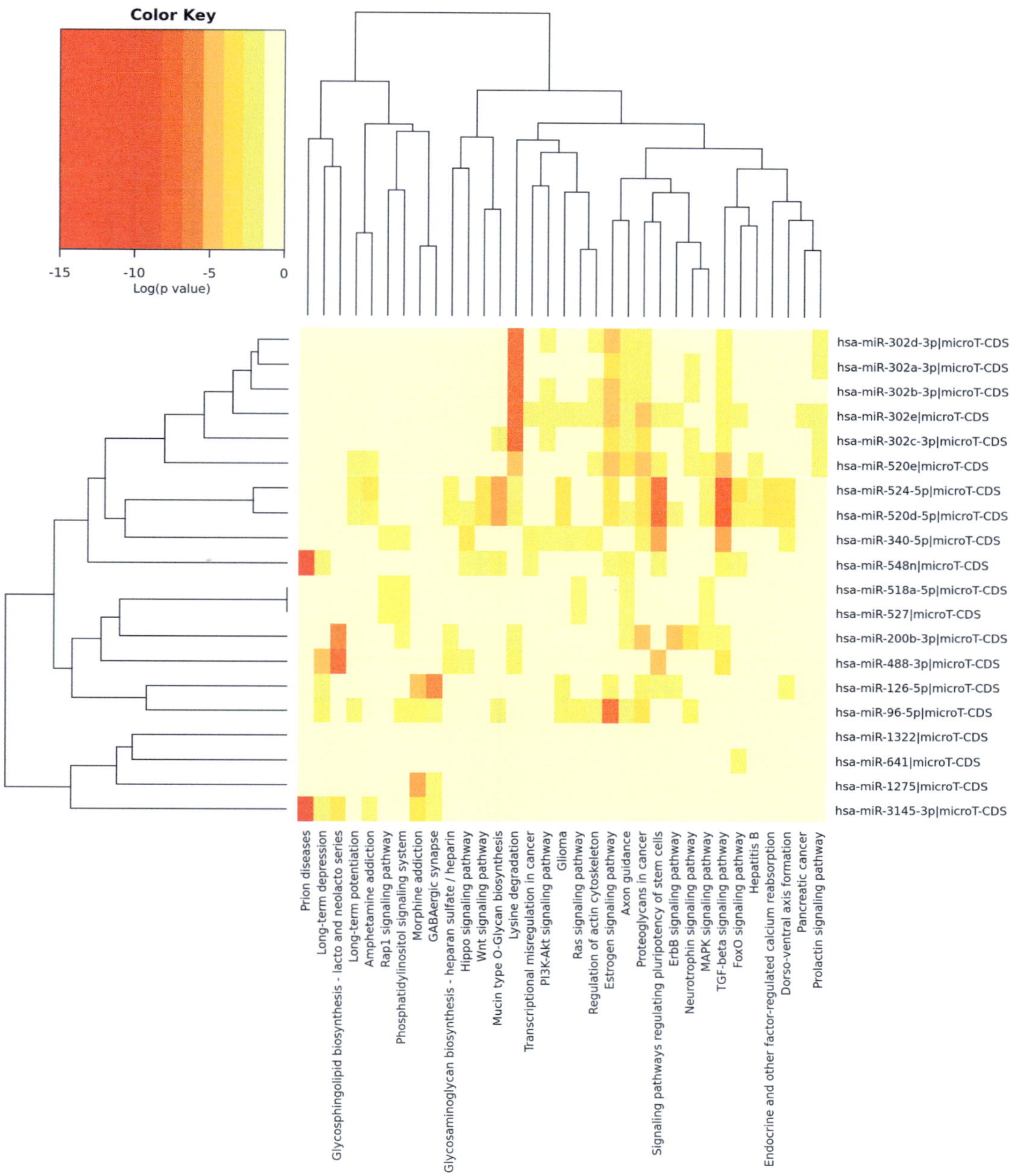


**Fig. 8** miRNAs vs Pathways heat map created by DIANA-miRPath v3.0. miRNA target enrichment *p*-values are used for clustering and for coloring the heat map. Lower enrichment *p*-values are marked with *orange* and *red*. miRNAs targeting similar pathways and pathways targeted by the same miRNAs are clustered together. This graph enables direct comparisons of miRNA functionality and the identification of molecules of interest

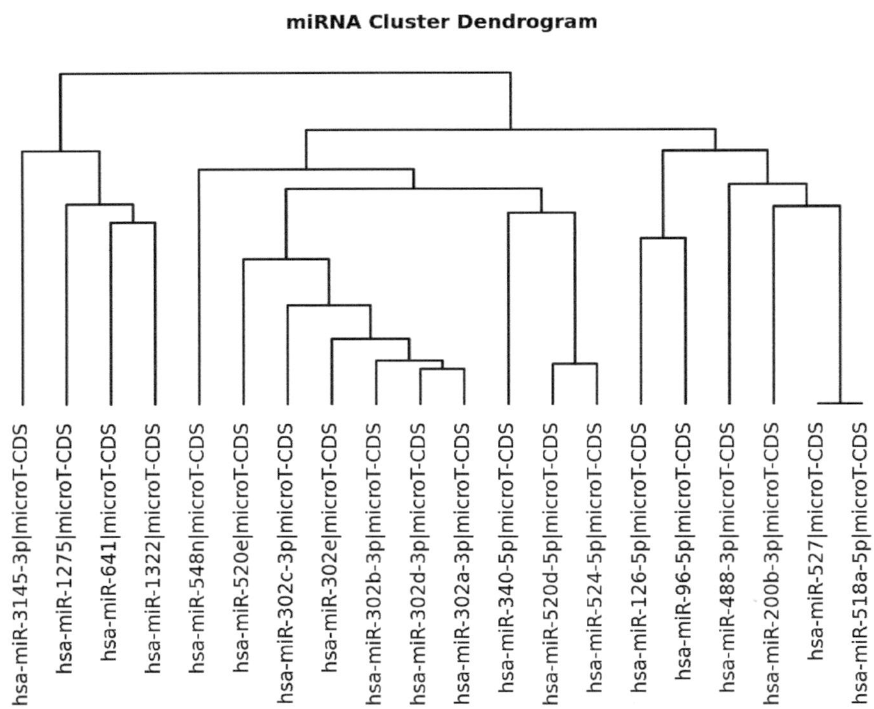


**Fig. 9** DIANA-miRPath v3.0 miRNA Cluster Dendrogram. miRNAs are clustered based on the pathways they control. miRNAs exhibiting similar functions are clustered together

13. All options available to the previous steps (genes/pathways union and intersection, thresholds, FDR correction, conservative statistics, empirical distributions, heat maps, and clustering) are also available to the GO analysis. However, the GO module offers also some specific options, including the selection of GO subsets (Biological Process, Cellular Component, Molecular Function) or the use of GOSlim, instead of GO.
14. For example, select GO analysis: GO and Subcategories: Biological Process. The results will be also automatically recalculated. In the top results, there are categories related to transcriptional control (e.g. "Transcription initiation from RNA polymerase II promoter" (GO:0006367). Therefore, many changes observed in the expression of Pol II transcribed entities (mRNAs and miRNAs) between the two examined states can be a result of perturbation in the expression of transcriptional regulators, such as transcription factors. We will investigate toward this end in Subheading 3.6.
15. All results from all analyses can be saved and downloaded for later reference by selecting the "download results" link.
16. DIANA-miRPath offers numerous tools to fine-tune our selections of candidate molecules. The initial list can be refined

repeatedly to keep only miRNAs exhibiting a targeting and functional profile relevant to the study. However, DIANA-miRPath v3.0 can also be used as an initial step in any analysis or to meta-analyze thousands of experiments and publications, in order to uncover miRNAs controlling molecular pathways or having specific functions. It is important to know that this analysis will remove any results we already have in miRPath. If all results have been saved and downloaded, select the "KEGG analysis" tab and then the "Reverse Search" link. Alternatively, open a new tab or window in the web browser; navigate to DIANA-miRPath v3.0 (http://www.microrna.gr/miRPathv3/) and select "Reverse Search", in order to keep also the previous analyses available.

17. In the Reverse Search module (Fig. 10), we search for miRNAs targeting specific pathways or having specific functionalities. These results can be based on predicted (DIANA-microT-CDS or TargetScan 6.2) or experimentally supported interactions (DIANA-TarBase v7.0). The latter meta-analyses thousands of publications and datasets and can identify patterns that are usually lost in individual manuscripts. Type: "Signaling pathways regulating pluripotency of stem cells" in the edit box or "hsa04550". Select microT-CDS and 0.8 as threshold and press "Find miRNAs". In the results list, we can examine which miRNAs are predicted to target this pathway,

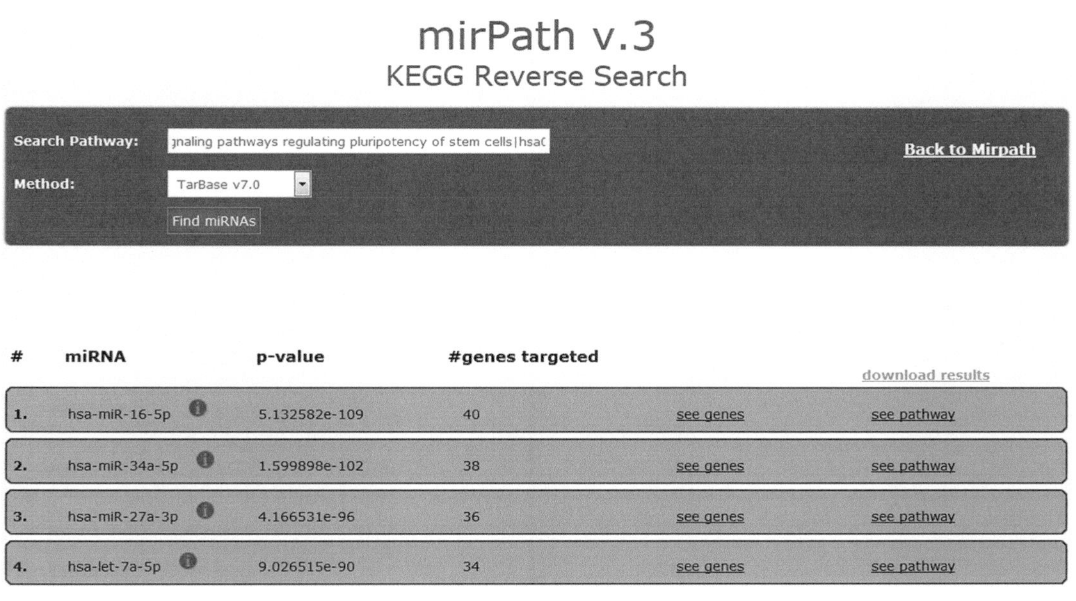


**Fig. 10** DIANA-miRPath v3.0 Reverse Search Module. Users can utilize this module to identify miRNAs targeting pathways of interest or that exhibit specific functionalities. The module can be used with in silico or experimental interactomes. The latter option is equivalent to meta-analyzing thousands of articles from the available literature

the enrichment *p*-values and the number of targeted genes. By selecting "see pathway" or "see genes", we access the pathway figure with targeted genes marked in yellow color or the list of targeted genes, respectively.

18. Select "TarBase v7.0" and press "Find miRNAs". These results are based on experimentally supported interactions and can have higher specificity, especially for well-studied miRNAs or miRNAs having average and above expression levels.
19. This analysis can also be performed for GO categories. In order to access the relevant module, select "Back to Mirpath", press the "GO analysis" tab and then select "Reverse Search". We can now perform similar analyses for GO categories. For instance, enter "GO:0006367" in order to see which miRNAs are predicted (microT-CDS or TargetScan) or are experimentally supported to control the "transcription initiation from RNA polymerase II promoter" GO category, which was found enriched in Subheading 3.5, **step 14**. The resulting miRNAs seem involved in transcriptional control by targeting genes belonging to this category.

### 3.6 Identifying TFs Controlling miRNA or mRNA Expression Between Two Conditions

1. Following the selection of the most important miRNAs, it is often useful to identify which TFs control miRNA expression or which TFs can also be regulating the changes observed in DE mRNAs between two conditions. Both analyses can be performed similarly to the analysis presented in this section by selecting "Find TFs controlling mRNAs" or "Find TFs controlling miRNAs" following a combined DE analysis or by directly selecting these options and importing the DE files as in Subheading 3.4, **step 1**.
2. The menu of these modules is similar to the "Find miRNAs with central roles by combining mRNA and miRNA expression" we saw in Subheading 3.4. The only differences are in the options menu, which are tailored to a TF-centered analysis. TF function can be selected (Activators, Repressors, Mixed Actions), as well as the promoter scanning window (upstream and downstream regions from the transcription start site (TSS)) and the familiar thresholds for up/downregulation.
3. To perform a medium sensitivity analysis to identify Activators, select Species: Human, Interactions based on: Activators, UpStream: 5000, DownStream: 5000, Threshold type: *p*Value, miRNAs Threshold value: 0.05, TFs Threshold value: 0.05.
4. As in Subheading 3.4, results for up- and downregulated TFs will be presented below along with the TF name and *p*-value. The most important regulators of miRNAs are expected to be on the top of these two lists.
5. All results can be downloaded by pressing the relevant "Download" or "Download all" buttons.

6. Press "Interactive Graph" to access the TF:miRNA regulation network graph (Fig. 11). Up/downregulated miRNAs and TFs are presented in different colors. Since the analysis was set to identify activators, upregulated TFs tend to target more upregulated miRNAs and the opposite for downregulated TFs (*see* **Note 11**).
7. This analysis expands the investigations performed in previous steps, since it gives an insight of which TFs can be responsible for the miRNAs changing expression between the two conditions.

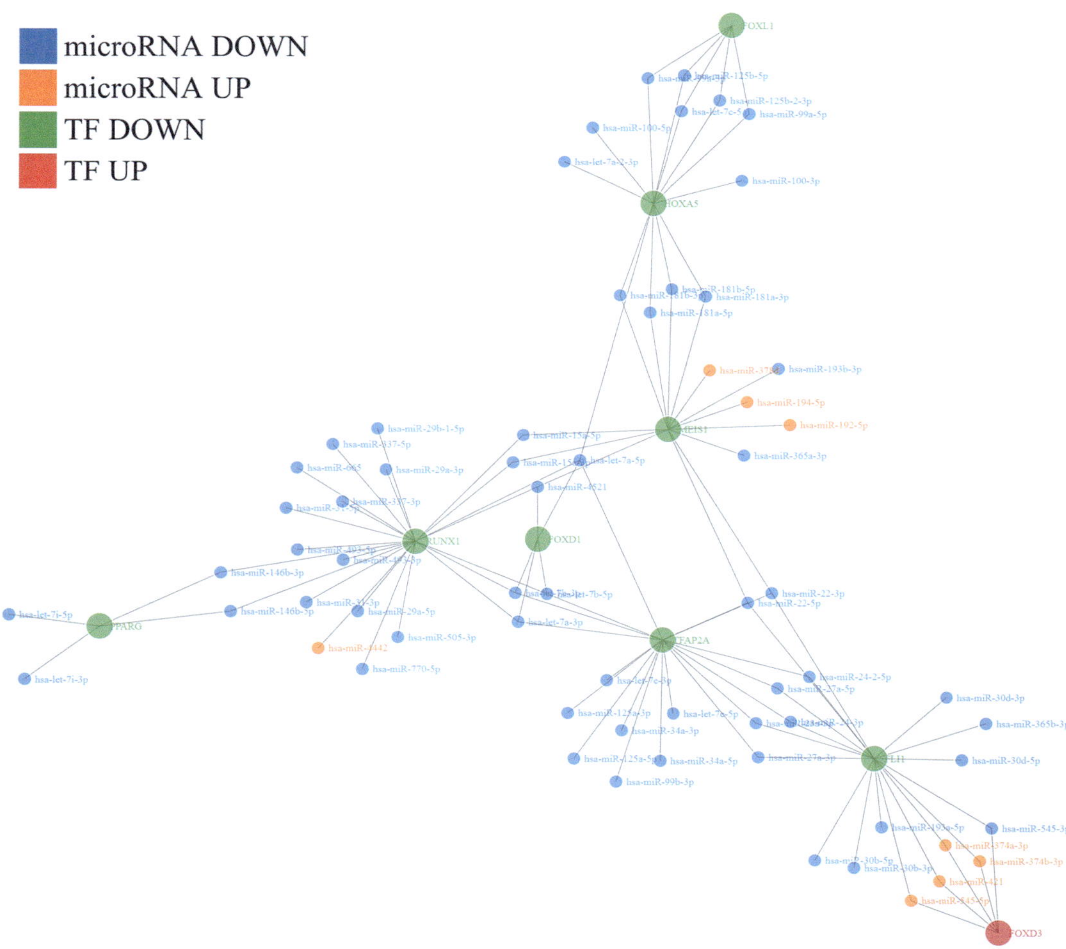


**Fig. 11** Transcription Factor vs miRNA interactive Network from DIANA-mirExTra v2.0. miRNAs and transcription factors are presented in different colors based on their differential expression. Since the performed analysis aimed in the identification of transcription factors activating miRNA transcription, upregulated transcription factors tend to control more upregulated miRNAs and vice versa

## 4 Notes

1. Creating a DIANA account can provide access to downloadable versions of various databases, history, and access to support by a ticketing system. The account can be created by using the relevant tab on the left of most tools and it is free for all users.
2. miRNA interactions can significantly change in different cell types, tissues, and conditions. Even when working in one organism, it is not always straightforward to transfer results from one cell type or tissue to another. Therefore, expression studies (miRNA or mRNA), and use of specific tools such as mirExTra, miRPath gene expression filter, TarBase cell type options, etc., can be really useful in identifying what is relevant to the studied samples.
3. In mirExTra, the produced homogeneity graphs can substantially assist in the identification of improper replicates or samples that do not behave as expected. Often, if an improper replicate is removed, there is a significant increase in the derived statistical power.
4. Selecting the best binding site (MRE) for validation is usually a complex process. We commonly start from MREs with higher degree binding types (e.g. 8mer or 9mer) that are also conserved between species. Certainly, MREs with non-canonical binding types or lacking conservation can also be functional but binding sites with strong seed signals tend to have a higher success rate in validation studies.
5. DIANA-microT-CDS scores can be a useful means to specifying the sensitivity of the algorithm. For instance, for analyses using human miRNAs and genes, a score threshold of 0.8 is slightly stringent (increased specificity), 0.7 is balanced and 0.6 (or below) exhibits high sensitivity but increases also the false-positive rate. For species other than human, these behaviors are similar to thresholds with slightly lower values (e.g. 0.05 or 0.1 lower than relevant human thresholds).
6. TarBase database cannot be directly downloaded as DIANA-microT-CDS or other DIANA tools. A license application must be sent first by using the DIANA account on the left pane. The database is free for bulk download to all research, academic, and non-profit organizations.
7. Experimental methods do not all have the same signal to noise ratio and robustness. TarBase methodology filters can be really useful in keeping only methods that are relevant to each type of analysis.
8. The number of replicates per condition is crucial for having adequate statistical power in mirExTra. Analyses without replicates (groups having one member) are of extremely low

statistical power and can be used only for investigative studies. Such studies should be enriched with more samples if possible, in order to increase the accuracy of the produced results.

9. Gene and miRNA groups should be properly matched in mirExTra in order to maximize the accuracy of the produced results. Groups A and B for both categories should be as similar as possible, optimally identical.
10. Thresholds for miRNAs and genes or TFs in mirExTra can many times uncover results that can be hidden with the default settings. Selecting the sets by using FDR levels often exhibits the highest specificity and fold changes the highest sensitivity. When there are no enriched results, then this is an indication that the regulator threshold (miRNA or TF) is set too strictly, while when there are too many targets that do not follow the expression patterns of their regulator (e.g. downregulated miRNAs controlled by an upregulated activator TF), this might mean that the target threshold is too lax.
11. The produced interactive graphs, especially when having too many members, might initially look complicated but after a few moments the molecules usually find a conformation that is easier to examine in 2D.

## Acknowledgments

The authors would like to thank Maria D. Paraskevopoulou, Dimitra Karagkouni, and Georgios Georgakilas for their helpful comments and suggestions.

This work has been supported from the project "NGS-infect" from Greek General Secretary of Research and Technology.

### References

1. Vlachos IS, Hatzigeorgiou AG (2013) Online resources for miRNA analysis. Clin Biochem 46(10-11):879–900. doi:10.1016/j.clinbiochem.2013.03.006
2. Alexiou P, Maragkakis M, Papadopoulos GL, Simmosis VA, Zhang L, Hatzigeorgiou AG (2010) The DIANA-mirExTra web server: from gene expression data to MicroRNA function. PLoS One 5(2), e9171. doi:10.1371/journal.pone.0009171
3. Vlachos IS, Paraskevopoulou MD, Karagkouni D, Georgakilas G, Vergoulis T, Kanellos I, Anastasopoulos IL, Maniou S, Karathanou K, Kalfakakou D, Fevgas A, Dalamagas T, Hatzigeorgiou AG (2015) DIANA-TarBase v7.0: indexing more than half a million experimentally supported miRNA:mRNA interactions. Nucleic Acids Res 43(Database issue):D153–D159. doi:10.1093/nar/gku1215
4. Paraskevopoulou MD, Georgakilas G, Kostoulas N, Vlachos IS, Vergoulis T, Reczko M, Filippidis C, Dalamagas T, Hatzigeorgiou AG (2013) DIANA-microT web server v5.0: service integration into miRNA functional analysis workflows. Nucleic Acids Res 41(Web Server Issue):W169–W173
5. Paraskevopoulou MD, Vlachos IS, Karagkouni D, Georgakilas G, Kanellos I, Vergoulis T, Zagganas K, Tsanakas P, Floros E, Dalamagas T, Hatzigeorgiou AG (2016) DIANA-LncBase v2: indexing microRNA targets on non-coding transcripts. Nucleic Acids Res 44(D1):D231–D238. doi:10.1093/nar/gkv1270

6. Georgakilas G, Vlachos IS, Zagganas K, Vergoulis T, Paraskevopoulou MD, Kanellos I, Tsanakas P, Dellis D, Fevgas A, Dalamagas T, Hatzigeorgiou AG (2016) DIANA-miRGen v3.0: accurate characterization of microRNA promoters and their regulators. Nucleic Acids Res 44(D1):D190–D195. doi:10.1093/nar/gkv1254
7. Vlachos IS, Zagganas K, Paraskevopoulou MD, Georgakilas G, Karagkouni D, Vergoulis T, Dalamagas T, Hatzigeorgiou AG (2015) DIANA-miRPath v3.0: deciphering microRNA function with experimental support. Nucleic Acids Res 2015:gkv403. doi:10.1093/nar/gkv403
8. Kiriakidou M, Nelson PT, Kouranov A, Fitziev P, Bouyioukos C, Mourelatos Z, Hatzigeorgiou A (2004) A combined computational-experimental approach predicts human microRNA targets. Genes Dev 18(10):1165–1178. doi:10.1101/gad.1184704
9. Georgakilas G, Vlachos IS, Paraskevopoulou MD, Yang P, Zhang Y, Economides AN, Hatzigeorgiou AG (2014) MicroTSS: accurate microRNA transcription start site identification reveals a significant number of divergent pri-miRNAs. Nat Commun 5:5700. doi:10.1038/ncomms6700
10. Garcia DM, Baek D, Shin C, Bell GW, Grimson A, Bartel DP (2011) Weak seed-pairing stability and high target-site abundance decrease the proficiency of lsy-6 and other microRNAs. Nat Struct Mol Biol 18(10):1139–1146. doi:10.1038/nsmb.2115
11. Kozomara A, Griffiths-Jones S (2014) miRBase: annotating high confidence microRNAs using deep sequencing data. Nucleic Acids Res 42(D1):D68–D73. doi:10.1093/nar/gkt1181
12. Barrett T, Wilhite SE, Ledoux P, Evangelista C, Kim IF, Tomashevsky M, Marshall KA, Phillippy KH, Sherman PM, Holko M, Yefanov A, Lee H, Zhang N, Robertson CL, Serova N, Davis S, Soboleva A (2013) NCBI GEO: archive for functional genomics data sets—update. Nucleic Acids Res 41(Database issue):D991–D995. doi:10.1093/nar/gks1193
13. Rosenbloom KR, Armstrong J, Barber GP, Casper J, Clawson H, Diekhans M, Dreszer TR, Fujita PA, Guruvadoo L, Haeussler M, Harte RA, Heitner S, Hickey G, Hinrichs AS, Hubley R, Karolchik D, Learned K, Lee BT, Li CH, Miga KH, Nguyen N, Paten B, Raney BJ, Smit AF, Speir ML, Zweig AS, Haussler D, Kuhn RM, Kent WJ (2015) The UCSC genome browser database: 2015 update. Nucleic Acids Res 43(Database issue):D670–D681. doi:10.1093/nar/gku1177
14. Consortium EP (2012) An integrated encyclopedia of DNA elements in the human genome. Nature 489(7414):57–74. doi:10.1038/nature11247
15. Anders S, Huber W (2010) Differential expression analysis for sequence count data. Genome Biol 11(10):R106. doi:10.1186/gb-2010-11-10-r106
16. Ritchie ME, Phipson B, Wu D, Hu Y, Law CW, Shi W, Smyth GK (2015) Limma powers differential expression analyses for RNA-sequencing and microarray studies. Nucleic Acids Res 43(7):47. doi:10.1093/nar/gkv007
17. Robinson MD, McCarthy DJ, Smyth GK (2010) edgeR: a bioconductor package for differential expression analysis of digital gene expression data. Bioinformatics 26(1):139–140. doi:10.1093/bioinformatics/btp616
18. Yates A, Akanni W, Amode MR, Barrell D, Billis K, Carvalho-Silva D, Cummins C, Clapham P, Fitzgerald S, Gil L, Giron CG, Gordon L, Hourlier T, Hunt SE, Janacek SH, Johnson N, Juettemann T, Keenan S, Lavidas I, Martin FJ, Maurel T, McLaren W, Murphy DN, Nag R, Nuhn M, Parker A, Patricio M, Pignatelli M, Rahtz M, Riat HS, Sheppard D, Taylor K, Thormann A, Vullo A, Wilder SP, Zadissa A, Birney E, Harrow J, Muffato M, Perry E, Ruffier M, Spudich G, Trevanion SJ, Cunningham F, Aken BL, Zerbino DR, Flicek P (2016) Ensembl 2016. Nucleic Acids Res 44(D1):D710–D716. doi:10.1093/nar/gkv1157
19. Kanehisa M, Goto S, Sato Y, Kawashima M, Furumichi M, Tanabe M (2014) Data, information, knowledge and principle: back to metabolism in KEGG. Nucleic Acids Res 42(Database issue):D199–D205. doi:10.1093/nar/gkt1076
20. Ashburner M, Ball CA, Blake JA, Botstein D, Butler H, Cherry JM, Davis AP, Dolinski K, Dwight SS, Eppig JT, Harris MA, Hill DP, Issel-Tarver L, Kasarskis A, Lewis S, Matese JC, Richardson JE, Ringwald M, Rubin GM, Sherlock G (2000) Gene ontology: tool for the unification of biology. The gene ontology consortium. Nat Genet 25(1):25–29. doi:10.1038/75556

# Chapter 3

# Non-nucleotide Modification of Anti-miRNA Oligonucleotides

Kim A. Lennox, Christopher A. Vakulskas, and Mark A. Behlke

## Abstract

MicroRNAs (miRNAs) are important modulators of gene expression. Synthetic anti-microRNA oligonucleotides (AMOs, or anti-miRs) are a form of steric-blocking antisense oligonucleotides (ASOs) that inhibit miRNA function through high-affinity binding and subsequent inactivation and/or degradation of the targeted miRNA. AMOs are a primary tool used to empirically determine the biological targets of a miRNA and can also be used therapeutically when overexpression of a miRNA contributes to a disease state. Chemical modification of synthetic AMOs enhance potency by protecting the oligonucleotide from nuclease degradation and by increasing binding affinity to the target miRNA. A new steric-blocking ASO modification strategy with favorable properties for use in AMOs was recently developed that combines use of high-affinity 2′-*O*-methyl RNA with terminally positioned non-nucleotide "ZEN" modifiers. This protocol describes use of ZEN AMOs in a dual-luciferase reporter assay as a simplified means to validate AMO performance or to quickly test putative miRNA binding sites in target sequences. This protocol also describes a method using Western blot analysis for quantifying the level of upregulation of proteins made from an mRNA that is thought to be under miRNA regulation, following inhibition of that miRNA by ZEN AMO treatment.

**Key words** microRNAs (miRNA, miR), Oligonucleotides, Inhibitors, Non-nucleotide modifier, ZEN, Chemical modifications, Knockdown, Western blot, miR-21, PTEN, MARCKS

## 1 Introduction

MicroRNAs (miRNAs) are a group of small non-coding RNAs that are evolutionarily conserved to regulate protein expression at the post-transcriptional level [1]. Since their discovery in the early 1990s, interest in miRNAs has steadily increased as their biological importance and clinical relevance has been documented in many different systems [2]. In humans, there are currently >2500 identified mature miRNA sequences (miRBase release 21, June 2014), each of which has context-dependent variable expression patterns depending on cell type, stage of development, and pathological conditions. MiRNA dysregulation has been associated with many disease states, including cancer, some hereditary diseases such as

Marco F. Schmidt (ed.), *Drug Target miRNA: Methods and Protocols*, Methods in Molecular Biology, vol. 1517,
DOI 10.1007/978-1-4939-6563-2_3, © Springer Science+Business Media New York 2017

hearing loss and growth defects, myocardial disease, kidney disease, immune-related diseases, and neurological disorders (reviewed in [3–5]). Given their clear importance in gene regulation and disease association, the ability to inhibit miRNA function is a useful tool.

MiRNA biogenesis is a tightly regulated process that begins in the nucleus and ends in the cytoplasm [6]. MiRNA genes are transcribed in the nucleus as long (generally over 1 kb) primary miRNAs (pri-miRNAs) that contain internal ~80 nucleotide (nt) stem-loop structures. These stem-loop structures are excised from the pri-miRNA by the nuclear endoribonuclease Drosha into a ~70 nt precursor microRNA (pre-miRNA) and exported out of the nucleus to complete maturation in the cytoplasm. In the cytoplasm, the pre-miRNA is further processed by the endoribonuclease Dicer into a small RNA duplex 18–25 nt long (average length is 22 nt) and is subsequently loaded onto an Argonaute protein to form the multi-protein miRNA-induced silencing complex (miRISC). Once loaded into miRISC, the "passenger" strand of the duplex is unwound and discarded, leaving the "guide" strand as the biologically active mature miRNA. This RISC-loaded mature miRNA base pairs imperfectly with target sites in an mRNA (which are often in the 3' untranslated region (UTR)) by hybridization nucleated from a critical 6–8 nt "seed region" at the 5'-end of the miRNA. Binding of the miRNA to the mRNA, either alone or in conjunction with other miRNAs, can lead to mRNA degradation or downregulate protein translation off the transcript [7].

The step-wise process of miRNA biogenesis from (1) pri-miRNA transcript to (2) pre-miRNA stem-loop structure to (3) single-stranded mature miRNA in miRISC provides three different stages in which miRNA function could theoretically be inhibited. The pri-miRNA transcript could be targeted for degradation using RNase H1 degradative antisense oligonucleotides (ASOs) [8]; however, these transcripts often contain polycistronic miRNA precursors or are associated with other RNA molecules which may lead to unintended degradation of non-targeted RNAs that are physically linked with the targeted miRNA [9]. In theory, the ~70 nt pre-miRNA stem-loop is an RNA target that could also be degraded using ASOs. In practice, the secondary structure in the stem-loop can be difficult for the ASO to invade [10]; importantly, the pre-miRNA is protein-bound during the maturation process which can block ASO accessibility [6]. The most accessible miRNA biogenesis stage to inhibit miRNA function is when the mature miRNA is miRISC-loaded in single-stranded form. Single-stranded steric-blocking ASOs (anti-miRNA oligonucleotides, or AMOs) complementary to the mature miRNA can prevent the miRNA from binding to its target and thereby inhibit miRNA function [11–13].

MiRNA inactivation requires that the AMO has a binding affinity (related to melting temperature, or $T_m$) to the targeted miRNA that is high enough for the inhibitor to outcompete the Watson-Crick interactions that normally occur between the miRNA guide strand/passenger strand in miRISC as well as between the miRNA and its natural target mRNA. It is generally observed that AMOs with a higher binding affinity have higher potency [11–13]. AMOs also need to survive exposure to endo- and exonucleases present in serum and the intracellular environment. Chemical modification can be made on the nucleotide base, the phosphate backbone, or by adding non-base modifiers singly or in combination to provide various levels of $T_m$ enhancement and nuclease protection.

One of the greatest challenges in designing oligonucleotides for RNA knockdown techniques, such as RNase H degradative ASOs, is site selection in highly structured long targets. Fortunately, mature miRNAs are relatively short (~22 nt), simplifying the design requirements. AMOs are typically designed to be the perfect reverse complement to the full-length mature miRNA [11]. Desirable characteristics of a chemically modified AMO include high potency, nuclease resistance, specificity, amenable to transfection, and low toxicity. We optimized AMO design and developed a strategy that combines modifications having the desired characteristics into "ZEN-AMOs" [13]. These compounds are perfectly complementary to the full-length miRNA, with one base removed from the 3' end. The ZEN AMOs comprise 2'OMe bases paired with two ZEN modifiers (Fig. 1). 2'OMe RNA resides are

A)

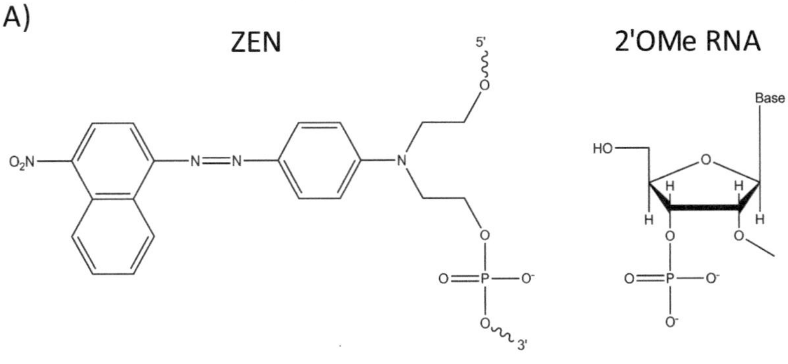


B)

| Target[a] | AMO Sequences (5' to 3')[b] |
|---|---|
| Negative Control | GzCGACUAUACGCGCAAUAUGGz |
| miR-21 | UzCAACAUCAGUCUGAUAAGCUz |

[a] This negative control is suitable for human, mouse and rat

[b] Uppercase black = 2'OMe; "z" = ZEN

**Fig. 1** ZEN AMO Chemical modification strategy. (**a**) Chemical modification structures for ZEN and 2'OMe RNA. (**b**) Hsa-miR-21 and the negative control ZEN AMO sequences

non-toxic, resistant to endonucleases, and increase binding affinity; however, 2'OMe residues are susceptible to exonuclease attack. "ZEN" is a napthyl-azo group (*N*,*N*-diethyl-4-(4-nitronaphthalen-1-ylazo)-phenylamine); it is a non-base modifier which is not recognized by exonuclease enzymes and so blocks exonuclease attack when placed at or near the ends of a nucleic acid sequence. It also increases binding affinity of the synthetic oligonucleotide to its natural target, presumably through hydrophobic stacking interactions with the nucleobases. The ZEN AMOs should be administered using a delivery tool, such as a cationic lipid, lipid nanoparticle or polymer system. It is not advised to use naked delivery of ZEN AMOs for either cell culture or in vivo.

This protocol first describes a method to verify that the miRNA knockdown reagents are working properly by targeting miR-21 using a reporter assay in cell culture with cationic lipid transfection. MiR-21 is highly expressed in HeLa cells, giving a large dynamic range of signal when effectively inhibited with an AMO, making it a good target to use as a positive control or to use in methods development work [12, 13]. Starting investigations into miRNA function using a reporter assay system provides experimental validation that the reagents are working and offers an important positive control to ensure that the miRNA is expressed in the cell line, that the putative miRNA target is actually regulated by the miRNA, and verifies that the transfection conditions are effective. Most researches remember to include negative controls in experimental design, but the positive control is frequently forgotten. In this protocol, we describe the use of the dual-luciferase PsiCHECK-2 plasmid, which expresses both firefly luciferase (FLuc) and *Renilla* luciferase (RLuc) from different promoters. The FLuc is used for normalization to control for transfection uptake and plasmid expression efficiency. The 3'UTR of RLuc is modified to contain either (1) a perfect match miRNA binding site, (2) one or multiple consecutive putative miRNA binding sites (imperfect match to the miRNA), or (3) the entire 3'UTR of the mRNA targeted by the miRNA (*see* Fig. 2). Each of these three strategies has its own utility and rationale for use. The RLuc RNA containing the perfect match binding site (perfectly complementary to the mature miRNA) in its 3'UTR will be cleaved via an Argonaute 2 (AGO2) mechanism, giving the highest dynamic range of luciferase signal between AMO-treated and untreated cells. This provides a good qualitative method to assess relative miRNA levels present in the cell line studied (to make sure an appropriate cell line is being used) and can help optimize the transfection efficiency of the AMO. For example, if miRNA levels are too low, there will not be much downregulation of RLuc compared to cells transfected with unmodified PsiCHECK-2 plasmid. If AMO transfection efficiency is suboptimal, there will not be much difference between AMO-treated and untreated cells. The second strategy incorporates 1–6

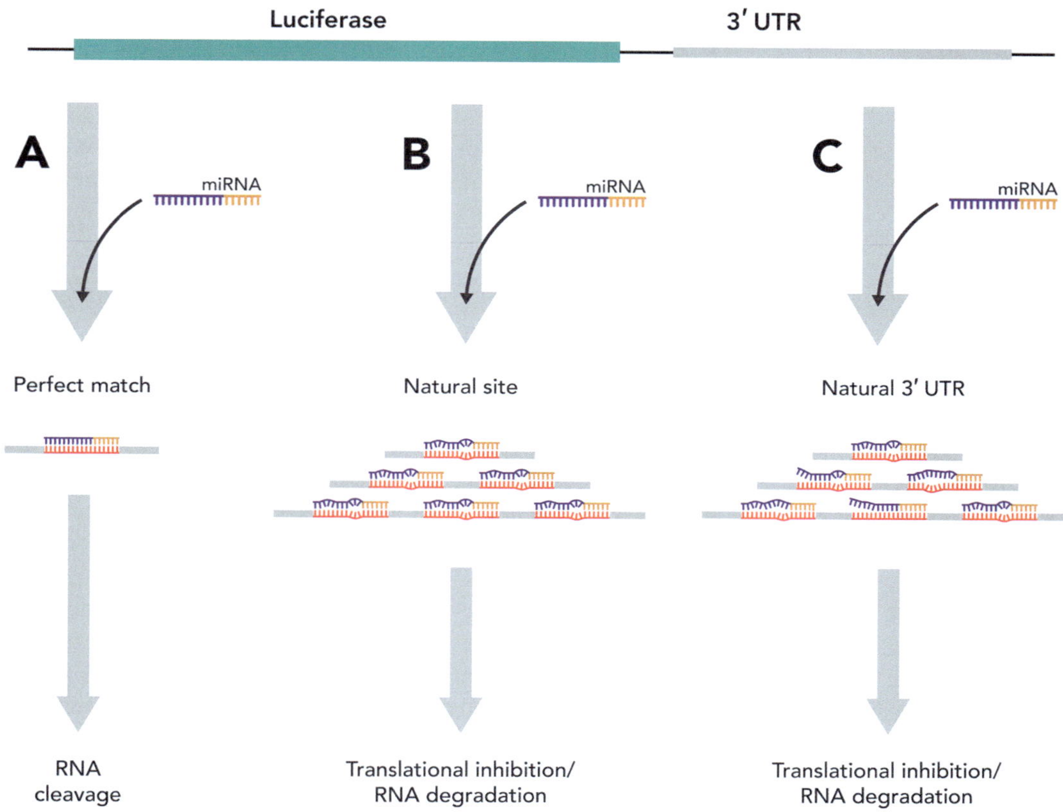


**Fig. 2** A schematic of the options for cloning miR-21 binding sites into the 3'UTR of *Renilla* luciferase. (**a**) A miRNA binding site that is a perfect match to the miRNA will induce AGO2-mediated RNA cleavage, giving the highest luciferase signal differential between AMO-treated and untreated cells. This option is preferred as a positive control used to validate experimental procedure. (**b**) One or multiple identical natural miRNA binding sites cloned consecutively will lead to translational inhibition, oftentimes with RNA degradation. This strategy is an effective method to verify unvalidated miRNA binding sites. (**c**) Assaying with the entire 3′UTR of the mRNA predicted to be regulated by a miRNA is the best method to test activity of predicted miRNA binding sites. These sites may or may not have the same sequence. This option provides the native sequence context surrounding the miRNA binding site which can influence secondary structure and RNA protein binding, potentially affecting the ability of a miRNA to bind. Yellow nucleotides depict the "seed region" of the miRNA

natural (predicted or validated) imperfectly complementary miRNA binding sites into the 3'UTR of RLuc. This method helps verify that the miRNA can regulate mRNA translation with the predicted binding site(s). Binding sites work cooperatively, and we have found that the use of multiple binding sites leads to higher protein downregulation. The third strategy, where the entire 3'UTR of the target mRNA is cloned into the 3'UTR of RLuc, is the best control to determine whether a particular miRNA is capable of regulating a particular mRNA through putative miRNA binding sites, and how effective this regulation can be (using a controlled reporter assay). This option includes the entire sequence context of the 3'UTR under investigation; having the natural 3'UTR secondary structure and RNA protein binding can better mimic if the miRNA can truly target this mRNA in the cell. Using one or all of these strategies is a good starting point for all anti-miRNA studies. Finally, this protocol describes a method of quantifying protein upregulation of an endogenous miRNA target after AMO treatment using Western blot analysis.

## 2 Materials

### 2.1 Nucleic Acid Reagents

1. Pre-designed target-specific and negative control (NC) ZEN-modified anti-miRNA inhibitors (ZEN AMOs) (Integrated DNA Technologies). The example protocol in this chapter uses the hsa-miR-21 ZEN AMO (UzCAACAUCAGUCUGAUAAGCUz, where all bases are 2'OMe RNA and "z" denotes ZEN, *see* Fig. 1).
2. PsiCHECK-2 vector (Promega) with appropriate miRNA target sequences cloned into the multiple cloning site in the 3'UTR of RLuc. The cloned miRNA target sequence can come in the form of one of the following options: the perfect complement to the mature miRNA sequence; the imperfectly complementary sequence of the natural miRNA binding site; or the entire 3'UTR of the target mRNA (*see* Subheading 1 for discussion of the function of each option and Fig. 2). For this hsa-miR-21 binding site example, the following two oligonucleotides were annealed and cloned into the XhoI/NotI restriction sites:/5phosTCGAGCGAGCCGGTCTCAACATC AGTCTGATAAGCTACCGGATCGCGGGCTGC; /5phos/GGCCGCAGCCCGCGATCCGGTAGCTT ATCAGACTGATGTTGAGACCGGCTCGC.
3. Sterile Tris-EDTA (TE) buffer: 10 mM Tris(hydroxymethyl) aminomethane hydrochloride (TRIS–HCL), 0.1 mM disodium ethylenediaminetetraacetic acid (EDTA), pH 8.0. This buffer may also be purchased (IDTE buffer, Integrated DNA Technologies).

### 2.2 Cell Culture and Transfection Reagents

All reagents and tools should be sterile and nuclease-free.

1. Cell line expressing the target miRNA. This specific protocol uses HeLa cells (ATCC). If the cell line employed does not express the miRNA of interest, then the experiments will fail to produce a quantifiable effect in the reporter assay.
2. Cell line-specific culture media and supplements recommended by ATCC. HeLa cells require Dulbecco's Modified Essential Medium (DMEM) containing 10% fetal bovine serum (FBS) (ThermoFisher Scientific).

3. 100 mm culture dishes.
4. 96-well tissue culture plates (for the Luciferase experiments).
5. 6-well tissue culture plates (for the Western Blot experiments).
6. Phosphate-buffered saline (1 X PBS) (ThermoFisher Scientific).
7. Opti-MEM® (ThermoFisher Scientific).
8. Optimal cell line-specific transfection reagent, such as Lipofectamine® 2000 or Lipofectamine® RNAiMAX (ThermoFisher Scientific).
9. 1.5 mL polypropylene microcentrifuge tubes.
10. 5 mL polypropylene round bottom tubes.

### 2.3 Luciferase Reagents

1. Dual-Luciferase® Reporter Assay System (Promega).
2. Corning® white 96-well plates, opaque bottom.
3. 15 mL polypropylene tubes [2].

### 2.4 Western Reagents

1. 2X Laemmli Sample Buffer [14]; 125 mM Tris–HCl pH 6.8, 4% sodium dodecyl sulfate (SDS), 20% glycerol, 10% 2-mercaptoethanol, and 0.004% bromophenol blue dye.
2. Precision Plus Protein™ Unstained Protein Standards (Bio-Rad).
3. Mini-PROTEAN® TGX™ Precast Gels (Bio-Rad). Alternatively, Tris–HCl or Bis-Tris gels can be made in-house using pre-established protocols [15].
4. SDS-PAGE Running Buffer (Tris–HCl or TGX™ gels only); 25 mM Tris–HCl pH 8.3, 192 mM glycine, and 0.1% SDS.
5. Trans-Blot® Turbo™ Mini Polyvinylidene fluoride (PVDF) Transfer Packs (Bio-Rad). Alternatively, Whatman™ 3MM chromatography paper, Nitrocellulose or PVDF membranes, and Western Blot Transfer reagents may be purchased or assembled separately.
6. SuperBlock™ T20 (TBS) Blocking Buffer (ThermoFisher). Alternatively, Western blocking buffer can be made in-house with TBST (20 mM Tris–HCl pH 7.5, 150 mM NaCl, and 0.1% Tween™ 20) containing either 5% nonfat dry milk, 1% casein, or 3% BSA.
7. Anti-PTEN mouse monoclonal antibody clone 6H2.1 (EMD Millipore).
8. Anti-β-ACTIN mouse monoclonal antibody clone 4C2 (EMD Millipore).
9. Anti-MARCKS mouse monoclonal antibody clone 2 F12 (EMD Millipore).

10. Western blot wash buffer; TBST (20 mM Tris–HCl pH 7.5, 150 mM NaCl, and 0.5% Tween™ 20). Tween™ 20 concentration may vary from 0.05-0.5% (or left out entirely), and the ideal wash buffer should be empirically determined for each antibody-antigen tested.
11. Amersham ECL Mouse IgG, HRP-linked whole antibody from sheep (GE Healthcare Life Sciences).
12. Precision Protein™ *Strep*Tactin-HRP Conjugate (Bio-Rad).
13. SuperSignal™ West Femto Maximum Sensitivity ECL Western Blot Substrate (ThermoFisher).

### 2.5 Equipment

1. Cell culture hood and 37 °C incubator.
2. GloMax® 96 Microplate Luminometer (Promega).
3. Mini-PROTEAN® Tetra Vertical Electrophoresis Cell (Bio-Rad).
4. Trans-Blot® Turbo™ Transfer System (Bio-Rad).
5. Rocker II Platform Rocker (Boekel™ Industries).
6. ChemiDoc™ Touch Gel Imaging System (Bio-Rad).

## 3 Methods

This procedure is partitioned into two steps: 1) experimental validation using a reporter assay, and 2) Western blot analysis of an endogenous target. The selected miRNA target for this protocol is hsa-miR-21, and knockdown will be performed in HeLa cells which are known to highly express this miRNA [12, 13, 16]. The reporter is a luciferase assay with the perfect match hsa-miR-21 binding site cloned into the 3'UTR of RLuc. For the endogenous studies, PTEN and MARCKS were selected as validated endogenous miR-21 targets for Western blot analysis [17–19]. Successful knockdown of miR-21 will increase protein levels for each assay.

### 3.1 Reporter Assay

Here we outline steps to transfect the psiCHECK-2 plasmid containing a perfectly matched miR-21 binding site in the 3'UTR of RLuc, followed by transfection of the AMOs. MiRNA inhibition directly correlates to an increase in RLuc expression.

#### 3.1.1 Nucleic Acids

1. A targeting and negative control ZEN AMO can be designed on the Integrated DNA Technologies website (http://www.idtdna.com/pages/products/mirna). Lyophilized AMOs should be centrifuged prior to opening, and reconstituted in TE or IDTE buffer at a stock concentration of 100 μM (e.g., add 50 μl TE to 5 nmoles AMO). Further working dilutions can be made in TE or IDTE buffer (*see* **Note 1**). For a 30, 10, and 3 nM dose–response experiment, prepare serial AMO dilutions of 3, 1 and 0.3 μM. AMOs should be stored at −20 °C.

2. The PsiCHECK-2 plasmids should be endotoxin-free and sterile prior to use in cell culture. Endotoxin removal can be done during the plasmid prep stage, or with an endotoxin removal kit (*see* **Note 2**). All plasmids should be filtered through a 0.2 μm filter to ensure sterility.

### 3.2 Cell Culture and Transfections

Here we outline the protocol for psiCHECK-2 plasmid transfection in a 100 mm cell culture dish, followed by transfection of the AMO in a 96-well plate format. If different sized dishes or plates are required, adjust the volumes accordingly by surface area. For example, all reagent volumes can be doubled if using a 48-well plate versus a 96-well plate. This protocol uses HeLa cells; if a different cell line is used, seed cells at the specified confluency. "PsiCHECK-2" denotes an unmodified plasmid, while "psiCHECK-miRNA" indicates the plasmid contains the miRNA binding site; testing both of these plasmids simultaneously is a recommended control.

1. Seed 2,000,000 HeLa cells in each 100 mm cell culture dish in 10 mL DMEM supplemented with 10% FBS. Include one 100 mm dish for the PsiCHECK-2 plasmid, and one 100 mm dish for the PsiCHECK-miRNA plasmid.
2. Incubate the cells at 37 °C and 5% $CO_2$ until cells are ~80–90% confluent (typically the next day).
3. Replace the growth media in each 100 mm dish with 15 mL fresh DMEM supplemented with 10% FBS.
4. Individually transfect the PsiCHECK-2 and PsiCHECK-miRNA plasmids into the cells. Dilute 5 μg plasmid in a total volume of 1.5 mL Opti-MEM®, and dilute 10 μL Lipofectamine® 2000 in a total volume of 1.5 mL Opti-MEM®. Combine the diluted plasmid and diluted Lipofectamine® 2000 (3 mL total volume). Mix gently, and incubate at room temperature for 20 min for complex formation.
5. Add the lipid complexes to the cells, and gently rock the dish to mix. Incubate the cells for 24 h at 37 °C and 5% $CO_2$. We recommend changing the growth media 6 h after the transfection to reduce cell toxicity.
6. Reverse transfect the PsiCHECK-2 and PsiCHECK-miR21 expressing cells with the negative control and miR-21 ZEN AMOs. Include a "reagent only" control in which only the transfection reagent (no ZEN AMO) is applied to the cells as a control to assess toxicity or contamination issues that might arise. We recommend starting with a dosing range of 30, 10, and 3 nM (*see* **Note 3**). All dilutions should be made in polypropylene tubes (such as 1.5 mL microcentrifuge tubes), and Opti-MEM® should be at room temperature. For a single well, dilute 0.5 μL Lipofectamine® RNAiMAX into 24.5 μL Opti-MEM® (total volume is 25 μL) (*see* **Note 4**). For triplicate transfections, multiply these values by 3.3 to account for pipet-

ting errors (e.g., combine 1.65 μL Lipofectamine® RNAiMAX with 80.9 μL Opti-MEM®), and multiply again by the total number of transfection conditions used. Next, dilute 1.5 μL of the appropriate AMO dilution (e.g., use the 3 μM dilution for 30 nM dose, *see* **Note 1**) into 23.5 μL Opti-MEM® (total volume is 25 μL). For triplicate transfections, multiply these values by 3.2 to account for pipetting errors (e.g., combine 4.8 μL AMO with 75.2 μL Opti-MEM® for a total volume of 80 μL). Add 80 μL of the diluted Lipofectamine® RNAiMAX to the diluted AMO (total volume now is 160 μL). Gently mix the complexes with a quick vortex or by pipetting up and down, and incubate at room temperature for 20 min.

7. During the 20 min incubation, trypsinize the HeLa cells and dilute to 20,000 cells per 100 μL (200,000 cells per 1 mL) in DMEM containing 10% FBS. Each well in the 96-well plate will be seeded with 100 μL of diluted cells. Scale up the volumes appropriately, accounting for pipetting errors. Cells are seeded to be ~90% confluent the next day (*see* **Note 5**).
8. After the 20 min incubation, add 50 μL of the AMO/lipid complex in triplicate wells in a 96-well plate, followed by 100 μL diluted HeLa cells for final volume of 150 μL. Incubate the cells at 37 °C and 5% $CO_2$ for 24 h. Gently rock the plate periodically for the first hour to allow cells to become adherent to the plate and evenly dispersed in a monolayer. After 24 h, visualize the cells to ensure there is no toxicity or contamination (*see* **Note 6**).

#### 3.2.1 Luciferase Analysis

1. Luciferase expression is measured 24 h after AMO transfection using the Dual-Luciferase® Reporter Assay System (Promega). Prepare a 1× solution of Passive Lysis Buffer (PLB) by adding one volume of 5× PLB to 4 volumes of $H_2O$. Enough PLB should be prepared to aliquot 45 μL per well in a 96-well plate, which is enough lysate for two runs/well on the luminometer. Remove media from transfected HeLa cells and wash with 100 μL 1× PBS. Aspirate PBS from the cells, add 45 μL 1× PLB to each well, and gently rock/nutate the plate for 15 min at room temperature to lyse cells (*see* **Note 7**).
2. Prepare the Luciferase Assay Reagent II (LAR II) by adding 10 mL Luciferase Assay Buffer II to the Luciferase Assay Substrate and mixing thoroughly. Prepare the Stop & Glo® Reagent by diluting the 50× Stop & Glo® Substrate to a 1× concentration in Stop & Glo® buffer. In 15 mL polypropylene tubes, prepare enough of these solutions to accommodate 50 μL each per well, and an additional 400 μL for luminometer priming (*see* **Note 8**).

3. Transfer 20 μL cell lysate to a white, opaque-bottomed 96-well plate.
4. Prime the GloMax® 96 Microplate Luminometer (Promega) auto-injector system with the LAR II and Stop & Glo® reagent according to the manufacturer's recommendations. Priming reagent can be recovered by placing the injector tip back into the appropriate 15 mL polypropylene tube to reduce waste. Set injectors to dispense 50 μL of each reagent per well, and run the luminometer.
5. Analyze the data. Firefly luciferase is used as an internal normalization control. The negative control AMO and "reagent only" treated cells should have similar ratios of RLuc/FLuc. If not, there might have been an off-target effect from the negative control AMO or some other toxicity that occurred during the transfection (*see* **Note 6**). Calculate the RLuc/FLuc values for all of the samples and average the biological triplicates. The average RLuc/FLuc negative control AMO values can be set to "1", and compared with the average RLuc/FLuc values of AMO-treated cells. An increase in RLuc/FLuc values for AMO-treated cells signifies derepression of RLuc, indicating successful miRNA inhibition (*see* Fig. 3). The dynamic range for the miRNA inhibition is defined by the RLuc/FLuc ratio

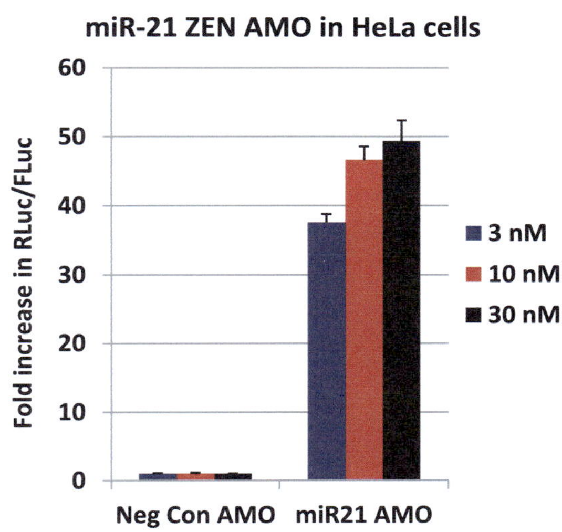


**Fig. 3** Mir-21 inhibition with a ZEN AMO using the Dual-Luciferase® Reporter Assay System. The perfect match miR-21 binding site was cloned into the 3′UTR of *Renilla* luciferase (RLuc) in the PsiCHECK-2 plasmid (psiCHECK-miR-21). The miR-21 ZEN AMO was transfected into HeLa cells expressing psiCHECK-miR-21 with Lipofectamine® RNAiMAX. After 24 h, cells were lysed and analyzed for luciferase activity. All RLuc values were normalized with the internal firefly luciferase (FLuc) control, and reported as a fold change in RLuc compared with a negative control AMO, which was set at 1

in the unmodified PsiCHECK-2 plasmid (representing maximum miRNA inhibition) and the RLuc/FLuc ratio of negative control AMO treatment in PsiCHECK-miR21 cells (as an indicator of no miRNA inhibition). By then comparing RLuc/FLuc values of AMO-treated cells expressing PsiCHECK-miR21 within this dynamic range, the degree of miRNA inhibition can be quantified.

### 3.3 Western Blot Analysis

1. Reverse transfect HeLa cells with the negative control and miR-21 ZEN AMOs. Include a "reagent only" control in which only the transfection reagent (no ZEN AMO) is applied to the cells as a control to assess toxicity or contamination issues that might arise. We recommend starting with a dosing range of 30, 10, and 3 nM (*see* **Note 3**). All dilutions should be made in polypropylene tubes (such as 5 mL round bottom tubes). For a single well, dilute 12.5 μL Lipofectamine® RNAiMAX into 237.5 μL Opti-MEM® (total volume is 250 μL) (*see* **Note 4**). For triplicate transfections, multiply these values by 3.3 to account for pipetting errors (e.g., combine 41.3 μL Lipofectamine® RNAiMAX with 783.8 μL Opti-MEM®), and multiply again by the total number of transfection conditions used. Next, dilute 25 μL of the appropriate AMO dilution (e.g., use the 3 μM dilution for 30 nM dose, *see* **Note 1**) into 225 μL Opti-MEM® (total volume is 250 μL). For triplicate transfections, multiply these values by 3.2 to account for pipetting errors (e.g., combine 80 μL AMO with 720 μL Opti-MEM® for a total volume of 800 μL). Add 800 μL of the diluted Lipofectamine® RNAiMAX to the diluted AMO (total volume now is 1600 μL). Gently mix the complexes with a quick vortex or by pipetting up and down, and incubate at room temperature for 20 min.
2. During the 20 min incubation, trypsinize the HeLa cells and dilute to 200,000 cells per 1 mL in DMEM containing 10% FBS. Each well in the 6-well plate will be seeded with 2 mL of diluted cells. Scale up the volumes appropriately, accounting for pipetting errors. Cells are seeded to be ~90% confluent the next day (*see* **Note 5**).
3. After the 20 min incubation, add 500 μL of the AMO/lipid complex in triplicate wells in a 6-well plate, followed by 2 mL diluted HeLa cells for final volume of 2.5 mL. Incubate the cells at 37 °C and 5% $CO_2$ for 48 h. Gently rock the plate periodically for the first hour to allow cells to become adherent to the plate and evenly dispersed in a monolayer. After 24 h, visualize the cells to ensure there is no toxicity or contamination (*see* **Note 6**), and replace the transfection media with fresh media.
4. After 48 h, aspirate growth media and wash cells with 1 mL ice-cold PBS.

5. Aspirate PBS and add 0.75 mL of 2× Laemmli sample buffer to each well (*see* **Note 9**). The lysates may be quite viscous, and light sonication or further dilution may be required prior to SDS-PAGE (*see* **Note 10**). Rock plates gently for 10 min at room temperature.
6. Transfer the resulting cell lysates to 1.5 mL microcentrifuge tubes. You can verify complete cell lysis by inspection of the original plate by microscopy.
7. Incubate lysates at 95 °C for 5 min, and bring to room temperature for SDS-PAGE or store at −80 °C indefinitely.
8. Load 5 μL of Precision Plus Protein™ Unstained Protein Standard (Bio-Rad) and 15 μL each sample onto Mini-PROTEAN® TGX™ Precast Gels (Bio-Rad), and run electrophoresis in SDS-PAGE running buffer at 200 V for 30 min (*see* **Note 11**). Tris–HCl or Bis-Tris gels prepared "in-house" should be electrophoresed for 60 min.
9. Gels should be carefully removed using new, protective gloves and assembled into a Trans-Blot® Turbo™ Transfer System (Bio-Rad) gel sandwich as per the manufacturer's instructions. If using PVDF or nitrocellulose membranes and a traditional Western Blot Transfer apparatus, proceed to **step 10a**; otherwise, proceed to **step 11**.
10. (a) Equilibrate SDS-PAGE gels in Western Blot Transfer buffer (25 mM Tris–HCl pH 8.3, 192 mM glycine, 20% methanol, and 0.1% SDS) for 15 min at room temperature.
    (b) Cut membrane roughly to the size of the SDS-PAGE gel. If PVDF membranes are used, incubate cut PVDF membrane in 100% methanol for 5 min and transfer immediately to Western Blot Transfer buffer until proceeding further. Nitrocellulose membranes can be immediately placed in transfer buffer.
    (c) Cut two pieces of Whatman 3MM chromatography paper to roughly the size of the gel and wet each in transfer buffer.
    (d) Assemble gel sandwich in the following order being careful to remove air bubbles by rolling each layer with a clean glass test tube: (bottom) one wet layer of 3MM paper, nitrocellulose or PVDF membrane, SDS-PAGE gel, one wet layer of 3MM paper (top).
    (e) Wet or semi-dry transfer apparatuses should be electrophoresed according to the manufacturer's instructions.
11. If using TGX™ precast gels, run the Trans-Blot® Turbo™ program "Mini-TGX", which will transfer for 3 min at 2.5 A and up to 25 V. Alternatively, standard SDS-PAGE gels may be transferred for 30 min at 1.0 A and 25 V (*see* **Note 11**).

12. Disassemble the transfer apparatus and immediately place the wet membrane in 50 mL of SuperBlock™ T20 (TBS) Blocking Buffer, in a clean tray that is just larger than the membrane. A pipette tips box lid with a flat bottom is often perfectly suited for this task. If using PVDF membranes and any portion of the membrane appears dried (white appearance), the membrane can again be wetted in 100% methanol prior to blocking with minimal loss in protein. Gently rock membrane in blocking buffer for 30 min at room temperature.
13. Prepare primary antibody solution with 10 mL of blocking buffer, 1:1000 dilution (10 μL) anti-β-ACTIN monoclonal antibody, and 1:1000 dilution (10 μL) of either the anti-MARCKS or anti-PTEN mouse monoclonal antibodies (*see* **Note 12**). If 10 mL is not sufficient to completely cover the membrane, larger volumes may be used.
14. Decant blocking buffer and add primary antibody solution to the gel tray, and incubate 1–4 h at room temperature. Gel trays should be covered in clear plastic wrap if incubation is longer than 1 h.
15. Decant primary antibody solution, and wash three times for 5–20 min with 50 mL Western washing buffer at room temperature with gentle rocking.
16. Prepare secondary antibody solution with 10 mL of blocking buffer, 1:10,000 dilution (1 μL) Amersham ECL anti-Mouse IgG, HRP-linked whole antibody from sheep (GE Healthcare), and 1:10,000 dilution (1 μL) of Precision Protein™ *Strep*Tactin-HRP Conjugate (Bio-Rad).
17. Decant final primary wash, and add 10 mL secondary antibody solution. Incubate for 30 min at room temperature with gentle rocking.
18. Decant secondary antibody solution, and wash three times for 5–20 min with 50 mL Western washing buffer at room temperature with gentle rocking.
19. Prepare SuperSignal™ West Femto working solution by adding an equal volume (1 mL each per membrane) of stable peroxide solution and luminol/enhancer solution, and gently mix.
20. Decant final secondary wash and pipette West Femto working solution directly onto the membrane ensuring that the entire membrane is covered with a thin layer of liquid.
21. Incubate 5 min at room temperature periodically pipetting working solution onto the membrane so that it does not dry.
22. Grab the corner of the membrane with clean forceps, briefly let residual liquid drip off the membrane, and place directly onto the glass bed of the ChemiDoc imager. At this point, the blot can be exposed for up to an hour without rewetting the membrane.

23. Perform several exposures of the membrane such that each band of interest (including the marker) has the maximum signal possible prior to saturation. Typically, β-ACTIN is a strong signal, and will require a separate exposure from PTEN, MARCKS, or other low-abundance proteins. An increase in protein expression directly correlates with miRNA inhibition (*see* Fig. 4).
24. Subsequent analysis and densitometry can be performed using Image Lab™ (Bio-Rad) or other software according to the manufacturer's instructions.

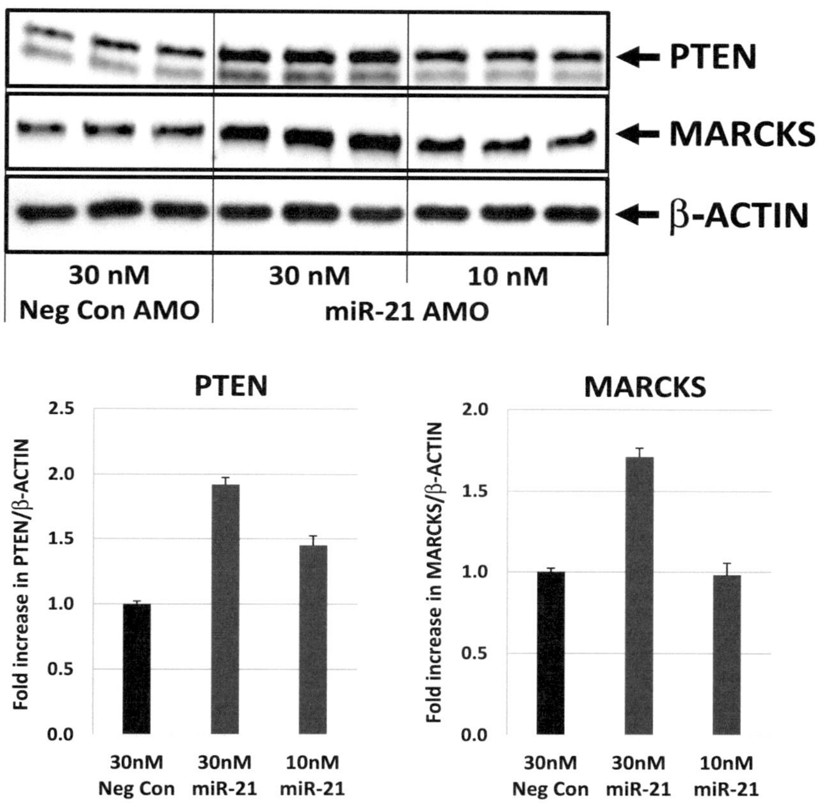


**Fig. 4** Mir-21 inhibition of endogenous PTEN and MARCKS protein in HeLa cells with a ZEN AMO. The miR-21 ZEN AMO was transfected into HeLa cells with Lipofectamine® RNAiMAX. After 48 h, cells were lysed directly in 2× Laemmli samples buffer and subjected to SDS-PAGE. Proteins were transferred to PVDF membranes and blotted with anti-β-ACTIN and anti-PTEN or anti-MARCKS antibodies. Western blots were performed using chemiluminescence on the ChemiDoc™ Touch Imaging System (Bio-Rad). Image Lab Software (Bio-Rad) was used for densitometry, and PTEN or MARCKS values were normalized with the β-ACTIN control, and reported as a fold change in PTEN or MARCKS compared with a negative control AMO, which was set at 1

## 4 Notes

1. For cell culture experiments, 5 nmol is sufficient material for ~370 transfections performed in biological triplicates in 96-well plates with 150 μL final volume at the maximum recommended dose (30 nM). It is important to quantify nucleic acids prior to use to ensure the correct concentration is used. Working dilutions should be made so that the same volume of AMO is added to the transfection mix, regardless of the dose. For example, for the recommended 30, 10, and 3 nM dose response, prepare AMO dilutions of 3, 1 and 0.3 μM respectively.
2. Some plasmid DNA preparation kits incorporate an endotoxin removal step. We recommend using the PureYield™ Plasmid Midiprep System (Promega) for the purification of plasmids for cell culture. If using a different plasmid DNA preparation kit that does not include an endotoxin removal step, we recommend using the MiraCLEAN® Endotoxin Removal Kit (Mirus) to treat the plasmid DNA prep prior to use.
3. The selected dose range may vary due to transfection efficiency of the individual cell line. For example, in cells difficult to lipofect, the AMO concentration may need to be higher. Alternatively, in cells easy to lipofect, the high dose may cause toxicity requiring the use of lower doses. We recommend starting with a 30, 10, and 3 nM dose–response study and to subsequently adjust concentrations up or down according to results and toxicity observed.
4. One effective reagent for transfecting ZEN AMOs into HeLa cells is Lipofectamine® RNAiMAX. However, Lipofectamine® 2000 is also a suitable transfection reagent (but shows higher toxicity); it should be used at 0.25–0.5 μL/well in a 96-well plate. If using a different cell line, an alternative transfection reagent may be more suitable; transfection conditions should be optimized for every cell line studied. In general, a transfection reagent that has high transfection efficiency of a similar small nucleic acid, such as an antisense oligonucleotide or a siRNA, in a particular cell line will also have high transfection efficiency for the ZEN AMOs. Optimal lipofection results are achieved when holding the volume of the lipid transfection reagent constant while titrating down the AMO for the dose response. For example, in a 96-well plate we will transfect AMOs at 30, 10, and 3 nM, all with 0.5 μL Lipofectamine® RNAiMAX/well.
5. Cell confluency can affect internal AMO concentration in the cells. We have observed that a lower cell confluency can have higher AMO activity, presumably because more AMO is available for uptake in the fewer number of cells. For inter-experiment consistency, ensure that the confluency is similar

between experiments. This same variable can impact toxicity levels as well. While ZEN AMOs are non-toxic, other chemically modified oligonucleotides can exhibit toxicity at higher doses. We have found that having a confluency of ~90% will mitigate toxicity of a wide variety of chemically modified oligonucleotides.

6. Bacterial contamination is evident if the media has a cloudy appearance, and often causes a change in media color due to a change in pH. Bacteria can be visualized by microscopy as tiny moving granules, but macroscopic examination should provide conclusive evidence. If this occurs, make sure all tools and equipment are sterile, and filter suspect nucleic acids through a 0.2 μm filter. Cell toxicity can sometimes result from residual chemicals during the AMO synthesis and/or purification process. Ethanol precipitating the AMOs can help remove trace toxic substances. If toxicity remains problematic, lowering the dose or increasing cell confluency (*see* **Note 5**) can help resolve the issue. Alternatively, miRNA knockdown itself could be the cause of toxicity if the targeted miRNA is involved in an important cellular pathway or cell viability.
7. After lyses, HeLa cells often do not completely disintegrate, and the outer cell structure is still visible by microscopy. However, RLuc and FLuc values are generally in the expected range even with incomplete lyses. If concerned, carefully tap the plates against a table or use a pipette tip to scrape the wells to further break up cells. We recommend using 45 μL/well of 1× PLB to lyse cells in a 96-well plate to provide extra lysate in case the experiment needs to be repeated.
8. Promega's protocol for the Dual Luciferase Assay recommends using 100 μL of the LAR II and Stop & Glo reagent per well. Optimization experiments have shown that in HeLa cells or Huh-7 cells, the same results are achieved when using 50 μL of each reagent. This may need to be optimized if using other cell lines. All Dual Luciferase Assay reagents should be handled according to Promega's recommendations.
9. Typically procedures for lysis of animal cells grown in tissue culture entails lysis in RIPA (*R*adio*I*mmuno*P*recipitation *A*ssay) buffer, followed by denaturation of proteins in Laemmli sample buffer. An advantage of the RIPA protocol is that you can determine total protein concentration and normalize loading prior to electrophoresis. A complication of this procedure is that RIPA buffer does not fully denature many proteases, and Western blot targets may be degraded prior to PAGE. In this protocol, we denature directly in denaturing Laemmli sample buffer and load using a uniform volume (15 μL). We did not observe significant fluctuations in extracted protein concentration as observed using the β-ACTIN control, and

small differences were normalized mathematically based on the concentration of β-ACTIN. If large differences in β-ACTIN concentration are detected, it is advisable to adjust loading based on a preliminary β-ACTIN test blot.

10. If the viscosity of lysates is too high for consistent gel loading, sonication may be required. A 1.5 mL microcentrifuge tube containing 0.25–0.5 mL of lysate should be sonicated with ten pulses (50% duty cycle or 0.5 s on and 0.5 s off) using a microtip attachment, with an amplitude of ~20–30% maximum. The tube can be held by hand with the tip just barely above the tube bottom. It may be helpful to test a blank 2× sample buffer to ensure that the conditions to not induce foaming.
11. Prestained molecular weight standards may be used to ensure efficient transfer of proteins to the blotting membrane. However, typically these standards are not detectable with the StrepTactin-HRP conjugate. Alternatively, gel transfer can be visualized with a 0.1% (w/v) Ponceau S solution in 5% acetic acid. Staining can be reversed with multiple washes in water.
12. Human β-ACTIN is ~42 kDa, and may need to be blotted separately if the target of interest is 35–50 kDa. Alternatively, the membrane may be stripped after a blotting using the Restore™ Western Blot Stripping Buffer (ThermoFisher).

## Acknowledgements

The authors thank Dr. Garrett Rettig for critical reading of the chapter and Todd Adamson for assistance in preparing Fig. 2.

### References

1. Bartel DP (2004) MicroRNAs: genomics, biogenesis, mechanism, and function. Cell 116:281–297
2. Lee RC, Feinbaum RL, Ambros V (1993) The C. elegans heterochronic gene lin-4 encodes small RNAs with antisense complementarity to lin-14. Cell 75:843–854
3. Li Y, Kowdley KV (2012) MicroRNAs in common human diseases. Genomics Proteomics Bioinformatics 10:246–253
4. Trionfini P, Benigni A, Remuzzi G (2015) MicroRNAs in kidney physiology and disease. Nat Rev Nephrol 11:23–33
5. Meola N, Gennarino VA, Banfi S (2009) MicroRNAs and genetic diseases. Pathogenetics 2:7
6. Ha M, Kim VN (2014) Regulation of microRNA biogenesis. Nat Rev Mol Cell Biol 15:509–524
7. Carthew RW, Sontheimer EJ (2009) Origins and mechanisms of miRNAs and siRNAs. Cell 136:642–655
8. Lima WF, Wu H, Crooke ST (2008) Antisense drug technology, principles, strategies, and applications, vol 2. CRC Press, Boca Raton, FL, pp 47–74
9. Baskerville S, Bartel DP (2005) Microarray profiling of microRNAs reveals frequent coexpression with neighboring miRNAs and host genes. RNA 11:241–247
10. Vickers TA, Wyatt JR, Freier SM (2000) Effects of RNA secondary structure on cellular antisense activity. Nucleic Acids Res 28:1340–1347
11. Lennox KA, Behlke MA (2011) Chemical modification and design of anti-miRNA oligonucleotides. Gene Ther 18:1111–1120
12. Lennox KA, Behlke MA (2010) A direct comparison of anti-microRNA oligonucleotide potency. Pharm Res 27:1788–1799
13. Lennox KA, Owczarzy R, Thomas DM, Walder JA, Behlke MA (2013) Improved performance of anti-miRNA oligonucleotides using a novel

non-nucleotide modifier. Mol Ther Nucleic Acids 2:e117

14. Laemmli UK (1970) Cleavage of structural proteins during the assembly of the head of bacteriophage T4. Nature 227:680–685
15. Graham DR, Garnham CP, Fu Q, Robbins J, Van Eyk JE (2005) Improvements in two-dimensional gel electrophoresis by utilizing a low cost "in-house" neutral pH sodium dodecyl sulfate-polyacrylamide gel electrophoresis system. Proteomics 5:2309–2314
16. Zhou JY, Ma WL, Liang S, Zeng Y, Shi R, Yu HL, Xiao WW, Zheng WL (2009) Analysis of microRNA expression profiles during the cell cycle in synchronized HeLa cells. BMB Rep 42:593–598
17. Meng F, Henson R, Wehbe-Janek H, Ghoshal K, Jacob ST, Patel T (2007) MicroRNA-21 regulates expression of the PTEN tumor suppressor gene in human hepatocellular cancer. Gastroenterology 133:647–658
18. Zhang JG, Wang JJ, Zhao F, Liu Q, Jiang K, Yang GH (2010) MicroRNA-21 (miR-21) represses tumor suppressor PTEN and promotes growth and invasion in non-small cell lung cancer (NSCLC). Clin Chim Acta 411:846–852
19. Li T, Li D, Sha J, Sun P, Huang Y (2009) MicroRNA-21 directly targets MARCKS and promotes apoptosis resistance and invasion in prostate cancer cells. Biochem Biophys Res Commun 383:280–285

# Chapter 4

# Quantification of Oligonucleotide Association with miRNA–Argonaute Complexes In Vitro

**Dimitrios G. Zisoulis**

## Abstract

A major challenge in the development of oligonucleotide-based microRNA (miRNA) inhibitors for therapeutic applications is the identification of candidate designs with strong affinity for the target miRNA in the context of the Argonaute complex. To this effect, distinct chemical modifications are employed along the length of the oligonucleotide aimed at strengthening the interactions with the target miRNA. However, the modification chemistry and placement can inadvertently affect the intrinsic ability of the oligonucleotide to pair with its target in the context of Argonaute. To facilitate the design of potent oligonucleotides, we developed a sensitive high-throughput methodology to compare anti-miR compounds for their ability to associate with the miRNA/Argonaute complex.

**Key words** Anti-miR, microRNA, microRNA inhibitors, Argonaute, Drug discovery, Oligonucleotide therapeutics

## 1 Introduction

microRNAs (miRNAs), the family of small non-coding RNA molecules, regulate diverse gene networks involved in a plethora of physiological functions and subsequently aberrant miRNA expression can lead to disease states [1, 2]. The emerging role of miRNAs in disease lead to fervent attempts by many academic labs to develop tools to identify miRNA targets in vivo [3, 4] and to development efforts by the biotech community to advance therapeutic interventions for miRNAs [5–10], with some of them reaching the clinic recently [11–13]. As our understanding of the mechanism of oligonucleotide-based miRNA inhibition expands, novel technologies arise to modulate the interaction of Argonaute (AGO) complexes with its targets and inhibitors.

A key aspect of miRNA-mediated gene regulation involves Argonaute-containing microRNA-induced silencing complexes (miRISC) that are guided to the target sites of target messenger RNAs (mRNAs) by mature miRNAs, typically 21–22 nucleotides

Marco F. Schmidt (ed.), *Drug Target miRNA: Methods and Protocols*, Methods in Molecular Biology, vol. 1517,
DOI 10.1007/978-1-4939-6563-2_4, © Springer Science+Business Media New York 2017

long. The interaction between the "seed" portion of the miRNA, nucleotides 2–8, and the target sequence, primarily in the 3′ untranslated region (3′UTR) of the target mRNAs leads to mRNA destabilization and translational repression [14]. Interestingly enough, few studies have focused on the relative strength of interaction of a specific miRNA with its potential targets, mostly using reporter systems or biophysical and computational models [15, 16]. miRNA inhibitors, termed anti-miRs or antagomiRs are synthetic oligonucleotides complementary to the target miRNA with modifications aimed at stabilizing the oligonucleotide, such as phosphorothioate and phosphodiester backbones, and at increasing the affinity to the target miRNA sequence, by modifications to the sugar molecules [17–19]. However, not all anti-miRs are created equally; evidence suggests that the Argonaute/miRNA/anti-miR interaction can be modulated by the chemical modifications and their placement in the anti-miR sequence [20].

To facilitate determining the effect of oligonucleotide chemical modifications and placement on ability of anti-miRs to engage miRNAs we developed a high-throughput, sensitive and specific methodology, the REvamped Biochemical/Binding Oligonucleotide Procedure (Rebop). In this biochemical competition-based assay, which can also be used to assay the relevant affinity of a miRNA for its mRNA targets, elecotrochemiluminescently labeled oligonucleotides compete with unlabeled test oligonucleotides for association with Argonaute complexes harboring the target miRNA. Briefly: (1) tissues or cells are lysed, (2) Argonaute complexes are immunocaptured on a plate coated with anti-Argonaute antibodies, (3) the purified Argonaute complexes are incubated with the tested anti-miR and increasing amounts of labeled, competing oligonucleotide probe, (4) excess probe and oligonucleotide compound is removed, and (5) luminescence levels are determined by an electrochemiluminescence plate reader (Meso Scale Discovery).

## 2 Materials

As with any procedure involving RNA-binding proteins, it is recommended that all buffer components are RNase-free.

### 2.1 Plate Preparation

1. High-bind, 96-well Meso Scale Discovery (MSD) plates.
2. Anti-Argonaute mouse monoclonal IgA antibody 4F9 (sc-53521, Santa Cruz Biotechnology).
3. Phosphate buffered saline, pH 7.4 (PBS).

### 2.2 Electro chemiluminescent Probe Preparation

1. 1 M sodium phosphate (98:2, dibasic:monobasic, pH 8).
2. Oligonucleotide with sequence complementary to target miRNA with two terminal amines containing 2′-*O*-methyl or phosphorothioate modifications (Integrated DNA Technologies).

3. Sulfo-Tag Reagent (Meso Scale Discovery).
4. 1 M glycine–HCl, pH 2.8.
5. Thermomixer.

### 2.3 Lysate Preparation

1. Liquid Nitrogen.
2. Mortar and pestle.
3. Hand-held tissue homogenizer.
4. Lysis Buffer: 20 mM Tris–HCl, pH 8.0, 140 mM KCl, 5 mM EDTA, 0.5 % NP-40, 1X Halt protease inhibitor cocktail (Pierce).

### 2.4 Argonaute Capture

1. Wash Buffer PBS-T: PBS with 0.05 % v/v Tween 20.
2. 96-well plate washer (Biotek plate washer) or multi-channel pipette for the washes.
3. Plate shaker.

### 2.5 Competitive Inhibition of Labeled Probes by Oligonucleotide Compounds

1. Dilutions of oligonucleotide anti-miRs to be tested; typically 1:10 dilutions of 1 pmol/μL (1 μM) in PBS.
2. MSD Read Buffer (2X).
3. MSD Reader.

## 3 Method

The Rebop methodology was developed to allow the direct comparison of multiple oligonucleotides with distinct chemical modifications in regards to their ability to target their cognate miRNA in the context of Argonaute. In the procedure outlined below we use as source of Argonaute and miRNAs rodent liver and other tissues or cell lines can be used as well as long as there is substantial expression of the target miRNA in the tissue. Briefly, the process is separated into four distinct stages (Fig. 1): (1) preparation of plate for Argonaute capture, (2) capture of Argonaute/miRNA complexes, (3) competition of compounds with the electrochemiluminescently labeled probe, and (4) detection of residual chemiluminescence and analysis.

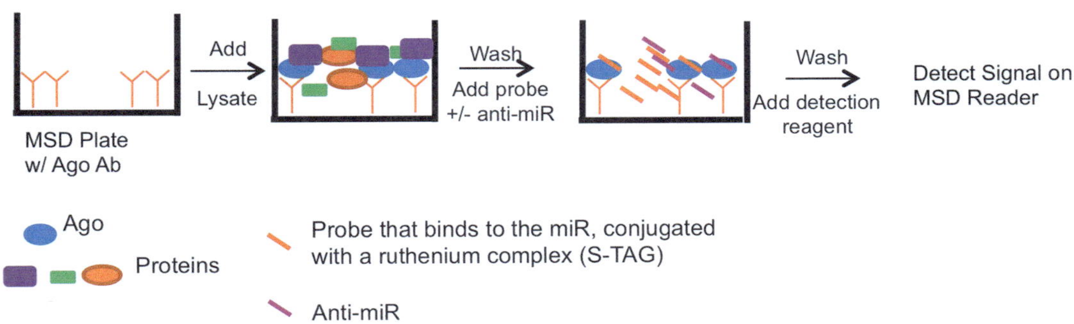


**Fig. 1** Overview of the experimental procedure

### 3.1 Preparation of MSD Plates for Argonaute Capture

1. Prepare solutions of 1 µg/mL of anti-Argonaute monoclonal IgA antibody and isotype control antibody in PBS.
2. Pipette 30 µL of anti-Argonaute or control antibody in the wells of a high-bind, 96-well MSD plate, resulting in approximately 30 ng/well of antibody (*see* **Note 1**).
3. Swirl plate to evenly distribute solution in the well.
4. Seal with self-adherent aluminum foil and place at −4 °C o/n. Keep the plates 2–3 weeks.

### 3.2 Electro chemiluminescent Probe Preparation

1. Resuspend the oligonucleotide with the terminal amine groups (probe) in appropriate volume to achieve 1 mM in 500 mM sodium phosphate buffer pH 8 (*see* **Notes 2** and **3**).
2. Reconstitute the Sulfo-Tag reagent (500 nmol) in 50 µL of ice-cold dd$H_2O$. Use within 10 min.
3. Incubate 25 µL of probe and 50 µL of S-TAG in small PCR tube at 50 °C in the dark with shaking for 2 h (Thermomixer)
4. Stop reaction by adding 40 µL of 1 M glycine-HCl, pH 2.8 and incubate at room temperature for 20 min.
5. The total volume is now ~120 µL which translates roughly to ~200 µM of probe.
6. Freeze in aliquots of 5 µL at −80 °C. Do not keep diluted final concentration probes (1 µM) after use.

### 3.3 Preparation of Tissue for Purification of Argonaute-Containing Complexes

1. Collect a piece of the Argonaute/miRNA source tissue, weigh and flash-freeze in liquid nitrogen. Store at −80 °C or proceed (*see* **Note 4**).
2. Crash frozen tissue using mortar and pestle pre-cooled with liquid nitrogen and make sure powder stays frozen.
3. Dissolve the tissue powder in Lysis Buffer (100 mg/mL) and lyse with the hand-held tissue homogenizer for 30 s, on ice. Let tissue sit on ice for 5 min to allow detergents to lyse the tissue.
4. Move lysate to 2 mL Eppendorf tubes and centrifuge at 16,000 × *g* for 10 min at 4 °C.
5. Remove supernatant, proceed or freeze in liquid nitrogen and store at −80 °C.

### 3.4 miRNA/Argonaute Capture

1. Equilibrate the MSD plates coated with the anti-Argonaute or control antibody to room temperature and tap out the antibody solution.
2. Wash 1X with PBS-T.
3. Add the miRNA/Argonaute source lysate and incubate for 1 h at room temperature with gentle shaking to capture Argonaute (*see* **Notes 5** and **6**).

4. Wash 3× with PBS-T using a plate washer or multi-channel pipette and move immediately to the next stage.

***3.5 Competition Between Oligonucleotide Compounds and Labeled Probe for the Argonaute Complexes and Quantification***

1. From the prepared series of 1:10 dilutions of compounds add 15 μL to each well.
2. Add 15 μL of the probe, diluted with PBS to 0.01 μM. It may be beneficial to test different amounts of the probe (Fig. 2 and *see* **Note 7**).
3. Incubate for 1 h at room temperature with gentle shaking, in the dark.
4. Wash plate with PBS-T (3×).

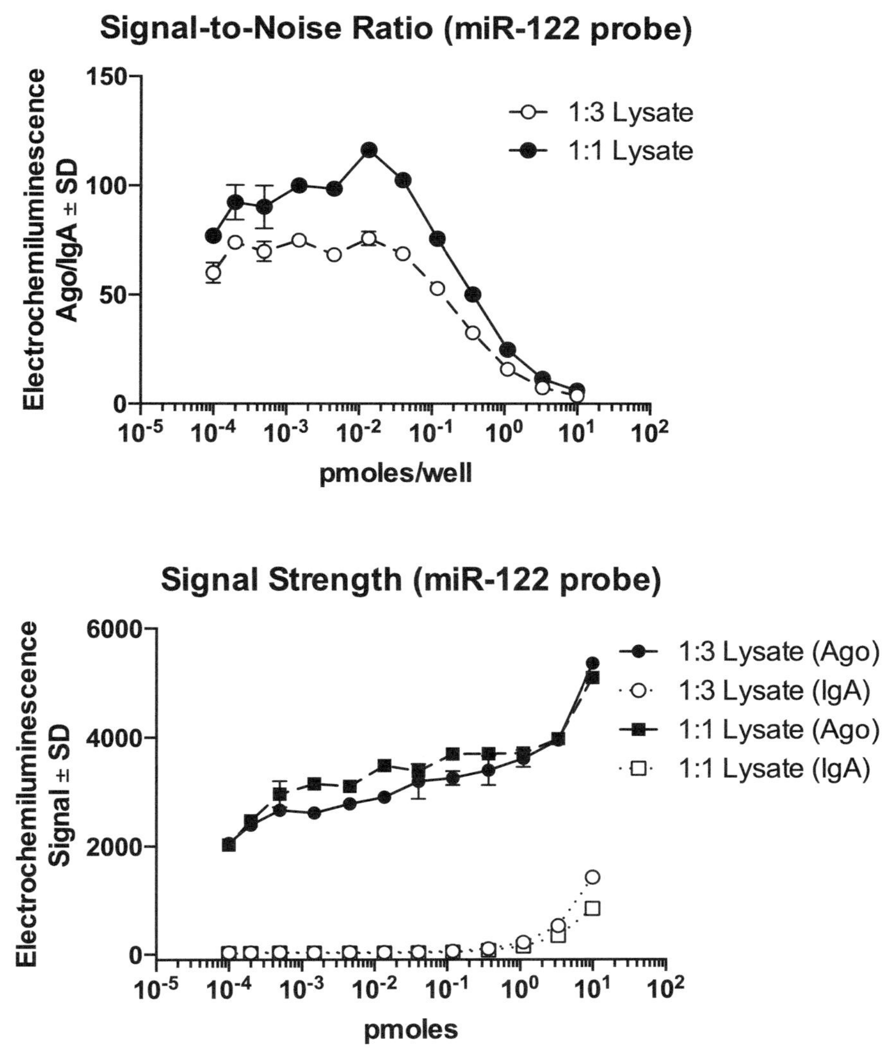


**Fig. 2** Calculation of signal-to-noise ratio for different concentrations of probe for miR-122 and liver lysate (*upper panel*) and signal strength from Argonaute and control IgA wells (*lower panel*)

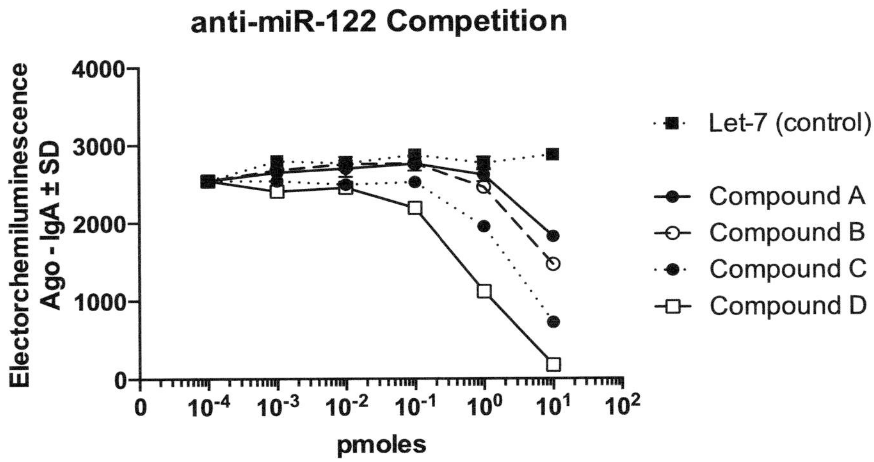


**Fig. 3** Results of the competition based assay for distinct compounds against miR-122. Anti-let-7 compound was used as a negative control

5. Tap out and add 150 μL of 2X MSD Read buffer.
6. Proceed to read the plate on the MSD Reader (*see* **Note 8**).
7. Processing of the raw data includes calculating signal-to-noise ratios by dividing the Argonaute signal with the control signal and calculating Argonaute-control signals for the quantification of competition (Fig. 3).

## 4 Notes

1. Different concentrations of antibody may need to be tested to ensure the highest signal-to-noise ratio (Ago signal/control signal).
2. General guidelines to achieve efficient conjugation of the Sulfo-Tag Reagent to oligonucleotide with primary amines for *N*-hydroxysuccinimide ester crosslinking reactions (Laure Moller, personal communication).
   (a) Oligonucleotide concentration should be relatively high (>0.5 mM).
   (b) Use higher molar excess of Sulfo-Tag to primary amines (>6X).
   (c) Keep the concentration of phosphate >25 times the concentration of Sulfo-TAG NHS ester.
   (d) Conjugating at higher temperature (e.g. 55 °C) improves the conjugation efficiency.

3. For all procedures involving oligonucleotide reagents ensure that the containers used (tubes, plates, etc.) are made of polypropylene and not other types of plastic that can absorb oligonucleotides.
4. It is possible to use cell lines expressing or overexpressing the miRNA. In this case make lysates using five times or more Lysis Buffer than the total volume of cells.
5. Alternatively, instead of capturing Argonaute and then adding the oligonucleotide/probe mix, the mix can be added at this stage (30 μL of lysate, 5 μL of compound, and 5 μL of probe).
6. Different lysate concentrations should be tested if using tissues other than liver as described here. For liver, the effective protein concentration of the lysate after all the centrifugations is diluted 1:3, resulting in ~1 mg/mL (Fig. 2).
7. Testing different concentrations of probe is recommended. The typical concentration used in these studies is 0.01 pmol/well.
8. Allow minimal time between adding MSD Read Buffer and reading the plate to avoid the establishment of new equilibrium of the probe in the buffer.

## References


1. Mendell JT, Olson EN (2012) MicroRNAs in stress signaling and human disease. Cell 148:1172–1187
2. Seyhan AA (2015) microRNAs with different functions and roles in disease development and as potential biomarkers of diabetes: progress and challenges. Mol Biosyst 11:1217–1234
3. Chi SW, Zang JB, Mele A, Darnell RB (2009) Argonaute HITS-CLIP decodes microRNA-mRNA interaction maps. Nature 460: 479–486
4. Zisoulis DG, Lovci MT, Wilbert ML, Hutt KR, Liang TY et al (2010) Comprehensive discovery of endogenous Argonaute binding sites in Caenorhabditis elegans. Nature structural & molecular biology 17:173–179
5. Hutvagner G, Simard MJ, Mello CC, Zamore PD (2004) Sequence-specific inhibition of small RNA function. PLoS biology 2, E98
6. Meister G, Landthaler M, Dorsett Y, Tuschl T (2004) Sequence-specific inhibition of microRNA- and siRNA-induced RNA silencing. RNA 10:544–550
7. Jopling CL, Yi M, Lancaster AM, Lemon SM, Sarnow P (2005) Modulation of hepatitis C virus RNA abundance by a liver-specific MicroRNA. Science 309:1577–1581
8. Krützfeldt J, Rajewsky N, Braich R, Rajeev KG, Tuschl T et al (2005) Silencing of microRNAs in vivo with 'antagomirs'. Nature 438:685–689
9. Davis S, Lollo B, Freier S, Esau C (2006) Improved targeting of miRNA with antisense oligonucleotides. Nucleic acids research 34:2294–2304
10. Esau C, Davis S, Murray SF, Yu XX, Pandey SK et al (2006) miR-122 regulation of lipid metabolism revealed by in vivo antisense targeting. Cell metabolism 3:87–98
11. Janssen HL, Kauppinen S, Hodges MR (2013) HCV infection and miravirsen. N Engl J Med 369:878
12. Janssen HL, Reesink HW, Lawitz EJ, Zeuzem S, Rodriguez-Torres M et al (2013) Treatment of HCV infection by targeting microRNA. N Engl J Med 368:1685–1694
13. Van Der Ree MLV, Stelma F, Willemse S, van der Valk M, Rietdijk S, Molenkamp R, Schinkel J et al (2015) A single subcutaneous dose of 2 mg/kg or 4 mg/kg of RG-101, a GalNAc-conjugated oligonucleotide with antagonist activity against MIR-122, results in significant viral load reductions in chronic hepatitis C patients. Journal of Hepatology 62:261
14. Bartel DP (2009) MicroRNAs: target recognition and regulatory functions. Cell 136:215–233
15. Breda J, Rzepiela AJ, Gumienny R, van Nimwegen E, Zavolan M (2015) Quantifying the strength of miRNA-target interactions. Methods 85:90–9

16. Hammell M, Long D, Zhang L, Lee A, Carmack CS et al (2008) mirWIP: microRNA target prediction based on microRNA-containing ribonucleoprotein-enriched transcripts. Nat Methods 5:813–819
17. Esau CC (2008) Inhibition of microRNA with antisense oligonucleotides. Methods 44:55–60
18. Stenvang J, Petri A, Lindow M, Obad S, Kauppinen S (2012) Inhibition of microRNA function by antimiR oligonucleotides. Silence 3:1
19. Crooke ST (2008) Antisense drug technology: principles, strategies, and applications. CRC Press, Boca Raton, FL, xvii, 825 p, 812 p. of plates p
20. Hogan DJ, Vincent TM, Fish S, Marcusson EG, Bhat B et al (2014) Anti-miRs competitively inhibit microRNAs in Argonaute complexes. PLoS One 9, e100951

# Chapter 5

# Determination of Anti-miR Association with miRNA/Argonaute Complexes In Vivo

**Dimitrios G. Zisoulis**


## Abstract

Aberrant expression of microRNAs (miRNAs) has been causatively linked to multiple disease pathologies while pharmacological inhibition of overexpressed miRNAs by modified oligonucleotides, termed anti-miRs, has been shown to ameliorate the disease phenotype. Anti-miRs are also widely used in academia to define miRNA-mediated regulation of gene networks in vitro and in vivo. Here, we describe a methodology that allows the determination of the physical association of miRNA inhibitors and their targets in the context of the Argonaute complex in vivo, providing unprecedented insight into the physiological interactions of anti-miRs and the miRNA machinery.


**Key words** Anti-miR, microRNA, microRNA inhibitors, Argonaute, Drug discovery, Oligonucleotide therapeutics

## 1 Introduction

microRNAs (miRNAs) are small genomically encoded RNA molecules that post-transcriptionally regulate gene networks critical in development and disease. First discovered more than 20 years ago in the *C. elegans* system [1, 2], they remained a "peculiarity" of the worm model organism until early 2000 when the *let-7* miRNA was shown to be conserved across animal phyla all the way to humans [3]. A few years later, the role of miRNAs in disease was established [4, 5] and the first attempts to modulate miRNAs as a means of therapeutic intervention were reported [6–11]. Following the "small RNA revolution", a number of chemically distinct antisense oligonucleotide platforms have been developed to inhibit miRNAs in vivo and two oligonucleotide compounds incorporating bicyclic nucleosides are already undergoing clinical trials [12–14]. Despite the promise, miRNA antagonists, termed anti-miRs, hold as therapeutic agents, the mechanism of oligonucleotide-based miRNA inhibition is still being clarified.

Marco F. Schmidt (ed.), *Drug Target miRNA: Methods and Protocols*, Methods in Molecular Biology, vol. 1517,
DOI 10.1007/978-1-4939-6563-2_5, 

The mature miRNA molecules are ~22 nt long and are loaded onto the Argonaute-containing miRNA-induced silencing complex (miRISC) guiding these complexes to target sites residing mostly in the 3′ untranslated region (3′UTR) of messenger RNAs (mRNAs) [15]. The interaction between mature miRNA and the target mRNA is mediated by the imperfect complementarity between miRNA and target mRNA; nucleotides 2–8, termed the "seed" bind with near-perfect complementarity to the target site, while nucleotides 9–18 exhibit small, if any, requirements for complementary base-pairing. Anti-miRs are modified oligonucleotides designed to be complementary to the target miRNA; modifications such as the phosphorothioate backbone stabilize the oligonucleotide protecting it from nucleases while modifications in the sugar base, e.g. constrained ethyl, 2′-O-methoxyethyl, etc., increase the affinity with the target sequence bases leading to stronger interaction with the target miRNA [16–18]. Mounting evidence suggested that anti-miRs associate with Argonaute leading to degradation or inhibition of the target miRNA depending on the chemical modification of the anti-miR [6, 7, 10, 19, 20], however no direct confirmation of direct anti-miR/miRNA/Argonaute interaction was reported until recently.

We recently published a study delineating the interaction between miRNA inhibitors and their target miRNA in the context of Argonaute and showed that this interaction may be highly influenced by the type and position of modifications in the anti-miR sequence [21]. Thus, it is beneficial for the development of anti-miR therapeutics to be able to determine which decorations and placement combinations lead to therapeutics with strong target engagement profiles. Furthermore, the number of academic labs employing commercially available oligonucleotides that act as miRNA inhibitors is increasing along with the need to verify that the provided oligonucleotides exhibit the proper target engagement. To contribute to these efforts, we developed an experimental methodology aimed at determining the potential of anti-miRs to interact and engage their miRNA target in the context of Argonaute in vivo.

We determine oligonucleotide compound association with Argonaute in vivo by immunopurifying Argonaute complexes and analyzing the oligonucleotide levels associated with the Argonaute protein. Briefly, the methodology entails: (1) administration of the anti-miR compound into animals, (2) isolation and lysis of the target tissue, e.g. liver, (3) immunopurification of Argonaute complexes by antibodies coupled to magnetic beads, (4) extraction of the immunopurified oligonucleotide, and (5) detection of the oligonucleotide by Northern Blot analysis. This approach also allows the direct comparison of two compounds for miRNA/Argonaute targeting assuming that the oligonucleotides under comparison have similar pharmacokinetic properties and thus are delivered to the target tissue.

## 2 Materials

As with any procedure involving RNA-binding proteins, it is recommended that all buffer components are RNase-free.

### 2.1 Lysis Preparation

1. Liquid Nitrogen.
2. Mortar and pestle.
3. Hand-held tissue homogenizer.
4. Buffer A: 20 mM Tris–HCl, pH 8.0, 140 mM KCl, 5 mM EDTA, 0.5% NP-40, 0.1% Deoxycholate, 1X Halt protease inhibitor cocktail, 100 U/mL RNaseout and 0.5 mM DTT.

### 2.2 Pre-clearing

1. Epoxy-coated magnetic beads (M-270 Dynabeads, Life Technologies).
2. Dimethylformamide (DMF).
3. Phosphate buffered saline (PBS), pH 7.4.
4. Buffer A: 20 mM Tris–HCl, pH 8.0, 140 mM KCl, 5 mM EDTA, 0.5% NP-40, 0.1% Deoxycholate, 1X Halt protease inhibitor cocktail, 100 U/mL RNaseout and 0.5 mM dithiothreitol (DTT).

### 2.3 Anti-Argonaute Antibody Conjugation to Epoxy-Coated Magnetic Beads

1. Anti-Argonaute mouse monoclonal IgA antibody 4F9 (sc-53521, Santa Cruz Biotechnology).
2. Epoxy-coated magnetic beads (M-270 Dynabeads, Life Technologies).
3. Dimethylformamide (DMF).
4. PBS Solution, 1X.
5. Magnetic beads stand.
6. 3 M ammonium sulfate solution.
7. 1 M sodium phosphate solution (98:2 dibasic:monobasic).
8. 1 M KCl solution.
9. 1 M Tris–HCl, pH 8.0.
10. 16 M ethanolamine.

### 2.4 Argonaute Complexes Immunopurification

1. Wash Buffer B: 20 mM Tris–HCl pH 8.0, 140 mM KCl, 5 mM EDTA, 40 U/mL Rnaseout, 1 mM DTT and 1X Halt protease inhibitor cocktail.

### 2.5 Western Analysis

1. Sample buffer, 30 μL per sample: 7.5 μL of 4X LDS Sample buffer (Invitrogen), 3 μL of 1 M DTT, 10 μL $dH_2O$.
2. 1 M DTT.
3. Pre-cast Protein Gels, 4–20%.

4. SDS-PAGE, transfer system and power supply (Bio-Rad).
5. SDS-Page running buffer (Bio-Rad).
6. PVDF membrane.
7. Methanol.
8. Western Transfer Buffer (Bio-Rad).
9. PBS Solution with 0.05 % Tween 20 detergent (PBS-T).
10. Mouse monoclonal Argonaute antibody (2E12-1C9, Sigma).
11. Secondary Goat Anti-mouse antibody conjugated to horseradish peroxidase.
12. Blocking solution of Non-Fat Dry Milk (5 % w/v) in PBS-T.
13. Enhanced Chemiluminescence Reagent (ECL).
14. Access to film and developer or CCD digital imaging system.

### 2.6 Oligonucleotide Extraction from Argonaute Complexes

1. Concentrated ammonium hydroxide $NH_4OH$ (~30 % on $NH_3$ basis).
2. Phenol:chloroform:isoamyl alcohol (25:24:1, v/v).
3. Phase-lock tubes to isolate the aqueous from organic phase.
4. Chloroform.
5. 3 M sodium acetate.
6. Glycoblue pellet indicator.
7. Isopropanol 100 % v/v.
8. 1 M HEPES buffer.
9. Ethanol 70 % (v/v).

### 2.7 Northern Analysis

1. 15 % Tris-borate-EDTA (TBE)-Urea precast gel.
2. Tris-borate-EDTA Solution (TBE, 1X).
3. Pre-cast gel system and power supply.
4. Hybridization solution: 3X saline-sodium citrate (SSC) solution with 0.1 % sodium dodecyl sulfate (SDS).
5. RNA sample loading buffer.
6. Washing solution: 2X saline-sodium citrate (SSC) solution with 0.1 % SDS.
7. N+ Nylon membrane (GE Healthcare).
8. A Starfire probe (Integrated DNA Technologies) for the sequence complementary to the anti-miR tested.
9. [$\gamma$-$^{32}$P]-dATP.
10. Phosphor imaging screen K (Bio-Rad) and Personal Molecular Imager FX Plus (Bio-Rad) or access to film and developer.
11. Hybridization oven for Northern blots.
12. Stratalinker 1800 UV crosslinker.

## 3 Method

The methodology is comprised of four distinct stages (Fig. 1): isolation and processing of tissue from in vivo experiments, immunopurification of Argonaute complexes, extraction and visualization of anti-miRs, and Western analysis of Argonaute proteins.

### 3.1 Preparation of Tissue for Purification of Argonaute-Containing Complexes from In Vivo Samples

Tissue samples from in vivo experiments are collected, lysed, centrifuged, and prepared for processing.

1. Dose animals and collect a lobe of the target tissue (e.g. liver) at desired time-point. Weigh target tissue and flash-freeze in liquid nitrogen. Store at −80 °C or proceed.
2. Crash frozen tissue using mortar and pestle pre-cooled with liquid nitrogen and make sure powder stays frozen.
3. Dissolve the tissue powder in Buffer A (100 mg of tissue per mL of buffer A) and lyse with the hand-held tissue homogenizer for 30 s, on ice. Let tissue sit on ice for 5 min to allow detergents to lyse the tissue.
4. Move lysate to 2 mL Eppendorf tubes and centrifuge at 1,000 × *g* in a table-top microcentrifuge for 10 min, at 4 °C.
5. Move supernatant to a new tube and centrifuge at 16,000 × *g* for 10 min at 4 °C.
6. Remove supernatant, proceed or freeze in liquid nitrogen and store at −80 °C.

### 3.2 Pre-clearing

To avoid non-specific immunopurification interactions, it is best to pre-clear the lysate with the magnetic beads to be used for the actual immunopurification.

1. Thaw lysates on ice (~20–30 min).
2. Resuspend the Epoxy-coated magnetic beads in DMF (15 mg of beads/mL of DMF, can be stored at 4 °C).
3. Wash the beads 3× with PBS using the magnetic stand.

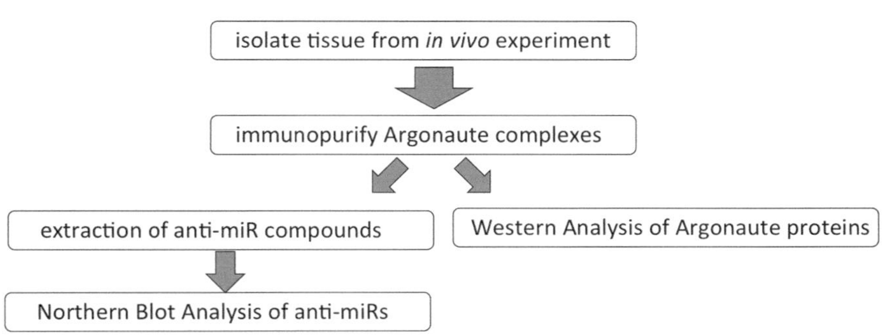


**Fig. 1** Overview of the experimental procedure

4. Equilibrate the beads 3× with 1 mL of ice-cold Buffer A per 100 μL of beads. You will need 100 μL of resuspended beads for pre-clearing per sample.
5. Measure protein concentration of samples and adjust concentration across all samples using ice-cold Buffer A.
6. Add 100 μL of equilibrated beads per mL of lysates and incubate at 4 °C on nutator for 30 min.
7. Collect and discard the beads (3×).

### 3.3 Anti-Argonaute Antibody Conjugation to Epoxy-Coated Magnetic Beads

The anti-Argonaute antibody is stably conjugated to the epoxy beads and free epoxy groups are quenched. This step should be performed in advance and the conjugated antibody can be stored at 4 °C for a couple of months.

1. Resuspend 15 mg of epoxy-coated magnetic beads in 1 mL of DMF. Resuspended beads can be stored at 4 °C.
2. Wash beads 3× in PBS using the magnetic stand in a 2 mL Eppendorf tube.
3. Add 1 mL (0.25 mg) of 4F9 anti-Argonaute antibody (at 0.25 mg/mL concentration).
4. Add 375 μL of 3 M ammonium sulfate.
5. Add 150 μL 1 M sodium phosphate (98:2, dibasic:monobasic).
6. Mix on nutator at 37 °C overnight.
7. Wash 3× in PBS.
8. Add 1 mL of 100 mM Tris–HCl, pH 8.0, 140 mM KCl and 100 mM ethanolamine.
9. Incubate at 37 °C for 1 h.
10. Wash 3× in PBS, resuspend in 1 mL of PBS and store at 4 °C.

### 3.4 Argonaute Immunopurification

At this step the actual immunopurification is performed, and aliquots are taken for subsequent analysis.

1. Take 5% of the lysate for anti-miR analysis (Subheadings 3.6 and 3.7) and 5% for protein analysis (Subheading 3.5) and store at −80 °C for later analysis.
2. Take 1 mL of the pre-cleared lysate per tube and add 100 μL of equilibrated antibody-conjugated magnetic beads per eppendorf tube (*see* **Note 1**).
3. Incubate at 4 °C on nutator for 1.5–2 h.
4. Wash 3× (5 min, nutator) with 1 mL of ice-cold Wash Buffer B, carefully not to lose beads.
5. Resuspend in 100 μL of ice-cold Wash Buffer B. Take a small aliquot (20 μL) for Western Analysis, and isolate the beads, removing the supernatant. Store at −80 °C or proceed to Western Analysis (Subheading 3.5).

6. Use the rest of the beads (80 μL) to extract and visualize the anti-miR (Subheadings 3.6 and 3.7).

### 3.5 Western Analysis (SDS-PAGE)

A typical SDS-PAGE methodology is used to visualize the levels of Argonaute protein in the lysates (input control) and to determine the Argonaute immunopurification efficiency (Fig. 2) (*see* **Note 2**).

1. Resuspend beads from Subheading 3.4 **step 5** in 30 μL of sample buffer.
2. Boil at thermomixer or in a water bath for 10 min at 99 °C with agitation (1,200 rpm). Quickly spin down.
3. Proceed with SDS-PAGE analysis using ½ of the boiled sample (15 μL). Vortex the tubes quickly, spin down and mix by pipetting, and place on magnetic stand (this will make the beads move away from the 30 μL of sample).
4. Fill with SDS-PAGE Running buffer and run at 180–200 V until the 102 kDa band that is close to Ago is in the middle of the gel (about 2–2.5 h).
5. Activate the PVDF membrane by dipping it into methanol for ~15 s, or until it becomes translucent.
6. Place the membrane into ~100 mL of water in a plastic tray and rock for 2 min, until the membrane submerges easily into the water.
7. Equilibrate the membrane by rocking for at least 5 min in Western Transfer Buffer.
8. Gently open the gel cassette, cut off the wells and the bottom of the gel and place in a plastic tray containing a small amount of Western Transfer Buffer and soak for ~5 min.

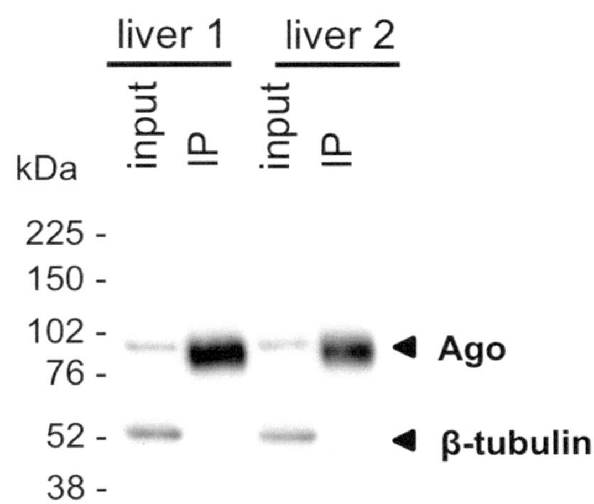


**Fig. 2** Detection of Argonaute and loading control protein in input and immunoprecipitation (IP) samples

9. Assemble the transfer sandwich, add ice-cold transfer buffer and run at 40 V for 240 min.
10. Disassemble the transfer apparatus and rinse blot in remaining transfer buffer, rocking at RT ~5 min.
11. Block for 30–60 min at RT in 5 % NFDM in PBS-T.
12. Incubate with primary antibody: Sigma 2E12-1C9 mouse Ab, 1:1500 in blocking solution at RT for 1 h (*see* **Note 3**).
13. Wash 3× with excess PBS-T.
14. Incubate with secondary antibody: Goat-anti-mouse 1:3,000 in blocking solution at RT for 1 h.
15. Wash 3× with excess PBS-T. Prepare ECL mix (50:50 of Solution A and B) for a total of 5 mL/blot and incubate for 5 min at RT. Reagents have to be at RT before you mix.
16. On a clean piece of saran wrap, lay the blot with protein side up (gently dab the edge of the blot on a Kimwipe to get rid of excess wash buffer) and carefully pipet the ECL mix over the entire blot and incubate for 5 min.
17. Proceed to expose to film or digitizer.

### *3.6 Oligonucleotide Extraction from Argonaute Complexes*

At this stage, input and IP samples are processed under conditions that allow the extraction of oligonucleotides from proteins and the complete hydrolysis of nucleic acids that may be present and could potentially interfere with the subsequent Northern analysis.

1. Bring all samples to 150 μL with distilled $dH_2O$ C.
2. Add 1/3 volume of concentrated $NH_4OH$ (50 μL) and mix.
3. Add equal volume of phenol/chloroform/isoamyl alcohol (200 μL) and vortex vigorously.
4. Prepare phase-lock tubes by spinning briefly.
5. Apply samples to phase lock tubes and spin for 5 min at 12,000 × *g*.
6. Remove aqueous phase and transfer to a new tube.
7. Add 200 μL chloroform, mix for 10 s and spin for 10 min at 12,000 × *g*.
8. Transfer aqueous phase to new tubes.
9. Add 22 μL 1 M NaOH to hydrolyze everything but the oligonucleotide. Incubate at 65 °C for 15 min and then place on ice.
10. Add 22 μL 1 M HEPES to neutralize the NaOH.
11. Precipitate by adding 25 μL of 3 M sodium acetate (NaOAc), 1 μL Glycoblue, and 1100 μL isopropanol.
12. Precipitate at −20 °C for 1 h (or O/N).
13. Spin 15 min at 4 °C.

14. Wash pellet with 500 μL cold 70% ethanol, spin 5 min, aspirate, dry.
15. Resuspend the pellet in 25 μL $H_2O$. Load all or 1/2 on Northern analysis gel (see below).

### 3.7 Northern Analysis of Oligonucleotides

A typical Northern Analysis coupled to high-efficiency DNA probes (Starfire, Integrated DNA Technologies) is used to visualize the anti-miR oligonucleotides. A standard curve comprised of known amounts of oligonucleotide can be used to quantify the results and ensure proper hybridization (Fig. 3).

1. Setup the Pre-cast TBE gel using the proper apparatus and pre-run gel in 0.5X TBE for 30 min at 150 V.
2. Add equal amount of loading buffer (typically 25 μL) to samples.
3. Denature at 70 °C for 5 min, spin and place quickly on ice.
4. Load samples onto the gel and run at 150 V for 45–60 min (*see* **Note 4**).
5. Remove gel and disassemble. Place gel in sandwich between Whatman wetted paper with 0.5X TBE, and add nylon membrane.
6. Transfer using semi-dry transfer apparatus (about 20 V for 30–45 min).
7. Remove membrane and place on dry Whatman paper. Crosslink in Stratalinker 1800 UV crosslinker (optimal setting).
8. Place membrane in hybridization solution at 37–42 °C for 1 h.
9. Prepare Starfire probe using the manufacturer's recommendations. Typically, in a 1.5 mL tube, add 1 μL of Starfire template, 1 μL of oligo and 1 μL of 10× buffer.
10. Heat at 95 °C for 1 min and quickly spin down.
11. Add 1 μL Klenow fragment, 6 μL of [$\gamma$-$^{32}$P]-dATP.

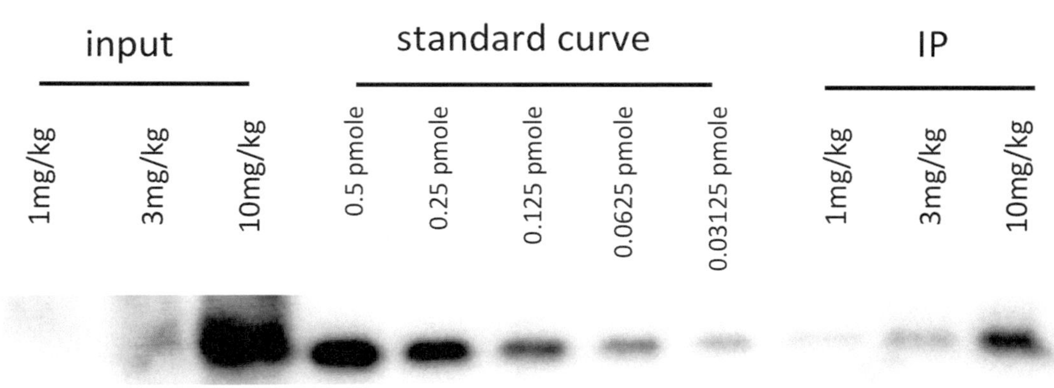


**Fig. 3** Northern analysis of Argonaute-associated oligonucleotides

12. Incubate at room temperature for 1–1.5 h.
13. Stop the reaction by adding 40 μL of STOP solution.
14. Add probe to membrane in the hybridization solution and rotate overnight at 42 °C.
15. Wash membrane 3 × 5 min, in washing solution.
16. Place membrane in sheet protector and expose on film or imager screen.

## 4 Notes

1. Magnetic beads, conjugated with the antibody not, tend to precipitate with time. Please make the effort to verify that the proper amount is dispensed every time by mixing the beads just before use to keep them in suspension.
2. It is important to establish that you can immunopurify Argonaute proteins before you investigate anti-miR association. It may be beneficial to perform a few IPs first.
3. During the antibody incubation stage, an additional antibody against a house-keeping gene, such as mouse α-tubulin can be used as a control (Fig. 2).
4. Since oligonucleotides are typically short, make sure you do not run them out of the gel by verifying the dye which runs at ~10 nt is not running off the gel (Fig. 3).

### References


1. Ambros V, Moss EG (1994) Heterochronic genes and the temporal control of C. elegans development. Trends Genet 10:123–127
2. Gottlieb S, Ruvkun G (1994) daf-2, daf-16 and daf-23: genetically interacting genes controlling Dauer formation in Caenorhabditis elegans. Genetics 137:107–120
3. Pasquinelli AE, Reinhart BJ, Slack F, Martindale MQ, Kuroda MI et al (2000) Conservation of the sequence and temporal expression of let-7 heterochronic regulatory RNA. Nature 408:86–89
4. Alvarez-Garcia I, Miska EA (2005) MicroRNA functions in animal development and human disease. Development 132:4653–4662
5. Soifer HS, Rossi JJ, Saetrom P (2007) MicroRNAs in disease and potential therapeutic applications. Mol Ther 15:2070–2079
6. Hutvagner G, Simard MJ, Mello CC, Zamore PD (2004) Sequence-specific inhibition of small RNA function. PLoS Biol 2, E98
7. Meister G, Landthaler M, Dorsett Y, Tuschl T (2004) Sequence-specific inhibition of microRNA- and siRNA-induced RNA silencing. RNA 10:544–550
8. Jopling CL, Yi M, Lancaster AM, Lemon SM, Sarnow P (2005) Modulation of hepatitis C virus RNA abundance by a liver-specific MicroRNA. Science 309:1577–1581
9. Krutzfeldt J, Rajewsky N, Braich R, Rajeev KG, Tuschl T et al (2005) Silencing of microRNAs in vivo with 'antagomirs'. Nature 438:685–689
10. Davis S, Lollo B, Freier S, Esau C (2006) Improved targeting of miRNA with antisense oligonucleotides. Nucleic Acids Res 34:2294–2304
11. Esau C, Davis S, Murray SF, Yu XX, Pandey SK et al (2006) miR-122 regulation of lipid metabolism revealed by in vivo antisense targeting. Cell Metab 3:87–98
12. Janssen HL, Kauppinen S, Hodges MR (2013) HCV infection and miravirsen. N Engl J Med 369:878
13. Janssen HL, Reesink HW, Lawitz EJ, Zeuzem S, Rodriguez-Torres M et al (2013) Treatment

of HCV infection by targeting microRNA. N Engl J Med 368:1685–1694
14. Van Der Ree MLV, Stelma F, Willemse S, van der Valk M, Rietdijk S, Molenkamp R, Schinkel J et al (2015) A single subcutaneous dose of 2 mg/kg or 4 mg/kg of RG-101, a GalNAc-conjugated oligonucleotide with antagonist activity against MIR-122, results in significant viral load reductions in chronic hepatitis C patients. J Hepatol 62:S261
15. Bartel DP (2009) MicroRNAs: target recognition and regulatory functions. Cell 136:215–233
16. Esau CC (2008) Inhibition of microRNA with antisense oligonucleotides. Methods 44:55–60
17. Stenvang J, Petri A, Lindow M, Obad S, Kauppinen S (2012) Inhibition of microRNA function by antimiR oligonucleotides. Silence 3:1
18. Crooke ST (2008) Antisense drug technology: principles, strategies, and applications. CRC Press, Boca Raton, FL, xvii, 825 p, 812 p. of plates p
19. Davis S, Propp S, Freier SM, Jones LE, Serra MJ et al (2009) Potent inhibition of microRNA in vivo without degradation. Nucleic Acids Res 37:70–77
20. Torres AG, Fabani MM, Vigorito E, Gait MJ (2011) MicroRNA fate upon targeting with anti-miRNA oligonucleotides as revealed by an improved Northern-blot-based method for miRNA detection. RNA 17:933–943
21. Hogan DJ, Vincent TM, Fish S, Marcusson EG, Bhat B et al (2014) Anti-miRs competitively inhibit microRNAs in Argonaute complexes. PLoS One 9:e100951

# Chapter 6

# Competitive Argonaute-Based RNA Immunoprecipitation for Investigation of Transcriptomic Response to Anti-miR

**John R. Androsavich**

## Abstract

Identification and validation of microRNA (miRNA) target genes is essential for gaining a better understanding of the many different functions miRNAs have in healthy and diseased cells. From a practical standpoint, validated target genes are also useful for monitoring pharmacological activity of developmental therapeutics that modulate miRNAs, such as anti-miRNA oligonucleotides (anti-miR). Here, we describe a method that uses changes in Argonaute 2-RNA immunoprecipitation in response to competition by anti-miR, titrated ex vivo, as physical evidence for target validation.

**Key words** microRNAs, Argonaute proteins, Immunoprecipitation, Anti-miR oligonucleotides, microRNAs/antagonists and inhibitors, microRNA target validation

## 1 Introduction

Anti-miRs are single-stranded, modified oligonucleotides designed to bind and inhibit complementary microRNAs (miRNAs). They have emerged as both a potential therapeutic and an important molecular tool for investigating the biological roles of miRNA [1, 2]. Introduction of an anti-miR into a biological system—be it a cell in culture or tissue in vivo—can have profound effects on gene expression at the messenger RNA (mRNA) level [3, 4]. Ensuing changes in the transcriptome stem from both primary and secondary effects of miRNA inhibition, as well as potential indirect effects.

Primary effects of miRNA inhibition can initially be identified using two basic criteria (Fig. 1a). First is direction of change in gene expression. miRNAs negatively regulate gene expression by destabilizing target mRNA through recruitment of RNA-binding proteins and deadenylation factors [5]. miRNA inhibition, therefore, is expected to cause gene *de*-repression or upregulation of expression. The second criterion is that upregulated genes should contain in their 3′UTR a seed-match site complementary to the 5′end of the inhibited miRNA, consistent with canonical principles

Marco F. Schmidt (ed.), *Drug Target miRNA: Methods and Protocols*, Methods in Molecular Biology, vol. 1517,
DOI 10.1007/978-1-4939-6563-2_6, © Springer Science+Business Media New York 2017

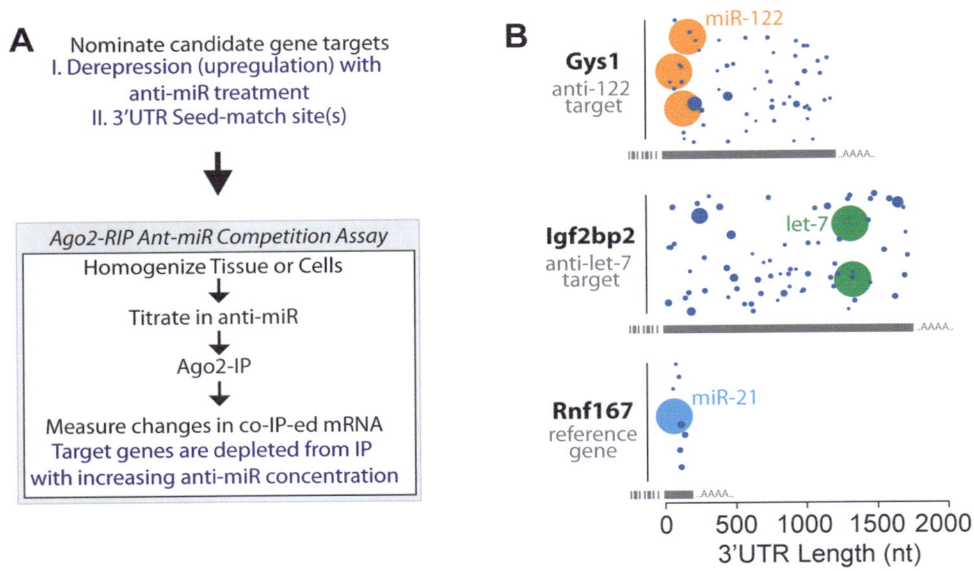


**Fig. 1** Candidate selection and validation of miRNA gene targets. (**a**) Flowchart of initial target identification and downstream validation by AGO2-RIP anti-miR competition assay, described in detail in this chapter. Gene candidates should be specifically upregulated in response to anti-miR treatment and should contain 3′UTR seed-match sites for the inhibited miRNA. Further empirical evidence is required to determine whether gene upregulation is a primary consequence of miRNA inhibition (due to change in AGO2 binding) or is a secondary/indirect effect. (**b**) Target gene candidates most responsive to anti-miR are typically those with "unilateral" miRNA regulation. That is, their 3′UTR contains multiple sites for the inhibited miRNA, but few sites for other miRNAs that are of similar or greater abundance. For example, Gys1 and Igf2bp2 have three or two sites for miR-122 or let-7, respectively. Both miR-122 and let-7 are highly expressed in mouse liver compared to other miRNAs thus making them strong repressors (circle radii represent relative miRNA expression in liver). Accordingly, Gys1 and Igf2bp2 both show robust upregulation and depletion from AGO2-RIP with respective anti-miR-122 or anti-let-7 treatment. If Gys1 hypothetically contained both miR-122 and let-7 sites, then inhibition of let-7 alone would likely lead to relatively weaker derepression due to persistent repression by miR-122. A third gene, Rnf167, is also depicted that contains few seed-match sites due to a short 3′UTR. This qualifies it as a suitable reference gene for most anti-miR treatments, except for anti-miR-21

of miRNA target recognition [6]. Numerous bioinformatic tools are available for finding these sites in annotated 3′UTR sequences (targetscan.org is recommended [7]).

Genes that meet these criteria are nominated as candidate miRNA targets. However, additional experimentation is required for validation in order to filter out false-positives (i.e. genes that coincidentally have a seed-match site, but are upregulated as a secondary/indirect effect).

RNA immunoprecipitation (RIP) has been useful for probing the physical interaction of miRNA factors and gene targets [8–10]. Transcripts pulled-down using antibodies against Argonaute 2 (AGO2), the central miRNA-induced silencing complex (miRISC) factor, are likely to be bound and regulated by one or more miRNA. Methods that combine RIP with RNA-sequencing, such as high-throughput sequencing of RNA isolated by cross-linked immunoprecipitation (HITS-CLIP), provide additional granularity, enabling single nucleotide resolution of specific miRNA–target interactions [11, 12].

Here, we describe a method that utilizes AGO2-RIP to validate target genes that are responsive to miRNA inhibition by anti-miR [13] (Fig. 1a). Anti-miR is titrated directly into tissue or cell lysates and changes in co-immunoprecipitated mRNA are assessed by reverse transcription quantitative polymerase chain reaction (RT-qPCR). Alternatively, high-throughput methods of detection such as Nanostring® profiling or RNA-sequencing can be used. The method is amenable to a number of different sample types, thus enabling context-specific target validation. This is a key feature since tissue-specific miRNA expression profiles seem to shape the transcriptomic response to anti-miR [13].

One distinction between this method and CLIP-type methods is that intact transcripts are detected and analyzed in the immunoprecipitate rather than fragmented miRNA binding sites. This appropriately accounts for the redundant and coordinated action of miRNA gene-regulatory networks that seemingly buffer against perturbations to a single miRNA [13, 14]. As a result, the most responsive target genes are those that have multiple binding sites for the inhibited miRNA and few binding sites for other miRNAs expressed in the system (Fig. 1b). In other words, responses are greatest for targets whose *total* AGO occupancy is primarily composed of the inhibited miRNA.

## 2 Materials

Prepare all solutions using ultrapure distilled water (0.1 μm filtered) that is RNase- and DNase-free. There is no need for diethylpyrocarbonate (DEPC) treatment. Prepare and store all reagents at room temperature unless indicated otherwise. Do not handle reagents with bare hands to avoid RNase contamination. Follow all local and federal waste disposal regulations when disposing waste materials.

### 2.1 Immuno precipitation

1. Dynabeads® M-270 Epoxy-coated magnetic beads (Life Technologies, Carlsbad, CA, USA). Resuspend 60 mg of beads in 4 mL DMF. Store at 4 °C.
2. Monoclonal 4F9 Anti-AGO2/eIF2C2 antibody (Santa Cruz Biotechnology, Dallas, TX, USA). Adjust to 200–250 mg/mL in PBS, if needed. Store at 4 °C (*see* **Note 1**).
3. Dimethyl formamide (DMF), molecular biology grade.
4. 3 M Ammonium sulfate (in water), molecular biology grade.

5. 1 M Sodium phosphate buffer, pH 7.4. Dissolve 2.62 g $NaH_2PO_4 \times H_2O$ (MW = 138) and 14.42 g $NaHPO_4 \times 2H_2O$ (MW = 178) in water. Adjust pH and bring up to 100 mL with water.
6. Quenching buffer: 100 mM Tris, pH 8.0, 140 mM KCl (*see* **Note 2**).
7. 16 M Ethanolamine (neat).
8. Lysis buffer (1×): 20 mM Tris, pH 7.4, 100 mM NaCl, and 2.5 mM $MgCl_2$ (*see* **Note 3**).
9. Halt® protease inhibitor cocktail, ethylenediaminetetraacetic acid (EDTA)-free (ThermoFisher). Store at 4 °C.
10. Glass Dounce homogenizer.
11. DC™ protein assay (BioRad, Hercules, CA, USA).
12. Anti-miR oligonucleotide miRNA inhibitor (*see* **Note 4**). Suspend in lysis buffer.
13. Ultrapure bovine serum albumin (BSA). Store in aliquots at −20 °C.
14. Wash buffer (1×): 20 mM Tris, pH 8.0, 140 mM KCl, and 5 mM ethylenediaminetetraacetic acid (EDTA) (*see* **Note 5**).
15. RNaseOut™ RNase inhibitor (Life Technologies, Carlsbad, CA, USA). Store at −20 °C.
16. 1 M dithiothreitol (DTT). Dissolve 1.5 g DTT in 8 mL of water. Adjust the volume to 10 mL for 1 M stock. Aliquot into 1 mL aliquots and store at −20 °C.
17. Deep (2 mL) 96-well plate (*see* **Note 6**).
18. 96-well PCR plates. For RT, any high-quality polypropylene plate will do. For qPCR, be sure to use a compatible optical plate.
19. Magnetic plate holder and magnetic tube rack (*see* **Note 7**).
20. Aluminum adhesive plate covers.
21. Hybridization oven or incubator with rotisserie. Set to 37 °C.
22. Phosphate buffered saline (PBS), pre-formulated (Corning brand) without calcium or magnesium.
23. Multichannel pipettes.
24. Cold room or refrigerator (4 °C) equipped with rotating mixer.
25. Fresh (preferably) or flash frozen mouse liver, intact.
26. Bench top centrifuge.
27. Bead preincubation buffer: 1 mg/mL BSA, 0.1 mg/mL yeast tRNA prepared in lysis buffer (*see* **Note 8**).
28. Ethanol, 95–100 % non-denatured.

#### 2.2 RNA Isolation and RT-qPCR

1. RNeasy® Micro kit with poly-A carrier RNA (Qiagen, Venlo, Netherlands). Dilute poly-A carrier RNA to 310 ng/μL in water and store in aliquots at −20 °C. Dilute to 2 ng/μL with water just before use.
2. Agilent 2100 Bioanalyzer with RNA 6000 Nano kit (Agilent, Santa Clara, CA, USA) (*see* **Note 9**).
3. PrimeTime® qPCR Assays (Integrated DNA Technologies, Coralville, IA, USA).
4. High-capacity cDNA reverse transcription kit (Life Technologies, Carlsbad, CA, USA).
5. TaqMan® Universal Master Mix II without UNG (Life Technologies, Carlsbad, CA, USA).
6. Thermal cycler.
7. Quantitative (real-time) PCR instrument, such as Viia7™.

## 3 Methods

#### 3.1 Conjugation of Antibody to Magnetic Beads

1. Transfer 1 mL of magnetic beads (15 mg total) suspended in DMF into a 15 mL centrifuge tube (*see* **Note 10**). Place tube on magnetic tube rack to pellet beads. Discard DMF supernatant. Wash beads three times, each with 1 mL of PBS (*see* **Note 11**). Remove all PBS after the final wash.
2. Resuspend beads in combination of 1 mL of anti-Ago2 antibody (200–250 mg/mL), 375 μL of 3 M ammonium sulfate, and 150 μL of 1 M sodium phosphate buffer. Tumble at 37 °C in hybridization oven or incubator overnight (12–24 h).
3. Remove antibody solution from beads and wash three times, each with 1 mL of PBS. Remove all PBS after final wash.
4. Quench free epoxy groups by adding to beads 1 mL of quenching buffer and 6.5 μL of ethanolamine. Tumble at 37 °C for 1 h.
5. Remove quenching buffer from beads and wash three times each with 1 mL of PBS. Resuspend in 1 mL of PBS. Store conjugated beads at 4 °C.

#### 3.2 Lysate Preparation

1. Place Dounce homogenizer on ice and add 3 mL of lysis buffer and 30 μL of protease inhibitor (*see* **Note 12**). After the apparatus has chilled, add liver tissue and homogenize with 20 strokes of the loose plunger followed by 20 strokes with the tight plunger (*see* **Note 13**).
2. Transfer homogenate to microcentrifuge tubes and spin at 1000 × *g* for 10 min at 4 °C. Transfer supernatant to new microcentrifuge tubes and centrifuge twice more at 16,000 × *g* at 4 °C for 10 min each, transferring the supernatant to fresh tubes after each spin. Label the final supernatant as "S16 lysate."

3. Measure S16 lysate protein concentration (*see* **Note 14**). Adjust protein concentration to 10 mg/mL with lysis buffer supplemented with protease inhibitor. Aliquots of S16 lysate can be flash frozen in liquid nitrogen and stored at −80 °C.

### 3.3 Anti-miR Competition and Immunoprecipitation

1. Pre-incubate antibody-conjugated beads in 1 volume of bead preincubation buffer, tumbling at 4 °C (*see* **Note 15**).
2. Meanwhile, in a 96-well plate prepare serial dilutions of anti-miR in lysis buffer (*see* **Note 16**). Anti-miR should be prepared in 50–100 μL volumes (depending on number of technical replicates) at 15× the desired final concentration.
3. Using a multichannel pipette, transfer 16.6 μL/well of each anti-miR dilution into a deep 96-well plate. Then to each well add 250 μL of S16 lysate, mixing with the anti-miR by gently pipetting (*see* **Note 17**). Cover the plate with an aluminum adhesive seal, briefly spin down to collect all liquid, and incubate for 30 min at room temperature on an orbital shaker at low speed.
4. Briefly spin down plate to collect liquid and carefully remove aluminum seal.
5. Remove bead preincubation buffer from beads and resuspend in 1 volume of fresh lysis buffer.
6. Add 25 μL of beads in lysis buffer to each well containing lysate. Carefully seal the plate with a new adhesive seal (*see* **Note 18**).
7. Incubate the samples at 4 °C, tumbling for 2 h (*see* **Note 19**). Meanwhile, chill wash buffer on ice. Once chilled add protease inhibitor, RNase inhibitor, and DTT (*see* **Note 20**).
8. Pellet beads and remove lysate, reserving 50 μL for checking RNA integrity. Wash beads three times, each with 0.5 mL of wash buffer tumbling for 5 min at 4 °C. After the final wash, remove as much wash buffer from beads as possible (*see* **Note 21**).
9. Immediately add 350 μL of Buffer RLT (included in RNeasy® kit) to the beads and vortex well. Then add 10 μL of 2 ng/μL poly-A carrier RNA plus 90 μL water to each sample. Samples can be stored at −20 °C if desired.

### 3.4 RNA Isolation

1. Mix RLT samples with 250 μL of 100% ethanol by pipetting. Place plate on magnet and transfer supernatant to spin-columns.
2. Purify RNA (*see* **Note 22**). Centrifuge spin-columns for 30 s at >8000 × *g* in a bench top centrifuge. Discard flow-through. Wash with 700 μL Buffer RW1. Spin at >8000 × *g* for 30 s. Discard flow-through and change to a fresh collection tube. Wash with 500 μL Buffer RPE. Spin >8000 × *g* for 30 s. Discard flow-through. Wash with 500 μL 80% ethanol. Spin >8000 × *g*

for 2 min. Discard flow-through and change to a fresh collection tube. Open lid of spin column and centrifuge at full speed for 5 min to dry the membrane. Discard flow-through and change to a fresh collection tube.

3. Elute RNA by adding 14 μL of water directly to the spin-column membrane. Incubate for 3 min. Collect by centrifuging at full speed for 1 min. Keep eluted RNA on ice at all times. RNA can be stored at −20 °C. Avoid repeated freeze/thaw.

### 3.5 Quantification of Pulled-Down mRNA by RT-qPCR

1. Prepare on ice 2× reverse transcription (RT) master mix containing 3.2 μL of water, 2.0 μL of 10× RT Buffer, 0.8 μL of 25× dNTP mix, 2.0 μL of 10× RT random hexamers, 1.0 μL of reverse transcriptase, and 1.0 μL of RNase inhibitor. Multiple reactions can be prepared in batch (*see* **Note 23**).
2. In a 96-well PCR plate (or similar tube setup), combine 10 μL of 2× RT master mix with 10 μL of IP'ed RNA. Spin down briefly to collect liquid. Place in thermal cycler programmed for: 25 °C for 10 min, 37 °C for 120 min, 85 °C for 5 min, and 4 °C infinite hold. After RT is complete, dilute cDNA by adding 80 μL of water.
3. Select target and reference genes to analyze (*see* **Note 24**).
4. In an optical 96-well qPCR plate, prepare qPCR reactions containing 5.0 μL of 2× Universal TaqMan Master Mix, 2.5 μL of water, and 0.5 μL of 20× primer/probe. Prepare multiple reactions in batch and aliquot 8.0 μL per well. Add 2.0 μL of each cDNA reaction. Spin-down briefly to collect liquid. Two to three technical PCR replicates are recommended to assess technical variation.
5. Process as "standard run" on Viia7 instrument or similar. Sample information can be inputted through the software or annotated post-run. At a minimum, we recommend including gene/primer information in the software's plate layout. Detailed technical information regarding qPCR is detailed in the corresponding Life Technologies literature [15].
6. Data files with CT values can be exported as *.xlsx or *.csv.

### 3.6 Data Analysis

1. Compute mean CT and standard deviation across PCR technical replicates. Standard deviations should be <0.5. If greater, qPCR should be repeated. Going forward, for each IP sample use mean CT of PCR technical replicates.
2. Check reference gene stability. For each reference gene, plot CT (*y*-axis) for each anti-miR dose (*x*-axis). Visually inspect plot to ensure reference gene CTs remain constant as a function of anti-miR concentration (Fig. 2b).

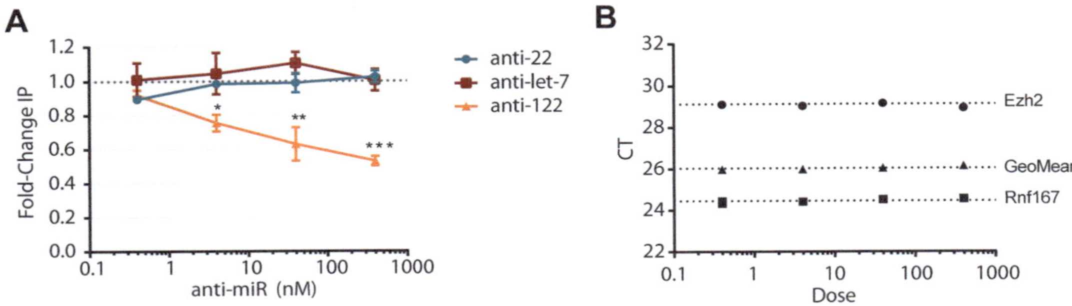


**Fig. 2** AGO2-RIP competition with Gys1. (**a**) Dose-dependent depletion of Gys1 from AGO2-RIP with anti-miR-122, but not controls. Stars represent significance using ANOVA with multiple comparisons for each dose relative to PBS, with Dunnett corrections. (**b**) Plot examining CT stability of reference genes Rnf167 and Ezh2 with increasing anti-miR. Use of multiple reference genes, using the geometric mean (GeoMean) CT, adds to assay robustness

3. Calculate relative change in target gene candidates immunoprecipitated between PBS and anti-miR treatments using comparative CT method ($\Delta\Delta$CT) (Fig. 2a).
4. Test for significance using *t*-test or ANOVA, being sure to correct for multiple comparisons if simultaneously testing >1 candidate gene. Significant depletion of candidate mRNAs in Ago-RIP in dose–response to anti-miR (but not control anti-miR), in combination with significant upregulation in vivo, can be taken as evidence for target validation (*see* **Note 25**).

## 4 Notes

1. In addition to the anti-Ago2 4F9 clone, we have achieved similar results with anti-AGO2 2A8 monoclonal antibody (EMD Millipore). For a slight twist on the protocol, antibodies can be used against RISC effector protein TNRC6A (Medical and Biological Laboratories Co., Nagoya, Japan). Nonspecific IgG should be used to assess specificity of the pull-down.
2. The simplest way to prepare this and other buffers in this protocol is to use purchased stock solutions. To prepare 100 mL of Quenching Buffer: combine 10 mL of Tris, pH 8.0 and 7 mL of 2 M KCl and adjust volume to 100 mL with water. Add ethanolamine just before use (100 mM final).
3. To prepare 1 L of 1× lysis buffer combine 20 mL of 1 M Tris, pH 7.4, 20 mL of 5 M NaCl, and 2.5 mL of 1 M $MgCl_2$. Make up to 1 L with water.
4. Commercial options are available through multiple vendors, such as Exiqon (Skelstedet, Denmark). Anti-miRs are typically designed with phosphorothioate backbones and other

nucleotide modifications to enhance stability and target binding affinity. Use of constrained ethyl or locked nucleic acid chemistries is recommended over lower affinity 2′O-methyl modifications. Anti-miR activity should always be independently confirmed by luciferase assay or alternative method. To test specificity of observed response in AGO2-RIP competition, a mismatch control anti-miR, such as one targeted against a miRNA not expressed in the sample tissue-type, should be used.

5. To prepare 1 L of 1× wash buffer combine 20 mL of 1 M Tris, pH 8.0, 70 mL of 2 M KCl, and 5 mL of 1 M EDTA. Make up to 1 L with water. Before use add protease inhibitor (1×), RNase inhibitor (40 U/mL), and DTT (0.5 mM).
6. We found the best plates to be deep 96-well (2 mL volume) plates with pyramid bottoms. When used with a peg-style magnetic plate holder, the pyramid bottoms provide adequate room for placing your pipet tip into the well to aspirate supernatant without disturbing the aggregated bead pellet. Always use high-quality polypropylene plastics. Polystyrene vessels should be avoided as they tend to cause nonspecific sticking of oligonucleotides to the vessel surface. Alternatively, for low-throughput applications, individual 2 mL non-stick microcentrifuge tubes can be used.
7. A peg-style (6×4) magnetic plate holder (Ambion/Life Technologies, Carlsbad, CA, USA) is preferred over a ring-style. The tube rack should be able to accommodate 15 mL volume centrifuge tubes.
8. To prepare 1.25 mL preincubation buffer: Mix 1.22 mL of lysis buffer, 25 μL of 50 mg/mL BSA, and 2.5 μL of 50 mg/mL yeast tRNA.
9. If bioanalyzer is unavailable, RNA integrity can be assessed using denaturing agarose electrophoresis with ethidium bromide staining.
10. This is sufficient for approximately 40 immunoprecipitations. Conjugation can be scaled according to need.
11. For each round of washing remove the tube from the magnet and completely resuspend the beads by gentle pipetting, then place the tube back on the magnet to pellet the beads before exchanging the buffer. Use this procedure for all bead washes.
12. Use 3 mL of lysis buffer for 1 g of liver tissue. Adjust buffer volume for smaller tissue pieces. Dilute protease inhibitor 1:100 in lysis buffer. If using fresh tissue, freeze single-use aliquots of lysate after adjusting protein concentration. If using frozen tissue, use lysates right away to avoid multiple freeze/thaws.
13. Lysate can also be prepared from other tissues or from cell lysates. For the latter, add 0.05 % NP-40 to the lysis buffer and

homogenize by passing through a 27-G needle. To yield enough lysate, we recommend growing cells on HYPERflasks® (Corning). Protein yields will vary depending on cell type.

14. Any protein assay can be used. Follow manufacturer's product sheet. We most frequently use Biorad's DC™ protein assay with BSA standards starting from 1 mg/mL and going to 0.008 mg/mL by 1:2 step dilutions. Expected lysate protein concentrations should be 20–60 mg/mL, therefore lysate should be diluted for input into protein assay.
15. Calculate total bead volume required for the experiment based on 25 μL of beads per sample. IP should be carried out in technical triplicate for all tested conditions. Be sure to include extra volume to account for pipetting error. Remove PBS storage buffer before adding bead preincubation buffer. Allow preincubation to continue while setting up downstream steps.
16. It is recommended that anti-miR concentration be titrated to test whether observed responses are dose-dependent, which aids interpretation of results. Effective concentrations will depend on the mRNA target and anti-miR potency. A good starting point is 0.4 nM to 4 μM by tenfold step dilutions. Dilutions should be prepared fresh since the effective concentration of dilute anti-miR solutions can change over time due to oligonucleotide adsorption to tube or plate walls.
17. If desired, reserve 2 × 12.5 μL (5 %) of lysate and set aside as "input" for Western blot and RNA analysis (RT-qPCR to determine baseline gene expression and bioanalyzer to check for RNA integrity). This is useful during initial method development/validation.
18. It is critical that the seal be pressed on tightly with an adhesive seal applicator or else the samples will leak while the plate is tumbling.
19. Check that the beads are fully dispersed during the IP incubation step. Tumbling is important to prevent the beads from settling.
20. Each sample will be washed with 3 × 0.5 mL of wash buffer. Prepare additional volume to account for pipetting error. For 12 samples, combine 25 mL of cold wash buffer, 250 μL of protease inhibitor, 25 μL of RNase inhibitor, and 12.5 μL of 1 M DTT.
21. IP efficiency can be assessed by Western blotting for Ago2. After the final wash resuspend beads in 250 μL wash buffer, and transfer 12.5 μL (5 %) to a new tube containing denaturing SDS or LDS loading buffer. Pellet remaining beads and remove remaining wash buffer. Little-to-no buffer should remain. Do not let beads dry out.

22. These steps follow closely with Qiagen's recommended procedure for RNeasy Micro kit. RNA purification can also be performed with RNeasy 96-well spin column plates for higher throughput, at the expense of some loss in signal. When doing so, it is important to include poly-A carrier RNA (20 ng per sample). Wash and spin according to RNeasy-96 instructions. Elute with 55 μL of water.
23. Alternative to RT-qPCR, higher throughput detection methods can be used. We have acquired consistent results using Nanostring® Gene Expression platform with custom-created CodeSets (Fig. 3a). To do so, directly use 5 μL of RNA, from 14 μL elution, as input. We have not tested Nanostring® with 96-well RNA isolation. Another alternative is RNA-seq. Although we have not carried out the full competition protocol using RNA-seq, a pilot study demonstrated similar detection of RIP mRNA with RNA-seq and Nanostring® suggesting that these detection methods are likely to produce similar results (Fig. 3b).
24. Use suggested criteria discussed in Fig. 1 as a starting point. Multiple reference genes should be tested for stability. Ultimately this is a trial and error process. Keep in mind that the presence of seed-match sites in annotated 3′UTRs does not guarantee an effect (or lack thereof). Due to low sequence specificity of seed-match sites (seven or eight nucleotides), there is a high-false positive rate associated with bioinformatic prediction of miRNA targets. Hence, the motivation to develop methods for biochemical validation.
25. Typical magnitude of significant effects range from 0.4- to 0.75-fold-change. One should not expect to see <0.4 depletion, except for unusual cases. For unknown reasons, a subpopulation of target mRNA appears to be insensitive to anti-miR under these conditions [13].

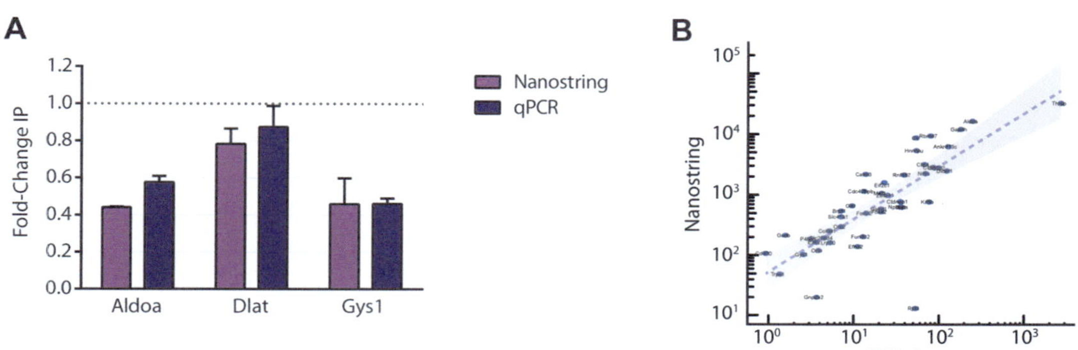


**Fig. 3** AGO2-RIP competition with different methods of mRNA quantification. (**a**) Comparison of qPCR and Nanostring® platforms for Aldoa, Dlat, and Gys1 AGO-RIP competition with anti-miR-122. (**b**) Scatter plot showing relative detection of miR-122 candidate genes in the same RIP sample analyzed with Nanostring® or RNA-seq

## Acknowledgement

This work was supported by Regulus Therapeutics Inc., which employed the author.

### References

1. Jackson A, Linsley PS (2010) The therapeutic potential of microRNA modulation. Discov Med 9(47):311–318
2. Stenvang J, Petri A, Lindow M, Obad S, Kauppinen S (2012) Inhibition of microRNA function by antimiR oligonucleotides. Silence 3(1):1. doi:10.1186/1758-907X-3-1
3. Lim LP, Lau NC, Garrett-Engele P, Grimson A, Schelter JM, Castle J, Bartel DP, Linsley PS, Johnson JM (2005) Microarray analysis shows that some microRNAs downregulate large numbers of target mRNAs. Nature 433(7027):769–773. doi:10.1038/nature 03315, nature03315 [pii]
4. Androsavich JR, Chau BN, Bhat B, Linsley PS, Walter NG (2012) Disease-linked microRNA-21 exhibits drastically reduced mRNA binding and silencing activity in healthy mouse liver. RNA 18(8):1510–1526. doi:10.1261/rna.033308.112
5. Bethune J, Artus-Revel CG, Filipowicz W (2012) Kinetic analysis reveals successive steps leading to miRNA-mediated silencing in mammalian cells. EMBO Rep 13(8):716–723. doi:10.1038/embor.2012.82
6. Bartel DP (2004) MicroRNAs: genomics, biogenesis, mechanism, and function. Cell 116: 281–297
7. Grimson A, Farh KK, Johnston WK, Garrett-Engele P, Lim LP, Bartel DP (2007) MicroRNA targeting specificity in mammals: determinants beyond seed pairing. Mol Cell 27(1):91–105. doi:10.1016/j.molcel.2007.06.017, S1097-2765(07)00407-8 [pii]
8. Wang W-X, Wilfred B, Hu Y, Stromberg A, Nelson P (2010) Anti-Argonaute RIP-Chip shows that miRNA transfections alter global patterns of mRNA recruitment to microribonucleoprotein complexes. RNA (New York, NY) 16(2):394–404. doi:10.1261/rna.1905910
9. Beitzinger M, Meister G (2011) Experimental identification of MicroRNA targets by immunoprecipitation of argonaute protein complexes. Methods Mol Biol 732:153–167. doi:10.1007/978-1-61779-083-6_12
10. Karginov FV, Conaco C, Xuan Z, Schmidt BH, Parker JS, Mandel G, Hannon GJ (2007) A biochemical approach to identifying microRNA targets. Proc Natl Acad Sci U S A 104(49): 19291–19296.doi:10.1073/pnas.0709971104, 0709971104 [pii]
11. Hafner M, Lianoglou S, Tuschl T, Betel D (2012) Genome-wide identification of miRNA targets by PAR-CLIP. Methods 58(2):94–105. doi:10.1016/j.ymeth.2012.08.006
12. Chi SW, Zang JB, Mele A, Darnell RB (2009) Argonaute HITS-CLIP decodes microRNA-mRNA interaction maps. Nature 460(7254):479–486. doi:10.1038/nature08170
13. Androsavich JR, Chau BN (2014) Non-inhibited miRNAs shape the cellular response to anti-miR. Nucleic Acids Res 42(11):6945–6955. doi:10.1093/nar/gku344
14. Ivanovska I, Cleary MA (2008) Combinatorial microRNAs: working together to make a difference. Cell Cycle 7(20):3137–3142
15. LifeTechnologies (2014) Real-time PCR handbook, 3rd edn. LifeTechnologies, Carlsbad, CA

# Chapter 7

# Assessing Anti-miR Pharmacology with miRNA Polysome Shift Assay

John R. Androsavich


## Abstract

Target engagement measurements are critical for evaluating developmental drug candidates and their pharmacological activity. microRNA (miRNA) Polysome Shift Assay enables measurement of anti-miR drug target engagement (i.e. extent of miRNA inhibition) without the need to pre-identify or pre-validate downstream miRNA-regulated genes. This makes it useful for assessing anti-miR activity in target tissues or cells where biology of the inhibited miRNAs may not be well understood. In addition, miRNA Polysome Shift Assay can be multiplexed to assess inhibition of multiple miRNAs by a single anti-miR, thus guiding drug optimization for enhancing or avoiding these activities as desired. This chapter outlines the miRNA Polysome Shift Assay technique, describes sample preparation and quality control, and how to calculate and interpret results.


**Key words** microRNAs, Polysomes, Anti-miR oligonucleotides, microRNAs/antagonists and inhibitors, Pharmacology

## 1 Introduction

microRNA Polysome Shift Assay (miPSA) is a direct measure of microRNA (miRNA) inhibition that was designed to complement conventional approaches that use downstream changes in gene expression [1]. miPSA takes advantage of the fact that miRNAs bind to target messenger RNAs (mRNA) while the transcripts are actively being translated in multiple ribosome complexes (i.e. polysomes) [2–5]. These polysome complexes can be isolated using rate zonal ultracentrifugation, wherein a lysate is layered on top of a continuous sucrose gradient that is then spun at high centrifugal force [6]. Due to their high molecular weight, polysomes sediment further than most other protein complexes toward the bottom of the gradient tube [7]. Under normal conditions, miRNAs sediment with polysomes—figuratively hitch-hiking their way to the bottom. This interaction requires that the miRNA can freely base-pair with polysome-bound mRNA [2, 3]. When a miRNA is inhibited by anti-miR, it is sterically blocked from binding mRNA [8, 9],

Marco F. Schmidt (ed.), *Drug Target miRNA: Methods and Protocols*, Methods in Molecular Biology, vol. 1517,
DOI 10.1007/978-1-4939-6563-2_7, © Springer Science+Business Media New York 2017

and thus is incapable of reaching the bottom portions of the gradient. This causes the miRNA to, in effect, 'shift' from the bottom heavy fractions to the top light fractions. The relative magnitude of this shift or displacement is measured in miPSA in order to determine the extent of miRNA inhibition.

The method can be broken down into five steps: (1) Tissue is homogenized in buffer containing cycloheximide, a translational inhibitor that preserves polysomes by preventing translational runoff. After a series of pre-clearing steps, the lysate is layered on top of a 5–60% continuous sucrose gradient. (2) The gradient is then spun in an ultracentrifuge at 274,000×$g$ for 1.5 h using a swinging bucket rotor. Next, (3) the gradient is fractionated into equal parts and polysome-containing fractions are identified based on ultraviolet (UV) absorbance trace. (4) Polysome fractions are then analyzed using reverse transcription quantitative polymerase chain reaction (RT-qPCR) to quantify relative levels of miR-of-interest (MOI; i.e. the miRNA(s) whose inhibition is to be evaluated) and a reference (REF) miRNA. (5) The relative displacement of the MOI(s) normalized to the REF is then calculated between treated and control samples, analogous to using a house keeping gene for gene expression analysis [10].

## 2 Materials

Prepare all solutions using ultrapure distilled water (0.1 μm filtered) that is RNase- and DNase-free. There is no need for diethylpyrocarbonate (DEPC) treatment. Prepare and store all reagents at room temperature unless indicated otherwise. Do not handle reagents with bare hands to avoid RNase contamination. Follow all local and federal waste disposal regulations when disposing waste materials.

### 2.1 Polysome Preparation

1. Sucrose gradient lysis buffer (SGLB): 100 mM Tris, pH 7.5, 100 mM NaCl, and 2.5 mM $MgCl_2$ (*see* **Note 1**)
2. 100 mg/mL (1000×) cycloheximide (CHX) solution: suspend 1 g CHX powder in 10 mL of DMSO. Store in aliquots at −20 °C (*see* **Note 2**).
3. 5% (w/v) and 60% (w/v) sucrose solutions in 1× SGLB containing 100 μg/mL CHX (*see* **Note 3**).
4. Syringe, 20 cc with Luer lock.
5. Gradient making accessories (*see* **Note 4**).
6. CoolRack® LV (Biocision, San Rafael, CA, USA) (*see* **Note 5**).
7. Open-top polyclear centrifuge tubes (Seton Scientific, Petaluma, CA, USA).
8. 1 M dithiothreitol (DTT). Dissolve 1.5 g DTT in 8 mL water. Adjust the volume to 10 mL for 1 M stock. Aliquot into 1 mL aliquots and store at −20 °C.

9. RNaseOut™ RNase inhibitor (Life Technologies, Carlsbad, CA, USA). Store at −20 °C.
10. Cell lysis buffer: 20 mM HEPES, pH 7.5, 125 mM KCl, and 5 mM $MgCl_2$. Store at room temperature.
11. 25% Nonidet P-40 solution. Mix 250 μL of NP-40 stock with 800 μL of 1× cell lysis buffer. Heat gently and vortex until detergent goes completely into solution.
12. Fast-Prep™ Tubes, Lysing Matrix D (MP Biomedicals, Santa Ana, CA, USA).
13. Samples to be analyzed (*see* **Note 6**).
14. Halt® Protease Inhibitor Cocktail, ethylenediaminetetraacetic acid (EDTA)-free (ThermoFisher). Store at 4 °C.
15. Mini-Beadbeater tissue homogenizer (Biospec Products, Bartlesville, OK, USA).
16. Benchtop centrifuges for microcentrifuge tubes, 15 mL conical tubes, and plates.
17. SW41 Swinging Bucket Rotor (Beckman Coulter, Indianapolis, IN, USA). Precooled in 4 °C refrigerator.
18. Ultracentrifuge, L-90K or equivalent (Beckman Coulter, Indianapolis, IN, USA).
19. Gradient Station™ (Biocomp Instruments, New Brunswick, Canada) with EM-1 UV monitor (BioRad, Hercules, CA, USA) and fraction collector (Gilson, Middleton, WI, USA).
20. Deep (2 mL) 96-well plates ("S-blocks").
21. Quant-IT™ Ribogreen® RNA Reagent and Kit (Life Technologies, Carlsbad, CA, USA). Store at −20 °C.
22. 96-well black, non-treated, clear-bottom plates.
23. Fluorescence microplate reader.

### 2.2 miRNA Detection

1. miRNeasy® 96-well Kit w/Qiazol (Qiagen).
2. Chloroform, molecular biology grade.
3. Multichannel pipettes.
4. Ethanol, 95–100% non-denatured.
5. TaqMan® MicroRNA Reverse Transcription Kit (Life Technologies, Carlsbad, CA, USA).
6. Thermal cycler.
7. TaqMan® Universal Master Mix II without UNG (Life Technologies, Carlsbad, CA, USA).
8. 20× TaqMan® miRNA RT-qPCR assays (Life Technologies, Carlsbad, CA, USA) (*see* **Note 7**).

9. 96- or 384-well PCR plates. For RT, any high-quality polypropylene plate will do. For qPCR, be sure to use a compatible optical plate.
10. Real-time PCR system, Viia7 or equivalent (Life Technologies, Carlsbad, CA, USA).

## 3 Methods

### 3.1 Preparing Sucrose Gradients

Sucrose gradient preparation and fractionation are carried out according to Biocomp Gradient Station, Model 153, Operator's Manual (*see* **Note 8**). It is recommended to prepare gradients 1 day before ultracentrifugation to allow for equilibration.

1. Mark the "half-full point" on centrifuge tubes by placing each tube in the SW40/41 marker block, then tracing a line with a broad-tipped marker along the upper lip of the marker block.
2. Using a syringe with attached cannula, transfer chilled 5% (w/v) sucrose solution to each centrifuge tube, filling just past the half-full point.
3. Next, fill syringe with 60% (w/v) sucrose solution. Place the cannula at the bottom of the centrifuge tube–below the 5% solution—and gently press down on the plunger to dispense the 60% solution. The heavy solution will displace the light solution and the two layers will be visibly distinct. Dispense enough 60% solution to fill the bottom half of the tube. *Total* volume should reach to the top of the tube.
4. Carefully seal tubes with caps (*see* **Note 9**).
5. Program Gradient Station™ for gradient mixing according to Table 1. Level Gradient Station platform and run program. After program is complete, carefully remove caps. Cover gradients with plastic wrap and store at 4 °C overnight or up to 1 week.

#### 3.1.1 Lysate Preparation (Tissue)

1. Pre-cool benchtop centrifuge to 4 °C.
2. To 10 mL of 1× SGLB add 10 μL of 1000× CHX stock and 100 μL of protease inhibitor. Chill on ice.
3. To frozen tissue samples, add 0.5 mL of SGLB (+CHX+protease inhibitor) without pre-thawing.
4. Homogenize samples at 2000 oscillations/min for 60–120 s in Mini-BeadBeater (*see* **Note 10**).
5. Transfer homogenate to microcentrifuge tubes and spin at 1000×*g* for 10 min at 4 °C. Transfer supernatant to new microcentrifuge tubes and centrifuge twice more at 16,000×*g* at 4 °C for 10 min each, transferring the supernatant to fresh tubes after each spin. Procedure should yield approximately 200 μL of final cleared lysate.

**Table 1**
**Parameters for gradient formation**

| Step | Time (s) | Angle | Spin (rpm) |
|---|---|---|---|
| S1 | 5 | 87 | 30 |
| S2 | 15 | 87 | 0 |
| S3 | 5 | 87 | 30 |
| S4 | 15 | 87 | 0 |
| S5 | 5 | 87 | 30 |
| S6 | 15 | 87 | 0 |
| S7 | 5 | 87 | 30 |
| S8 | 15 | 87 | 0 |
| S9 | 5 | 87 | 30 |
| S10 | 15 | 87 | 0 |
| S11 | 19 | 80 | 20 |

#### *3.1.2 Lysate Preparation (Cultured Cells)*

1. Pre-cool benchtop centrifuges to 4 °C, one for microcentrifuge tubes and the other for 15 mL conical tubes.
2. Combine 12.5 mL of 1× cell lysis buffer, 130 μL of protease inhibitor, 13 μL of 1000× CHX stock, 32.5 μL of RNase inhibitor, 26 μL of 1 M DTT, and 260 μL of 25 % NP-40 solution (0.5 % final). Chill on ice.
3. Incubate cells at 37 °C for 10–15 min in growth media containing 100 μg/mL CHX.
4. Rinse cells twice with ice-cold PBS supplemented with 100 μg/mL CHX.
5. Add 500 μL of supplemented cell lysis buffer directly to cells.
6. Incubate cells on ice for 10 min, shaking frequently.
7. Pipet lysates up and down to collect material from growth surface, and transfer to new microcentrifuge tubes.
8. Spin lysates at 16,000 ×*g* for 10 min at 4 °C. Collect supernatant for ultracentrifugation.

### 3.2 Ultra centrifugation and Fractionation

1. Place sucrose gradients into chilled SW41 swinging buckets.
2. Gently layer 150 μL (tissue) or 350 μL (cells) of lysate over sucrose gradient (*see* **Note 11**).
3. Cap buckets and carefully attach each to SW41 rotor, making sure both arms are attached. Place rotor in ultracentrifuge and run at 274,000 ×*g* for 1 h 30 min at 4 °C.

4. After the run is complete, transfer gradients to CoolRack® on ice.
5. Turn on and let EM-1 UV monitor warm up for 15–20 min.
6. Program Gradient Station™ for fraction collection: SPED = 0.3; DIST = 9.85; NUMB = 07; Total = 68.95.
7. Run a blank sample of SGLB through the Gradient Station™ fractionator, and zero the UV monitor mid-way through collection of the blank sample. Blank fractions can be collected in a waste beaker.
8. Fractionate sample gradients into seven fractions and collect in a deep 96-well plate (*see* **Note 12**).
9. Inspect UV traces for polysome containing fractions (Fig. 1). For more quantitative quality control, measure RNA abundance in each fraction of each gradient using Ribogreen® (*see* **Note 13**).
10. Transfer 200 μL of each fraction to a Collection Microtube Rack (from Qiagen miRNeasy-96 kit). Fractionated samples can be stored at −80 °C (*see* **Notes 14** and **15**).

### 3.3 RNA Isolation

These steps follow closely with Qiagen's recommended procedure for miRNeasy-96 kit.

1. To Collection Microtube Rack containing 200 μL of each fraction, add 700 μL of Qiazol and 150 μL of chloroform.
2. Securely cap Microtube Rack with Collection Microtube Caps. Mix by inverting several times and vortex for 30 s using a plate shaker. Let stand at room temperature for 3–5 min.
3. Centrifuge at 5600 × *g* for 15 min at 4 °C.

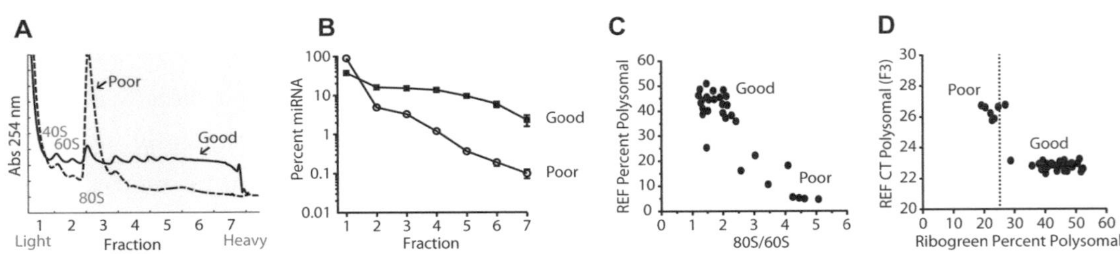


**Fig. 1** Quality control (QC) of polysomes. (**a**) Representative UV traces from good (*solid line*) and poor (*dashed line*) quality polysome preparations. Good traces have easily identifiable 40S, 60S, 80S, and polysome (>80S) peaks. Fractions typically taken as polysome-containing are shaded in *grey*. Poor sample quality, in this case due to RNase degradation, results in loss of signal in heavy fractions and often elongation of the 80S peak. (**b–d**) Loss of miRNA in heavy fractions confirms poor polysome yields. (**b**) Percent let-7d REF detected in each fraction from gradients whose UV traces are shown in **a**. (**c**) Relationship between let-7d REF detected in polysomes vs ratio of 80S:60S peak absorbance in UV traces. (**d**) Ribogreen is a convenient reagent for QC. Based on our experience a minimum cutoff of >25 % polysomal RNA is recommended. Samples with lower polysomal RNA often have high REF CTs and give inconsistent miPSA results

4. Using a multichannel pipette, transfer 300 μL of aqueous layer to a new S-block (*see* **Note 16**).
5. Add 450 μL of 95–100% ethanol to each well, mix by pipetting, and transfer entire volume to miRNeasy plate.
6. Centrifuge at 5600 × *g* for 4 min at room temperature. Discard flow through.
7. Wash plate with 800 μL of Buffer RWT, followed by 800 μL of Buffer RPE. Between each wash centrifuge plate at 5600 × *g* for 4 min at room temperature, discarding flow through.
8. Wash a second time with 800 μL of Buffer RPE. Centrifuge plate at 5600 × *g* for 10 min at room temperature in order to dry the membrane.
9. Elute into Elution Microtubes by adding 50 μL of water per well, incubating 3–5 min at room temperature, then spinning at 5600 × *g* for 4 min at room temperature.

### 3.4 Quantification of polysomal miRNA by RT-qPCR

1. Prepare on ice 2× reverse transcription (RT) master mix containing 2.1 μL of water, 1.0 μL of 10× RT Buffer, 0.1 μL of dNTP mix, 0.5 μL of 20× MOI RT primer, 0.5 μL of 20× REF RT primer, 0.13 μL of RNase inhibitor, and 0.66 μL of reverse transcriptase. Multiple reactions can be prepared in batch.
2. In a 96-well PCR plate (or similar tube setup), combine 5 μL of 2× RT master mix with 5 μL of RNA sample. Spin down briefly to collect liquid. Place in thermal cycler programmed for: 16 °C for 30 min, 42 °C for 30 min, 85 °C for 5 min, and 4 °C infinite hold. After RT is complete, dilute cDNA by adding 20 μL of water.
3. In an optical 96- or 384-well qPCR plate, prepare separate qPCR reactions for MOI and REF, each containing 5.0 μL of 2× Universal TaqMan Master Mix, 2.5 μL of water, and 0.5 μL of 20× primer/probe. Prepare multiple reactions in batch and aliquot 8.0 μL per well. Add 2.0 μL of each cDNA reaction. Spin-down briefly to collect liquid. Two to three technical PCR replicates are recommended to assess technical variation (*see* **Note 17**).
4. Process as "standard run" on Viia7 instrument or similar. Sample information can be inputted through the software or annotated post-run. At a minimum, we recommend including miRNA/primer information in the software's plate layout. Detailed technical information regarding qPCR is detailed in the corresponding Life Technologies literature.
5. Data files with CT values can be exported as *.xlsx or *.csv.

### 3.5 Data Analysis

1. Compute mean CT and standard deviation across PCR technical replicates. Standard deviations should be <0.5. If greater, qPCR should be repeated. Going forward, for each sample/fraction use mean CT of PCR technical replicates.

2. Calculate percent MOI and REF in each fraction, for each treatment:

$$\%\mathrm{miR}_n = \left( \frac{2^{-\mathrm{CT}_n}}{\sum_{i=1}^{m} 2^{-\mathrm{CT}_i}} \right)$$

where $n$ is fraction and $m$ is number of fractions collected. Check that REF miRNA distribution does not change with anti-miR treatment (*see* **Note 18**, Figs. 1 and 2).

3. Calculate displacement ($D$) for each fraction as:

$$D_n = \left[\mathrm{CT}_{\mathrm{MOI}_n} - \mathrm{CT}_{\mathrm{REF}_n}\right]_{\mathrm{Treatment}} - \left[\mathrm{CT}_{\mathrm{MOI}_n} - \mathrm{CT}_{\mathrm{REF}_n}\right]_{\mathrm{PBS}}$$

When calculated in this manner, positive displacement values indicate loss of miRNA from that fraction, while negative displacement values indicate enrichment or gain of miRNA from that fraction in $\log_2$ scale.

4. Summarize each gradient by taking mean displacement of polysomal fractions (typically fractions 3–7). Use these values for comparing effects between each treatment group (*see* Fig. 2).

$$D = \frac{\sum_{n=3}^{m=7} D_n}{(m - n + 1)}$$

5. Calculated percent inhibition (CPI) can be estimated as (*see* **Note 19**):

$$\mathrm{CPI} = \left(1 - \frac{1}{2^D}\right) \times 100$$

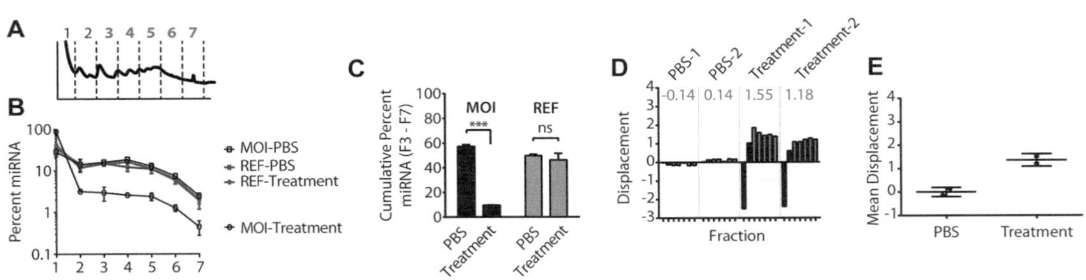


**Fig. 2** Example miPSA data. (**a**) UV trace showing good quality polysomes in fractions 3–7. (**b**) Percent MOI and REF miRNA detected in each fraction of samples treated with anti-miR treatment or PBS. (**c**) REF miRNA in polysome fractions does not significantly change with anti-miR treatment, unlike MOI. (**d**) Fractional displacement from duplicate samples treated with PBS or anti-miR. Mean polysome displacement for each sample is shown in grey. (**e**) Comparison of mean polysome displacement for PBS vs treatment (summarized data from **d**)

## 4 Notes

1. The simplest way to prepare this and other buffers in this protocol is to use purchased stock solutions. For 10× solution: Add 50 mL of 1 M Tris (pH 7.5), 100 mL of 5 M NaCl and 12.5 mL of 1 M $MgCl_2$ to 337.5 mL water. Dilute to 1× before use. Store at room temperature.
2. Cycloheximide (CHX) is harmful; avoid exposure. Work in hood when handling powdered CHX. Always wear nitrile gloves when handling CHX solutions.
3. Pre-heat a water bath to 60 °C. Prepare 5% (w/v) sucrose solution by adding 25 g of sucrose (molecular biology grade) to a 500 mL capped bottle with volume markings. Fill to 500 mL volume line with 1× SGLB. Mix well until sucrose goes into solution. Set aside. Prepare 60% (w/v) sucrose solution by adding 300 g of sucrose to a 500 mL capped bottle with volume markings. Fill to 500 mL volume line with 1× SGLB. Mix well and place in 60 °C water bath. Incubate for ~10 min, vigorously mixing at regular intervals until sucrose goes into solution. Chill both 5 and 60% sucrose solutions in ice-water bath for ~10 min. Add 500 μL 1000× CHX to each. Solutions can be stored at 4 °C for up to 1 week or −80 °C for long term.
4. Includes 4 mm rate zonal SW40/41 tube caps, SW40/41 marker block, bubble level, and cannula from Biocomp Instruments, Inc. (New Brunswick, Canada).
5. Optional, but highly recommended for storing and transporting gradients on ice.
6. Harvested tissues should be sectioned into 100–200 mg pieces, placed into Fast-Prep™ tubes, and flash frozen in liquid nitrogen as quickly as possible. Store frozen samples at −80 °C. Optimal tissue weights must be determined empirically. The protocol can potentially be adapted for any tissue. In our hands, we have tried and have had success with liver, kidney, adipose, and brain tissue. For cultured cells, a minimum of ~500,000 are needed (approximately one well of 6-well plate at 70–80% confluence).
7. A minimum of two assays are required: one for the miR of interest (MOI) and the other for the reference miRNA (REF). Multiple MOIs can be tested to assess anti-miR cross-reactivity. For instance, to test whether anti-miR-130a is equipotent against all family members: miR-130a, miR-130b, miR-301a, or miR-301b.
8. There are many ways to make sucrose gradients. Most importantly, any chosen method must be consistent from gradient-to-gradient.
9. Avoid capturing air bubbles underneath the cap by inserting the cap at an angle into the tube. Filling the tubes with additional

sucrose solution such that the surface tension holds the liquid just above the top of the tube will also help minimize air bubbles.

10. Alternatively, samples can be homogenized using a chilled glass Dounce homogenizer.

11. To make room for lysate, remove an equivalent volume of sucrose from the top of the gradient. For optimal results, dispense lysate slowly at an angle along the wall of the centrifuge tube.

12. If fractionating several samples, place an ice pack underneath the fraction collector's metal plate holder (if available) to keep the samples chilled. Set the fraction collector to collect down the columns of each plate, such that one column is filled with one gradient. Only seven fractions are collected and the eighth well of the column is left empty to maintain this plate format.

13. Dilute 55 μL of Ribogreen® reagent in 20 mL of 1× Buffer TE. Mix 180 μL of dilute reagent with 20 μL of each fraction in black, clear-bottom 96-well plate. Incubate at room temperature for 5 min, protected from light. Measure fluorescence in microplate reader with 480 nm excitation and 520 nm emission. Cumulative percent RNA in polysomal fractions should be >25 %.

14. It is recommended to transfer an aliquot of each fraction to the Microtube Rack for quicker thawing before RNA extraction. Larger volumes in deep 96-well plate take a long time to thaw.

15. One or two polysomal fractions are sufficient for miPSA analysis. Typically we analyze only fractions 3 and 4. For a first trial, however, it is useful to analyze all gradient fractions to get a sense of miRNA distribution and displacement across the entire gradient. Consider that target miRNA in top (non-polysomal) fractions of anti-miR-treated samples may not be reliably quantifiable due to interference from anti-miR.

16. Work column-by-column (strip-by-strip) from one side of the plate rack to the other. It is difficult to see the aqueous/organic interface of inner strips. An easy way to deal with this is to temporarily remove the strip, place it on top of the previously extracted strip, remove the aqueous layer, and replace the strip back into the plate. Repeat this process for remaining columns/strips.

17. For example: 12 gradients × 8 fractions × 2 primer/probes (1 for MOI; 1 for REF) × 2 technical replicates = 384 reactions.

18. Changes in percent REF miRNA in polysomes may be a result of poor polysome quality (nonspecific effect) or cross-reactivity with anti-miR (specific effect). If the latter is suspected, test additional miRNAs as possible REFs. It is best to select REF miRNAs that are well-expressed, have mid-to-high (≥40 %) basal polysome occupancy, and have highly dissimilar seed sequences from the designed target miRNA.

19. We recommend reporting displacement values, while using CPI only as a frame of reference. CPI compresses data on the high end and exaggerates noise on the low end. In general, displacement scores ≥4 are interpreted as strong drug target engagement (>94 % inhibition).

## Acknowledgement

This work was developed by Regulus Therapeutics Inc., which employed the author.

### References

1. Androsavich JR, Sobczynski DJ, Liu X, Pandya S, Kaimal V, Owen T, Liu K, MacKenna DA, Chau BN (2015) Polysome shift assay for direct measurement of miRNA inhibition by anti-miRNA drugs. Nucleic Acids Res 2015:gkv893. doi:10.1093/nar/gkv893
2. Androsavich JR, Chau BN, Bhat B, Linsley PS, Walter NG (2012) Disease-linked micro RNA-21 exhibits drastically reduced mRNA binding and silencing activity in healthy mouse liver. RNA 18(8):1510–1526. doi:10.1261/rna.033308.112
3. Maroney PA, Yu Y, Fisher J, Nilsen TW (2006) Evidence that microRNAs are associated with translating messenger RNAs in human cells. Nat Struct Mol Biol 13(12):1102–1107, doi:nsmb1174 [pii] 10.1038/nsmb1174
4. Nottrott S, Simard MJ, Richter JD (2006) Human let-7a miRNA blocks protein production on actively translating polyribosomes. Nat Struct Mol Biol 13(12):1108–1114, doi: nsmb1173 [pii] 10.1038/nsmb1173
5. Molotski N, Soen Y (2012) Differential association of microRNAs with polysomes reflects distinct strengths of interactions with their mRNA targets. RNA 18(9):1612–1623. doi:10.1261/rna.033142.112
6. Gandin V, Sikström K, Alain T, Morita M, McLaughlan S, Larsson O, Topisirovic I (2014) Polysome fractionation and analysis of mammalian translatomes on a genome-wide scale. J Vis Exp 87:PMID:24893926. doi:10.3791/51455
7. Noll H (2008) The discovery of polyribosomes. Bioessays 30:1220–1234
8. Stenvang J, Petri A, Lindow M, Obad S, Kauppinen S (2012) Inhibition of microRNA function by antimiR oligonucleotides. Silence 3(1):1. doi:10.1186/1758-907X-3-1
9. Krützfeldt J, Rajewsky N, Braich R, Rajeev KG, Tuschl T, Manoharan M, Stoffel M (2005) Silencing of microRNAs in vivo with 'antagomirs'. Nature 438(7068):685–689. doi:10.1038/nature04303
10. Schmittgen TD, Livak KJ (2008) Analyzing real-time PCR data by the comparative C(T) method. Nat Protoc 3(6):1101–1108

# Chapter 8

# Evaluating Synergistic Effects of miR-34a Mimics in Combination with Other Therapeutic Agents in Cultured Non-Small Cell Lung Cancer Cells

**Jane Zhao and Andreas G. Bader**

## Abstract

Tumor suppressor miRNAs such as miR-34a inhibit tumor growth by simultaneously regulating the expression of multiple important oncogenes across multiple oncogenic pathways and, therefore, provide a strong rationale for developing therapeutic miRNA mimics in combination with other therapeutic cancer agents to augment drug sensitivity. Here, we describe the experimental approach for evaluating miRNA and drug combinations using the "fixed ratio" method in cultured non-small cell lung cancer cells.

**Key words** miRNA therapeutics, miR-34a, MRX34, Combination index, Dose reduction index, Combination therapy

## Abbreviations

| | |
|---|---|
| CI | Combination index |
| DRI | Dose reduction index |
| $IC_{50}$ eq | $IC_{50}$ equivalent |
| miRNA | microRNA |
| NSCLC | Non-small cell lung cancer |

## 1 Introduction

The most common forms of current cancer treatment involve either conventional cytotoxic chemotherapy or targeted therapy. While targeted therapy often results in fewer side effects due to its focused mechanism of action, both types of treatment frequently yield limited effectiveness due to either intrinsic drug resistance or the inevitable development of secondary resistance [1, 2]. Despite much progress in recent years, the need remains

Marco F. Schmidt (ed.), *Drug Target miRNA: Methods and Protocols*, Methods in Molecular Biology, vol. 1517, DOI 10.1007/978-1-4939-6563-2_8, © Springer Science+Business Media New York 2017

for new therapeutic strategies that are safer and more efficacious. Some miRNAs, such as miR-34a, as well as its corresponding mimics, are known to suppress tumor formation and growth via the regulation of multiple cancer pathways [3, 4]. Tumor suppressor miRNAs may also play a role in suppressing the viability and propagation of cancer stem cells, a cancer cell subpopulation known to be more resilient to cancer therapies [3, 5]. Another potential tumor-suppressive effect may come from inhibiting tumor mechanisms of immune evasion, including PD-L1 expression [6]. Thus, mimics of tumor suppressor miRNAs may be used as promising candidates in combination with other cancer treatments, to counteract drug resistance mechanisms and potentially provide synergistic antitumor activity. For example, tumor-suppressive miR-34a produced strong synergy in cultured non-small cell lung cancer (NSCLC) cells in combination with Erlotinib, a small-molecule tyrosine kinase inhibitor of epidermal growth factor receptor (EGFR) currently used to treat types of NSCLC and advanced-stage pancreatic cancer [7]. An explanation for this enhanced therapeutic effect is provided by the observation that miR-34a directly represses both MET and AXL which are oncogenes that can render cancer cells refractory to Erlotinib (Fig. 1) [13–16]. Here, we describe (1) the experimental approach to assess miRNA-drug combinations in cultured non-small cell lung cancer cells following the "fixed ratio" method and (2) data interpretation in the form of combination index values, isobolograms and curve shift analysis to distinguish between additive, antagonistic, and synergistic drug combination effects.

Erlotinib: $C_{22}H_{23}N_3O_4 \cdot HCl$ (M.W. 429.90)

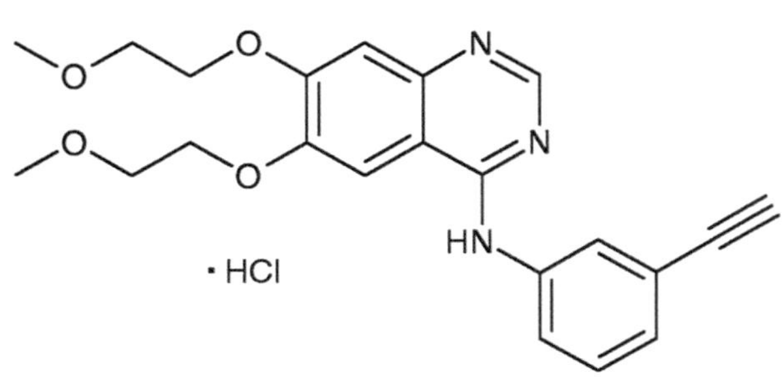


**Fig. 1** Structure of FDA-approved drug tyrosine kinase inhibitor Erlotinib

## 2 Materials

### 2.1 Cell Culture Medium and Supplies

1. Non-small cell lung cancer cell lines (ATCC).
2. RPMI-1640 culture media (Life Technologies), store at 4 °C.
3. Fetal Bovine Serum (FBS) (Life Technologies), store at −20 °C.
4. Phosphate-buffered saline (PBS) (Life Technologies), store at room temperature.
5. 0.25 % Trypsin/EDTA (Life Technologies), store at −20 °C.
6. Opti-MEM Reduced Serume Media (Life Technologies), store at 4 °C.
7. Lipofectamine RNAiMAX (Life Technologies), store at 4 °C.
8. AlamarBlue (Life Technologies), store at 4 °C.
9. Forma Series II water jacketed $CO_2$ incubator (Thermo Electron Corporation).
10. Forma Class II, A1 Biological Safety Cabinet (Thermo Electron Corporation).
11. Clear bottom 96-well cell culture plates.
12. White solid bottom 96-well plate.
13. T75 cell culture flask.
14. Adjustable single and multichannel precision pipettes for dispensing 1–20, 20–200 and 200–1000 μL.
15. Multichannel pipette reservoir.

### 2.2 Oligonucleotide and Chemo- Drugs

1. Nuclease-free water (not Diethylpyrocarbonate: DEPC treated).
2. Dimethylsulfoxide (DMSO: molecular biology grade).
3. miRNA mimics, here: a blunt-ended and double-stranded mimic of hsa-miR-34a comprising the following sequence: 5′-UGGCAGUGUCUUAGCUGGUUGUU-3′.
4. Chemotherapeutic compounds; here: Erlotinib, $C_{22}H_{23}N_3O_4 \cdot HCl$, MW = 429.9.

### 2.3 Instruments

1. Z1 single threshold particle counter (Beckman Coulter).
2. PolarStar Optima plate reader (BMG Labtech).
3. Eppendorf centrifuge 5810R.
4. 37 °C warm bath (VWR).

### 2.4 Data Analysis

Prism Graphpad, MS Excel, or comparable data software.

## 3 Methods

### 3.1 Cell Culture

Human non-small cell lung cancer cell lines used in this protocol were purchased from ATCC. Cells are maintained in their complete growth medium supplemented with 10% fetal bovine serum (*see* **Note 1**) at 37 °C in a humidified incubator of 95% air and 5% $CO_2$. All cell culture work is carried out in a biological safety cabinet following standard sterile techniques. For subculture, cells are cultured in T75 flasks, split regularly at 1:4–1:8 ratios and replenished with fresh medium twice a week.

### 3.2 Determine $IC_{50}$ of miR-34a Mimic by Reverse Transfection in Cells Cultured in 96-Well Plates

All experiments are carried out using a biological safety cabinet that has been wiped with 70% ethanol before use. All experiments are done in 96-well plates at room temperature in triplicates, and each experiment is repeated at least three times.

1. Warm up all culture medium to room temperature and spray bottles with 70% ethanol before use.
2. Prepare a 600 nM stock solution of miR-34a in nuclease-free water. If not used immediately, store at −20 °C.
3. Prepare a miR-34a dilution series starting with the 600 nM miR-34a stock solution in a 1:3 ratio in nuclease-free water to make the following concentrations: 0, 0.6, 2, 6, 20, 60, 200, and 600 nM.
4. To mix the oligonucleotides and the transfection reagent (lipofectamine RNAiMAX), add 5 μL of miR-34a mimic to 10 μL of OptiMEM in tube 1; add 0.2 μL of lipofactamine RNAiMAX to 10 μL of OptiMEM in tube 2. Combine the two together and mix well (total of 25 μL), incubate at room temperature for 15–20 min (*see* **Note 2**).
5. Meanwhile, remove the cells from the incubator and wash with 1× PBS once. Add 3–4 mL of Trypsin/EDTA per T75 flask, and put the cells back in the incubator for about 1–2 min. Remove Trypsin/EDTA, gently tab the bottom of the flask to detach the cells. Add 6–8 mL of complete medium onto the cells and pipette up-down 8–10 times to resuspend the cells into the medium (*see* **Note 3**).
6. To count cells, transfer 100 μL of resuspend cells into a cuvette containing 10 mL isotonic diluent, and count the cells using Z1 single threshold particle counter with aperture tube size of 100 μM, $K_d$ of 60.14 and lower threshold of 8.0 μM. Typically, the cell counter provides cell concentrations as cell number per mL (*see* **Note 4**).
7. Dilute the cells with complete culture medium to reach a concentration of 2500–3500 per 75 μL (volume required per 96-well). Prepare enough cells to cover all assay plates.

8. Add 25 μL of oligonucleotide and lipofectamine RNAiMAX mixture to each well using the multichannel pipet. Then, add 75 μL of cells. The final concentrations of miR-34a mimic are 0, 0.03, 0.1, 0.3, 1, 3, 10, and 30 nM (*see* **Note 5**). As controls (the wells with no miR-34a mimic), cells are also transfected with RNAiMAX alone in OptiMEM (mock).
9. To measure miRNA-induced inhibition of cellular proliferation, 4 days after transfection, remove media, add 70 μL AlamarBlue reagent per well (prepared in a 10-fold dilution in complete medium before use), and incubate for 1–4 h at 37 °C.
10. When the control wells (cells transfected with RNAiMAX, "mock") turn pink, transfer 50 μL from each well to a white solid bottom 96-well plate and measure fluorescence intensity on the PolarStar Optima plate reader with the following instrument settings: Ex = 544 nm, Em = 590 nm and gain 900 (*see* **Note 6**).
11. Cell proliferation data as fluorescence intensity are normalized to mock-transfected cells, and dose–response curves and $IC_{50}$ values are generated using the nonlinear regression method (four parameter variable slope) provided by the Graphpad (Prism) software. An appropriate cut-off for the goodness of fit is represented by the coefficient of determination $R^2 \geq 0.9$.

### 3.3 Determine $IC_{50}$ of Chemo-Drug Compound

1. To prepare cell suspension in culture medium, trypsinize and count the cells as described in Subheading 3.2 **steps 5** and **6**.
2. Dilute the cells in culture medium to reach the required concentration.
3. Seed cells in a 96-well plate at 2500–3500 cells per well and 100 μL per well and let cells settle overnight.
4. The next day, prepare dilution series of the second therapeutic compound in tenfold higher concentrations of the final concentrations (0, 1, 3, 10, 30, 100, 300, and 1000 μM) in DMSO (*see* **Note 7**).
5. Remove the media, add fresh media onto the cells at 90 μL per well, and then add 10 μL of diluted compound per well. The final concentrations are 0, 0.1, 0.3, 1, 3, 10, 30, and 100 μM. As controls (no compound), cells are treated with solvent alone, such as 1 % DMSO (mock) (*see* **Note 8**).
6. Three days post drug treatment, cellular proliferation is measured by AlamarBlue assay as fluorescence intensity described in Subheading 3.2 **steps 9** and **10**. Proliferation data are normalized to mock-DMSO alone cells. Nonlinear regression trendlines and $IC_{50}$ values are generated using four-parameter variable slope by Graphpad (Prism) software. A recommended cutoff for the goodness of fit is an $R^2 \geq 0.9$.

### 3.4 Evaluate Synergist Effects Using the "Fixed Ratio" Method

In 96-well plates, cells are treated with seven concentrations of compound each in combination with seven concentrations of miR-34a mimic. Each drug is used at a concentration approximately equal to its $IC_{50}$ and at multiple concentrations twofold (*see* **Note 9**) above or below (see schematic below). Combinations that are based on the same $IC_{50}$-derived concentrations (e.g. $IC_{50}+IC_{50}$ and $IC_{25}+IC_{25}$) contain drug concentrations in a fixed ratio (hence, the name of this method). Thus, this matrix yields a total of 49 different combinations representing 13 different ratios. Each drug is also used alone at these concentrations. As controls (no compound or miR-34a mimic), the wells contain transfection reagent and compound solvent, such as 1 % DMSO (mock) (*see* Table 1).

1. Cells are seeded at 2500–3000 cells per well and reverse transfected with miR-34a mimic in a serial dilution as described in Subheading 3.2 **steps 1–8** (*see* **Note 10**).
2. The following day, the compound is added onto the cells in a serial dilution as described in Subheading 3.3 **steps 4** and **5** (*see* **Note 10**).
3. To determine the cellular proliferation inhibition, fluorescence intensity is measured 3 days post drug treatment by AlamarBlue assay. All data are normalized to mock wells that contain DMSO and transfection reagent only. The single agent and six combination dose–response curves and $IC_{50}$ values are generated using Graphpad software, and these values are used to calculate combination index (CI) values (*see* Fig. 2) (*see* **Note 11**).

### 3.5 Data Analysis Methods

1. Calculation of combination index (CI) values.
   CI values based on Loewe's additivity model are determined to assess the nature of drug–drug interactions that can be additive

**Table 1**
**Experimental set-up to determine synergistic effects of miR-34 mimic and Erlotinib**

| | | miR-34a Mimic | | | | | | |
|---|---|---|---|---|---|---|---|---|
| | | 8×IC50 | 4×IC50 | 2×IC50 | 1×IC50 | 0.5×IC50 | 0.25×IC50 | 0.125×$IC_{50}$ |
| Drug | Mock | C1 | C2 | C3 | C4 | C5 | C6 | C7 |
| 8×IC50 | C1 | | | | | | | |
| 4×IC50 | C2 | | | | | | | |
| 2×IC50 | C3 | | | | | | | |
| 1×IC50 | C4 | | | | | | | |
| 0.5×IC50 | C5 | | | | | | | |
| 0.25×IC50 | C6 | | | | | | | |
| 0.125×IC50 | C7 | | | | | | | |

(CI = 1), antagonistic (CI > 1), or synergistic (CI < 1) for various drug–drug concentrations and effect levels (Fa, fraction affected; inhibition of cancer cell proliferation) [9–11]. CI values derived from nonlinear regression trendlines are calculated using Eq. 1 in which $C_{A,x}$ and $C_{B,,x}$ are the concentrations of drug A and drug B, respectively, in the combination to produce effect X (Fa). $IC_{x,A}$ and $IC_{x,B}$ are the concentrations of drug A and drug B used as a single agent to produce that same effect (*see* **Note 12**).

$$\mathrm{CI} = \frac{C_{\mathrm{A}},\mathrm{x}}{\mathrm{ICx}_{,\mathrm{A}}} + \frac{C_{\mathrm{B}},\mathrm{x}}{\mathrm{ICx}_{,\mathrm{B}}}. \quad (1)$$

Drug concentrations required in Eq. 1 to determine CI values ($C_{A,x}$, $C_{B,,x}$, $IC_{x,A}$, and $IC_{x,B}$) are calculated using the Hill equation (Eq. 2), $IC_{50}$, and Hill slope value ($n$) derived from nonlinear regression trendlines in Graphpad (*see* **Note 13**). If we assume $E_{max} = 100$, the drug concentration ($C$) used alone or in combination can be calculated at any effect level.

$$E = E_{\mathrm{max}} \times \frac{C^n}{\mathrm{IC}_{50}{}^n + C^n}. \quad (2)$$

2. Isobolograms.

   To describe the dose-dependent interaction of drug and miR-34a mimic, isobolograms at effect levels of 50 and 70–80% inhibition of cancer cell proliferation are created. Since the single agents—alone or in combination—usually inhibit cancer cell proliferation by at least 50%, the $IC_{50}$ isobologram (isobologram showing drug concentrations to inhibit cancer cell proliferation by 50%) provides an actual comparison of the single use vs. the combination. The 70–80% isobolograms are used to illustrate the utility of the combination at a high effect level that have practical implications in oncology is likely more clinically relevant if data can be produced within the actual dose–response curve and are not extrapolated. In each of these, additivity is determined by calculating the dose requirement for each drug in combination from its single use ($IC_{50}$, $IC_{80}$). Data points above or below the line of additivity indicate antagonism or synergy, respectively. In addition, dose reduction index values (DRI) are calculated to indicate by how much the concentration of each drug in the combination can be reduced (compared to its use as a monotherapy) to produce the same effect (e.g. $IC_{50}$) (*see* **Note 14**).

3. Curve shift analysis.

   To allow a direct comparison of the dose–response curves derived from the single agents alone or in combination, and to identify synergistic drug–drug interaction, nonlinear regression trendlines of each drug alone or of the combination ($IC_{50}$:$IC_{50}$ ratio or other ratios where indicated) are normalized to its own $IC_{50}$ value at any giving effect level, and referred to as $IC_{50}$ equivalents ($IC_{50}$ eq). This allows a visualization of mono and combination data in the same graph independent of drug concentrations (since drug concentrations have been normalized by the respective $IC_{50}$ values). $IC_{50}$ equivalents of the combination were calculated using Eq. 3 and described in [12]. $C_{A,x}$ and $C_{B,x}$ are the concentrations of drug A and drug B in the combination to produce effect X (Fa). $IC_{50,A}$ and $IC_{50,B}$ are the concentrations of drug A and drug B used as a single agent to produce 50% effect. When the drug is used as single agent, one of column equals to 0. Data of the single agents and in combination are graphed in the same diagram to illustrate lower drug concentrations required to achieve any given effect relative to the single agents. This is represented in a left-shift of the dose–response curve and indicates synergy. A right-shift relative to curves of the single agents indicates antagonism (*see* **Note 15**).

$$IC_{50}eq = \frac{C_A, x}{IC_{50,A}} + \frac{C_B, x}{IC_{50,B}} \quad (3)$$

4. Statistical analysis.

   Statistical analysis was done using the Excel (Microsoft) and Graphpad softwares. Averages and standard deviations are calculated from triplicate experiments. Goodness of fit of nonlinear regression trendlines are described by $R^2$ (Graphpad) values.

## 4 Notes

1. The complete medium is only supplemented with 10% FBS. We recommend omitting antibiotics, which are typically added to cultured cells, because it can affect the transfection efficiency of miRNA mimics.
2. Since multiple wells require transfection, the oligonucleotide-transfection solution is set up as a master mix such that the amount of reagent per well is multiplied by the number of wells with an additional 10% overage to avoid shortage.
3. Always check the cells before removing Trypsin/EDTA. When the cells become rounded up, it is time to remove the Trypsin/EDTA solution. If the cells are already detached before removing Trypsin/EDTA, add 10 mL of complete medium onto the cells, and pipette up-down a couple of times. Spin down the cells at 800 rpm at room temperature for 3–5 min. Discard the medium and add fresh culture medium.

4. Before counting the cells, be sure to completely resuspend cells in medium. If not done so, clumps of cells will affect the actual cell count and may also clog the instrument. Alternately, a hemocytometer can also be used to determine cell count. However, using a consistent method to count the cells is highly recommended to avoid variation from experiment to experiment.
5. Under certain circumstances, a given cell line cannot be used for combination studies using the "fixed ratio" method. (a) If a cell line is completely resistant to any of the therapeutic agents, the "fixed ratio" method is not suitable for assessing drug–drug combinations. Instead, we recommend assessing combinations following the "fixed concentration" method [7]. (b) Sometimes, however, certain cell lines are not susceptible to lipid-based transfection and, consequently, the transfection efficiency of the miRNA mimic is poor. To optimize and determine experimental conditions of lipid transfection in a given cell model, Kif11 or PLK1 siRNAs can be used as surrogates for inhibiting cellular proliferation. Typically, the maximal concentration of transfected oligonucleotide is 50 nM. If transfection efficiency remains too low, then this cell line cannot be used for combination studies, and we recommend using an alternative cell model.
6. The incubation time with AlamarBlue varies from cell line to cell line. Based on our experience, read the assay plate as soon as "mock" wells change from blue to pink. If waited too long, all wells could turn pick, and a measurable difference between controls and test cells is lost. The fluorescence intensity determined in "mock" wells should not exceed 20,000. However, this maximal value depends on the plate reader and instrument settings used.
7. If the compound is not dissolved in $H_2O$, the stock concentration of compound is normally prepared as a 10 mM stock solution in DMSO. Consequently, the final concentration of DMSO in cell cultures is 1 %. If some cell lines are sensitive to DMSO, prepare the compound as a 20 mM DMSO stock solution so that the final concentration of DMSO can be reduced to 0.5 %.
8. In general, use 100 μM as the highest concentration in the dose–response curve for a newly tested compound. If the compound is very potent or has a narrow therapeutic range, reduce the top concentration and/or increase the bottom concentration and prepare a dilution series in smaller dose increments. Sometimes, a repeat of the dose response is necessary to find the proper dose range.
9. $IC_{50}$ values determined for the single agents are used as a guide to design the concentrations of each drug in the combination study. In general, twofold of serial dilution is recommended,

however, 2.5- or 3-fold serial dilution can also be used depending on the compound.

10. In general, the highest concentration of each drug used in the combination study should be 70–80 % effective as single agent. The lowest concentration of each drug used in the combination study should be 10–20 % effective as a single agent.
11. There are a total of 13 different drug ratios which represent 13 combination dose–response curves. Due to the setup of this matrix, some of these dose–response curves have merely a few data points. We recommend analyzing the six combination ratios that contain four or more data points in each dose–response curve.
12. In general, lower CI values indicate stronger synergy. Synergy described by a $CI < 1$ at an effect level at or above 50 % inhibition of cancer cell growth is likely more clinically relevant. Depending on the robustness of data, the confidence interval for CI values can vary. We recommend considering CI values of 0.7 or lower indicative for synergy.
13. $IC_{50}$ values of each single agent alone and in combination, as well as hill slope values ($n$) are required to determine CI values using Eq. 1. The goodness of fit for dose–response curves should produce $R^2$ values ≥0.9. Compounds that are not potent enough to reach an effect of 50 % or greater will produce approximated, predicted $IC_{50}$ values based on an extrapolation of the dose–response curve. The accuracy of the predicted $IC_{50}$ values depends on the degree of extrapolation.
14. Conclusions drawn from isobolograms are similar to CI plots such that they both can predict synergy. For example, if the $CI < 1$ at 50 % of Fa, the concentration of each drug in combination is also below additivity line in the $IC_{50}$ isobologram. However, the two methods also provide complementary information: isobolograms show actual drug concentrations for one given effect level (e.g. $IC_{50}$) and, therefore, can be used to derive DRI values. For example, a $DRI \geq 2$ indicates that the drug can be reduced by twofold in the combination compared to the concentration necessary as a monotherapy to produce the same effect. CI plots indicate the level of synergy across multiple effect levels but not provide drug concentrations (nor DRIs).
15. Curve shift analysis is another alternative method to evaluate synergistic drug–drug interactions, similar to CI plots and isobolograms. For example, at 50 % effect level, if $CI < 1$, the combination isobole data point should be below the additivity line and $IC_{50eq}$ values of in combination should shift to the left toward single dose curve. Data analysis by multiple means provides confidence in data interpretation and conclusion.

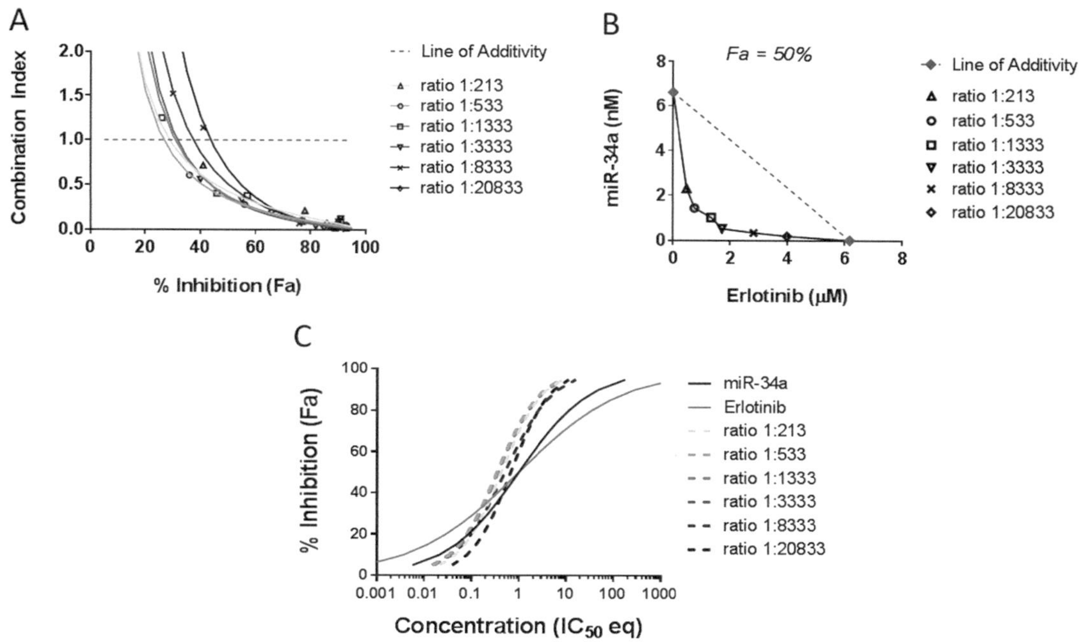


**Fig. 2** Synergistic effects between miR-34a and Erlotinib at multiple drug ratios in H460 non-small cell lung cancer cells. Cells were treated with seven concentrations of Erlotinib (100, 40, 16, 6.4, 2.56, 1.024, and 0.4096 μM) each in combination with seven concentrations of miR-34a mimic (30, 12, 4.8, 1.92, 0.768, 0.3072, and 0.12288 nM). Erlotinib or miR-34a alone was also used at these concentrations. This matrix yielded a total of 49 different combinations representing 13 different ratios; six different ratios (miR-34a: Erlotinib = 1:213, 1:533, 1:1333, 1:333, 1:8333, and 1:20833) were used for data analysis. (**a**) Combination index curve analysis demonstrates synergistic effect (CI < 1) for all six drug ratios at effect levels (Fa) approximately greater than 50 %. Different shades of *grey* represent the CI trend lines of the six drug ratios; *symbols* represent actual data points. (**b**) Isobologram at 50 % cancer cell inhibition. *Diamond shape symbols* represent the concentrations of drug used as single agent to produce 50 % inhibition of proliferation. *Other symbols* represent concentrations of each drug when used in combination to produce 50 % inhibition (six drug ratios). The *black line* represents the aligned isobole of the miR-34a + Erlotinib combination at various ratios to produce 50 % inhibition. The combination isobole is below the additive line which indicates synergistic effects for all six drug ratios. (**c**) Curve shift analysis of the dose–response curves derived from the single agents and the miR-34a + Erlotinib combination for all six combinations in the same graph. At an effect level of 50 % or above, the combination curves shift toward the left relative to the single agent curves indicating synergy (similar to CI plot)

## References

1. Ohashi K, Maruvka YE, Michor F et al (2013) Epidermal growth factor receptor tyrosine kinase inhibitor-resistant disease. J Clin Oncol 31:1070–1080
2. Sharma SV, Bell DW, Settleman J et al (2007) Epidermal growth factor receptor mutations in lung cancer. Nat Rev Cancer 7:169–181
3. Bader AG, Brown D, Winkler M (2010) The promise of microRNA replacement therapy. Cancer Res 70:7027–7030
4. Wiggins JF, Ruffino L, Kelnar K et al (2010) Development of a lung cancer therapeutic based on the tumor suppressor microRNA-34. Cancer Res 70:5923–5930
5. Liu C, Kelnar K, Liu B et al (2011) The microRNA miR-34a inhibits prostate cancer stem cells and metastasis by directly repressing CD44. Nat Med 17:211–215
6. Cortez MA, Ivan C, Valdecanas D et al (2015) PDL1 regulation by p53 via miR-34. J Natl Cancer Inst 108:djv303

7. Zhao J, Kelnar K, Bader AG (2014) In-depth analysis shows synergy between erlotinib and miR-34a. PLoS One 9, e89105
8. Bader AG (2012) miR-34 – a microRNA replacement therapy is headed to the clinic. Front Genet 3:120
9. Chou TC (2010) Drug combination studies and their synergy quantification using the Chou-Talalay method. Cancer Res 70:440–446
10. Tallarida RJ (2001) Drug synergism: its detection and applications. J Pharmacol Exp Ther 298:865–872
11. Tallarida RJ (2006) An overview of drug combination analysis with isobolograms. J Pharmacol Exp Ther 319:1–7
12. Zhao L, Au JL, Wientjes MG (2010) Comparison of methods for evaluating drug-drug interaction. Front Biosci (Elite Ed) 2:241–249
13. Engelman JA, Zejnullahu K, Mitsudomi T et al (2007) MET amplification leads to gefitinib resistance in lung cancer by activating ERBB3 signaling. Science 316(5827):1039–1043
14. He L, He X, Lim LP et al (2007) A microRNA component of the p53 tumor suppressor network. Nature 447(7148):1130–1134
15. Kaller M, Liffers ST, Oeljeklaus S et al (2011) Genome-wide characterization of miR-34a induced changes in protein and mRNA expression by a combined pulsed SILAC and microarray analysis. Mol Cell Proteomics 10(8):M111.010462
16. Zhang Z, Lee JC, Lin L et al (2012) Activation of the AXL kinase causes resistance to EGFR-targeted therapy in lung cancer. Nat Genet 44(8):852–860

# Chapter 9

# Assessing the Off-Target Effects of miRNA Inhibitors on Innate Immune Toll-Like Receptors

**Geneviève Pépin, Jonathan Ferrand, and Michael P. Gantier***

## Abstract

MicroRNAs (miRNAs) are involved in most cellular processes and are deregulated in several diseases. Antisense miRNA oligonucleotides (AMOs) therefore present novel therapeutic opportunities. Currently, in vivo delivery of AMOs often relies on high doses of nucleic acids, with nonspecific uptake by most tissues. Critically, AMOs accumulate in phagocytic cells where they can interfere with immune functions, such as the activation of Toll-Like Receptors (TLRs). In this chapter, we describe a method to assess the possible off-target effects of AMOs on TLR7, 8, and 9 sensing.

**Keywords** AMO, microRNA, Toll-like receptors, TLR7, TLR8, TLR9

## 1 Introduction

MicroRNAs (miRNAs) are short single-stranded RNAs of 19–24 nucleotides that bind to partially complementary messenger RNAs (mRNAs) to control their translation. Endogenous miRNAs result from the stepwise processing of structured primary stem-loop precursors [1, 2]. Following final cleavage of the stem-loop by the endonuclease Dicer and its cofactor TAR RNA-binding protein 2 [3], proteins including Argonaute (AGO) are recruited to the mature miRNA to form the RNA-induced silencing complex (RISC) [4, 5]. Due to loose complementarity with target mRNAs, a single miRNA can regulate several hundred targets [6]. As such, miRNAs are involved in the control of most cellular processes and are deregulated in several infections and pathologies including cancer [7–9].

Inhibition of miRNA function relying on steric antisense miRNA oligonucleotides (AMOs) has been used for more than a decade as a research tool to help inform on their biological activities [10–13]. In addition, AMOs present novel therapeutic

*Author contributed equally with all other contributors.

Marco F. Schmidt (ed.), *Drug Target miRNA: Methods and Protocols*, Methods in Molecular Biology, vol. 1517,
DOI 10.1007/978-1-4939-6563-2_9, © Springer Science+Business Media New York 2017

opportunities as evidenced with Miravirsen, a microRNA-122 (miR-122) AMO currently in clinical trial to treat Hepatitis C [14]. Several AMO chemistries have been developed over the years, with 2′-O-Methyl(2′OMe)-modified RNAs being one of the most common tools used to date [15, 16]. Importantly, what happens to miRNA/AMO duplexes following binding remains poorly understood. Previous reports indicate that the resulting ~20 bp duplexes would be stable and compete with processing of other miRNAs, leading to the de-repression of endogenous miRNAs [17, 18]. Nonetheless, the relatively high affinity for target miRNAs, lack of significant toxicity and low cost of synthesis, mean that AMOs are widely routinely used for in vitro and in vivo studies [16].

Current approaches of in vivo delivery of AMOs rely on very high dose of nucleic acids (adding up to 30–80 mg $kg^{-1}$), which penetrate most tissues (liver, kidney, lung, heart, skeletal muscle, colon, fat, skin, ovaries, adrenal glands, and bone marrow), with possible exception of the brain [19]. While such a strategy can probably be applied in disease contexts where tissue-specific miRNAs are targeted, as with the liver-specific miR-122 [14], it will be more problematic when targeting ubiquitously expressed miRNAs. In addition, in vivo administration of AMOs has the potential to interfere with phagocytic immune cells activation/function. Indeed, after systemic administration, AMOs preferentially accumulate in the macrophages from the bone marrow, the spleen, and the liver [20–22].

Besides their role in regulating homeostasis, macrophages provide an early line of defense against pathogens such as bacteria, fungus, or viruses. Toll-like Receptors (TLRs) expressed in these cells recognize pathogen-associated molecular patterns (PAMPs), such as bacterial lipopolysaccharide by TLR4, single-strand RNA (ssRNA) by TLR7/8, or unmethylated DNA with CpG motifs by TLR9 [23–26]. While most of the TLRs are expressed at the cell surface, TLR3, TLR7, TLR8, and TLR9 sensing of nucleic acids is restricted to the endosomal/lysosomal compartments to avoid the detection of self nucleic acids. Nonetheless, these receptors can thereby be affected by endocytosed AMOs, with the potential to interfere with their natural ligands [22, 27, 28].

Our laboratory and others have previously demonstrated that AMOs and other oligonucleotides with various modification patterns (e.g. 2′OMe-modified, LNA/DNA and phosphorothioate) have different affinity for TLR7/8 and 9 and can have off-target effects by inhibiting or potentiating their activation [29–33]. In light of the critical role of TLRs in infectious and autoimmune diseases, it is essential to test for the possible interplay between AMOs and these TLRs before embarking on preclinical in vivo studies. In this chapter, we describe a simple method to assess the possible off-target effects of AMOs on TLR7, 8, and 9 signaling. We illustrate our method with the use of an AMO targeting microRNA-16 (miR-16)—previously proposed to regulate the inflammatory transcription factor NF-kB [34]—which displays different effects on TLR7, 8, and 9.

## 2 Materials

### 2.1 Cell Culture

1. 293XL/hTLR7-HA (hTLR7), 293XL/hTLR8-HA (hTLR8) and 293XL/hTLR9-HA (hTLR9) cells (InvivoGen).
2. Dulbecco's Modified Eagle's Medium (DMEM; Life Technologies) supplemented with 10% sterile fetal bovine serum (FBS; Life Technologies), 1× antibiotic/antimycotic (Life Technologies); referred to as complete DMEM.
3. Blasticidin selective antibiotic (InvivoGen).
4. Dulbecco's Phosphate-Buffered Saline (DPBS; Life Technologies).
5. Versene non-enzymatic cell dissociation solution (Life Technologies).
6. Tissue culture plastic wares: 100 mm sterile tissue culture dishes; 6- and 96-well sterile tissue culture plates (BD Falcon).
7. 96-well solid white flat bottom plate (Corning).

### 2.2 Cell Transfections

1. Lipofectamine 2000 transfection reagent (Life Technologies).
2. Opti-Minimal Essential Medium (Opti-MEM; Life Technologies).
3. pNF-kB-Luc4 reporter, expressing the NF-kB response element (5′-GGGAATTTCCGGGAATTTCCGG GAATTTCCGGGAATTTCC-3′) upstream of the Firefly luciferase reporter (Clontech).
4. R848 (TLR7/8 agonist): stock solution at 1 mg/mL (2.8 mM) in endotoxin-free sterile $H_2O$ (InvivoGen).
5. Class B CpG oligonucleotide (ODN) 2006 (human TLR9 agonist): stock solution at 80 μM in endotoxin-free sterile water. 5′-TCGTCGTTTTGTCGTTTTGTCGTT-3′ (with full phosphorothioate backbone) (InvivoGen).
6. *N*-[1-(2,3-Dioleoyloxy)propyl]-*N*,*N*,*N*-trimethylammonium methylsulfate (DOTAP) (Roche).
7. miR-16 AMO LNA/DNA [31] (also referred to as "miR-16 DNA/LNA PS" [16]; 5′-c*g* ± $\underline{\text{C}}$*c*a* ± $\underline{\text{A}}$*t*a* ± $\underline{\text{T}}$*t*t* ± $\underline{\text{A}}$ *c*g* ± $\underline{\text{T}}$*g*c* ± $\underline{\text{T}}$*g*c* ± $\underline{\text{T}}$*a-3′, where lowercase is for DNA, ± *underlined* for LNA, with the asterisks for phosphorothioate linkages (Integrated DNA Technologies). Stock solution at 4 μM in sterile RNase-free TE buffer (Life Technologies).

### 2.3 Luciferase Assay

1. Glo Lysis Buffer (GLB, Promega).
2. Luciferase Assay System (Promega).
3. Microplate luminometer.

## 3 Methods

This section details a method to assess the effect of AMOs on TLR7, 8, and 9 signaling. The volumes provided in the method are sufficient to perform three conditions (non-stimulated cells, TLR agonist-stimulated/mock-transfected cells, and TLR agonist-stimulated/miR-16 AMO-transfected cells) in biological triplicate for one cell line.

### Cell Culture

1. Grow hTLR7, hTLR8, and hTLR9 293XL in complete DMEM at 37 °C in 5% $CO_2$ until the cells reach a 70–80% confluence (*see* **Note 1**).
2. Replace medium with 2 mL Versene and detach the cells by tapping the flasks and gentle pipetting. Transfer the cells into a 15 mL tube containing 5 mL of complete DMEM and spin down at 250 × *g* for 3 min (*see* **Note 2**).
3. Resuspend the cells in 5 mL of complete DMEM and count the cells with a hemocytometer. Prepare a suspension containing 500,000 cells in 1.9 mL of DMEM with 10% FCS without antibiotic/antimycotic.

### 3.1 Reverse-Transfection of the NF-kB Reporter Construct

The protocol and volumes given below are for one cell line.

1. Dilute 0.6 μL of Lipofectamine 2000 in 50 μL of Opti-MEM.
2. Dilute 200 ng of pNF-kB-Luc4 reporter in 50 μL of Opti-MEM (*see* **Note 3**).
3. Incubate the Lipofectamine 2000 and the DNA solutions at room temperature for 5 min.
4. Add the Lipofectamine solution to the DNA solution, and mix by gentle tapping before incubating for 20 min at room temperature.
5. Add 100 μL of the resulting Lipofectamine 2000/DNA/Opti-MEM solution directly into a well of a 6-well plate and subsequently add the 1.9 mL cell suspension, giving a final volume of 2 mL per well.
6. Incubate the cells overnight (approximately 16 h) at 37 °C in 5% $CO_2$.

### 3.2 AMO Transfection

1. The next morning, discard the medium and add 300 μL of Versene directly into the 6-well plate and incubate 5 min at 37 °C in 5% $CO_2$ (*see* **Note 4**).
2. Add 1660 μL of DMEM with 10% FCS without antibiotic/antimycotic into the well and break cluster of cells by vigorous pipetting (avoiding bubbles).

3. Plate 150 μL of the cell suspension into nine wells of a 96-well plate and incubate 6 h at 37 °C in 5% $CO_2$ (*see* **Note 5**).
4. In the afternoon, once the cells have adhered, dilute 11 μL of DOTAP in 140 μL of DMEM for the mock transfection (*see* **Note 6**).
5. Dilute 60 μL of AMO at 4 μM in 80 μL of DMEM and add 11 μL of DOTAP for the AMO transfection.
6. Incubate the solutions for 5 min at room temperature.
7. Add 50 μL of the mock solution into three wells ("Mock" condition) (*see* **Note 7**).
8. Add 50 μL of the miR-16 AMO/DOTAP solution into another three wells, giving a final concentration of 400 nM ("miR-16 AMO" condition).
9. Add 50 μL of DMEM into the remaining three wells—as untreated controls (*see* **Note 8**).
10. Incubate for 30 min at 37 °C in 5% $CO_2$.
11. For hTLR7 and hTLR8 cells: dilute 2 μL of R848 stock in 100 μL of DMEM, and add 7 μL of this solution into three wells of mock-transfected, and into three wells of AMO-transfected hTLR7 or hTLR8 cells, giving a final concentration of ~2 μM (700 ng/mL).
12. For hTLR9 cells: directly add 1 μL of ODN 2006 stock per well of mock-transfected, and AMO-transfected hTLR9 cells, giving a final concentration of 400 nM.
13. Incubate the cells overnight (approximately 16 h) at 37 °C in 5% $CO_2$.

### 3.3 Luciferase Assay

1. Discard the supernatants carefully avoiding to detach the cells, and lyse the cells with 40 μL of Glo lysis buffer (*see* **Note 9**).
2. Prepare Luciferase Assay Reagent by adding 10 mL of Luciferase Assay Buffer to the vial of lyophilized Luciferase Assay Substrate (*see* **Note 10**).
3. Dispense 15 μL of lysates into a solid white flat bottom 96-well plate (or an appropriate tube if not using a plate reader format) and add 40 μL of Luciferase Assay Buffer.
4. Immediately measure luminescence with a luminometer/plate reader.
5. To determine the effect of AMO transfection on TLR7/8/9 sensing, divide each luminescence value measured by the average luminescence obtained for the untreated condition (i.e. not transfected and not stimulated) (*see* Fig. 1).

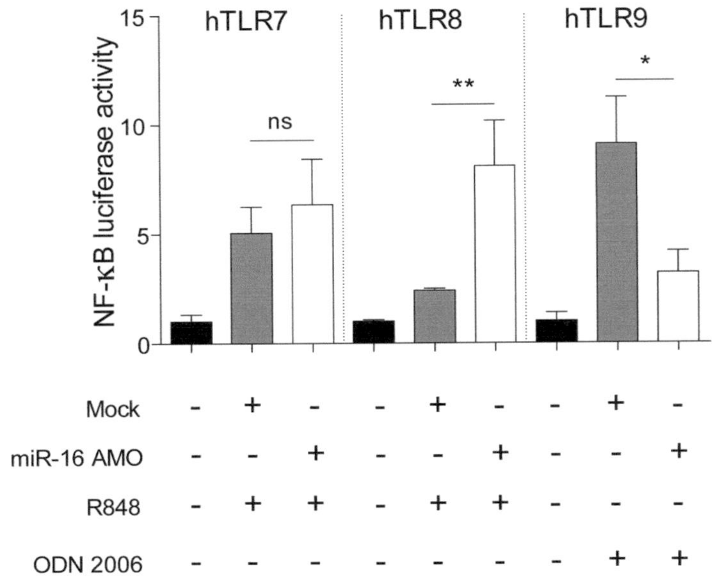


**Fig. 1** Modulation of TLR7, TLR8, and TLR9 sensing by miR-16 AMO. TLR7, TLR8, and TLR9 expressing 293XL cells were transfected with pNF-kB-Luc4 reporter construct prior to transfection with 400 nM miR-16 AMO and stimulation with 2 μM TLR7/8 agonist (R848) or 400 nM TLR9 agonists (ODN 2006). Each treatment was carried out in biological triplicates and the data are representative of two independent experiments, shown relative to the unstimulated condition. Two-tailed unpaired **t**-tests and standard deviation are shown (ns = non significant, $^{*}\mathbf{p} < 0.05$, $^{**}\mathbf{p} < 0.01$). The data suggest that the miR-16 AMO used here potentiates TLR8 signaling, while inhibiting TLR9 signaling and having no effect on TLR7 signaling. These effects are therefore unlikely related to miR-16 inhibition, but rather indicate an off-target effect on TLR8/9 sensing of their respective ligands. Mock condition refers to DOTAP control (without AMO)

## 4 Notes

1. Cells should be passaged at least once before use for the assay. Blasticidin-selective antibiotic should be added only when cells have been passaged twice after being brought back from frozen stocks.
2. The response of 293XL cells can be altered by the action of trypsin. Cells should be detached in non-enzymatic cell dissociation solution, such as Versene. Note that the cells do not need to be rinsed with PBS before adding the Versene—this avoids loosing cells when rinsing (the cells are poorly adherent).
3. pNF-kB-Luc4 transfection will result in the expression of firefly luciferase upon activation of TLR7/8/9. In this set up, there is no need to co-transfect a second reporter (such as

*Renilla* luciferase), given that all subsequent conditions will use the same parental transfection of pNF-kB-Luc4.

4. After overnight incubation, cells should reach a 50% confluence.
5. Incubation can be shortened, but cells have to be adherent. The cells should reach around 50% confluence per well in the 96-well format.
6. DMEM used during DOTAP/AMO complexation should be free of serum and antibiotics as these factors could impact lipid/AMO complexation.
7. These cells are poorly adherent; hence the 50 μL added should be added to the side of the well with care to avoid that the cells detach from the bottom of the well.
8. All the wells should have a final volume of 200 μL.
9. Make sure that there is no supernatant left in the wells, as this would affect the total amount of lysate. Lysates can be used fresh or stored at −80 °C for later use.
10. Luciferase assay reagent should be dispensed into working aliquots and store at −80 °C. Multiple freeze–thaw cycles should be avoided.

## Acknowledgments

The authors thank Frances Cribbin for her help with the redaction of this chapter. The authors are supported by funding from the Australian NHMRC (1062683 and 1081167 to M.P.G.); the Australian Research Council (140100594 Future Fellowship to M.P.G.); and the Victorian Government's Operational Infrastructure Support Program.

### References

1. Ha M, Kim VN (2014) Regulation of microRNA biogenesis. Nat Rev Mol Cell Biol 15(8):509–524. doi:10.1038/nrm3838
2. Erhard F, Haas J, Lieber D, Malterer G, Jaskiewicz L, Zavolan M, Dolken L, Zimmer R (2014) Widespread context dependency of microRNA-mediated regulation. Genome Res 24(6):906–919. doi:10.1101/gr.166702.113
3. Ketting RF, Fischer SE, Bernstein E, Sijen T, Hannon GJ, Plasterk RH (2001) Dicer functions in RNA interference and in synthesis of small RNA involved in developmental timing in C. elegans. Genes Dev 15(20):2654–2659. doi:10.1101/gad.927801
4. Rose SD, Kim DH, Amarzguioui M, Heidel JD, Collingwood MA, Davis ME, Rossi JJ, Behlke MA (2005) Functional polarity is introduced by Dicer processing of short substrate RNAs. Nucleic Acids Res 33(13):4140–4156. doi:10.1093/nar/gki732
5. Filipowicz W (2005) RNAi: the nuts and bolts of the RISC machine. Cell 122(1):17–20. doi:10.1016/j.cell.2005.06.023
6. Selbach M, Schwanhausser B, Thierfelder N, Fang Z, Khanin R, Rajewsky N (2008) Widespread changes in protein synthesis induced by microRNAs. Nature 455(7209):58–63. doi:10.1038/nature07228
7. Hartig SM, Hamilton MP, Bader DA, McGuire SE (2015) The miRNA interactome in metabolic homeostasis. Trends Endocrinol Metab. doi:10.1016/j.tem.2015.09.006

8. Yang Q, Zhang RW, Sui PC, He HT, Ding L (2015) Dysregulation of non-coding RNAs in gastric cancer. World J Gastroenterol 21(39):10956–10981. doi:10.3748/wjg.v21.i39.10956
9. Mizuguchi Y, Takizawa T, Yoshida H, Uchida E (2015) Dysregulated microRNAs in progression of hepatocellular carcinoma: a systematic review. Hepatol Res 46(5):391–406. doi:10.1111/hepr.12606
10. Hutvagner G, Simard MJ, Mello CC, Zamore PD (2004) Sequence-specific inhibition of small RNA function. PLoS Biol 2(4), E98. doi:10.1371/journal.pbio.0020098
11. Meister G, Landthaler M, Dorsett Y, Tuschl T (2004) Sequence-specific inhibition of microRNA- and siRNA-induced RNA silencing. RNA 10(3):544–550
12. Baigude H, Rana TM (2014) Strategies to antagonize miRNA functions in vitro and in vivo. Nanomedicine (Lond) 9(16):2545–2555. doi:10.2217/nnm.14.162
13. Beavers KR, Nelson CE, Duvall CL (2015) MiRNA inhibition in tissue engineering and regenerative medicine. Adv Drug Deliv Rev 88:123–137.doi:10.1016/j.addr.2014.12.006
14. Janssen HL, Kauppinen S, Hodges MR (2013) HCV infection and miravirsen. N Engl J Med 369(9):878. doi:10.1056/NEJMc1307787
15. Lennox KA, Behlke MA (2011) Chemical modification and design of anti-miRNA oligonucleotides. Gene Ther 18(12):1111–1120. doi:10.1038/gt.2011.100
16. Lennox KA, Owczarzy R, Thomas DM, Walder JA, Behlke MA (2013) Improved performance of anti-miRNA oligonucleotides using a novel non-nucleotide modifier. Mol Ther Nucleic Acids 2:e117. doi:10.1038/mtna.2013.46
17. Elmen J, Lindow M, Schutz S, Lawrence M, Petri A, Obad S, Lindholm M, Hedtjarn M, Hansen HF, Berger U, Gullans S, Kearney P, Sarnow P, Straarup EM, Kauppinen S (2008) LNA-mediated microRNA silencing in non-human primates. Nature 452(7189):896–899. doi:10.1038/nature06783
18. Khan AA, Betel D, Miller ML, Sander C, Leslie CS, Marks DS (2009) Transfection of small RNAs globally perturbs gene regulation by endogenous microRNAs. Nat Biotechnol 27(6):549–555. doi:10.1038/nbt.1543
19. Krutzfeldt J, Rajewsky N, Braich R, Rajeev KG, Tuschl T, Manoharan M, Stoffel M (2005) Silencing of microRNAs in vivo with 'antagomirs'. Nature 438(7068):685–689. doi:10.1038/nature04303
20. Butler M, Stecker K, Bennett CF (1997) Cellular distribution of phosphorothioate oligodeoxynucleotides in normal rodent tissues. Lab Invest 77(4):379–388
21. Lendvai G, Velikyan I, Bergstrom M, Estrada S, Laryea D, Valila M, Salomaki S, Langstrom B, Roivainen A (2005) Biodistribution of 68Ga-labelled phosphodiester, phosphorothioate, and 2′-O-methyl phosphodiester oligonucleotides in normal rats. Eur J Pharm Sci 26(1):26–38. doi:10.1016/j.ejps.2005.04.017
22. White PJ, Anastasopoulos F, Pouton CW, Boyd BJ (2009) Overcoming biological barriers to in vivo efficacy of antisense oligonucleotides. Expert Rev Mol Med 11, e10. doi:10.1017/S1462399409001021
23. Diebold SS, Kaisho T, Hemmi H, Akira S, Reis e Sousa C (2004) Innate antiviral responses by means of TLR7-mediated recognition of single-stranded RNA. Science 303(5663):1529–1531. doi:10.1126/science.1093616
24. Heil F, Hemmi H, Hochrein H, Ampenberger F, Kirschning C, Akira S, Lipford G, Wagner H, Bauer S (2004) Species-specific recognition of single-stranded RNA via toll-like receptor 7 and 8. Science 303(5663):1526–1529. doi:10.1126/science.1093620
25. Bauer S, Kirschning CJ, Hacker H, Redecke V, Hausmann S, Akira S, Wagner H, Lipford GB (2001) Human TLR9 confers responsiveness to bacterial DNA via species-specific CpG motif recognition. Proc Natl Acad Sci U S A 98(16):9237–9242. doi:10.1073/pnas.161293498
26. Hemmi H, Takeuchi O, Kawai T, Kaisho T, Sato S, Sanjo H, Matsumoto M, Hoshino K, Wagner H, Takeda K, Akira S (2000) A Toll-like receptor recognizes bacterial DNA. Nature 408(6813):740–745. doi:10.1038/35047123
27. Chuang TH, Ulevitch RJ (2000) Cloning and characterization of a sub-family of human toll-like receptors: hTLR7, hTLR8 and hTLR9. Eur Cytokine Netw 11(3):372–378
28. Juliano R, Bauman J, Kang H, Ming X (2009) Biological barriers to therapy with antisense and siRNA oligonucleotides. Mol Pharm 6(3):686–695. doi:10.1021/mp900093r
29. Barrat FJ, Meeker T, Gregorio J, Chan JH, Uematsu S, Akira S, Chang B, Duramad O, Coffman RL (2005) Nucleic acids of mammalian origin can act as endogenous ligands for Toll-like receptors and may promote systemic lupus erythematosus. J Exp Med 202(8):1131–1139. doi:10.1084/jem.20050914
30. Hamm S, Latz E, Hangel D, Muller T, Yu P, Golenbock D, Sparwasser T, Wagner H, Bauer S (2010) Alternating 2′-O-ribose methylation is a universal approach for generating non-stimulatory siRNA by acting as TLR7 antago-

nist. Immunobiology 215(7):559–569. doi:10.1016/j.imbio.2009.09.003

31. Sarvestani ST, Stunden HJ, Behlke MA, Forster SC, McCoy CE, Tate MD, Ferrand J, Lennox KA, Latz E, Williams BR, Gantier MP (2015) Sequence-dependent off-target inhibition of TLR7/8 sensing by synthetic microRNA inhibitors. Nucleic Acids Res 43(2):1177–1188. doi:10.1093/nar/gku1343
32. Gorden KK, Qiu X, Battiste JJ, Wightman PP, Vasilakos JP, Alkan SS (2006) Oligodeoxynucleotides differentially modulate activation of TLR7 and TLR8 by imidazoquinolines. J Immunol 177(11):8164–8170
33. Ferrand J, Gantier MP (2015) Assessing the inhibitory activity of oligonucleotides on TLR7 sensing, vol Toll-like receptors. Methods Mol Biol 1390:79–90
34. Zhou R, Li X, Hu G, Gong AY, Drescher KM, Chen XM (2012) MiR-16 targets transcriptional corepressor SMRT and modulates NF-kappaB-regulated transactivation of interleukin-8 gene. PLoS One 7(1):30772. doi:10.1371/journal.pone.0030772

# Chapter 10

# Design of Multimodal Small Molecules Targeting miRNAs Biogenesis: Synthesis and In Vitro Evaluation

Duc D. Vo and Maria Duca

## Abstract

microRNAs (miRNAs) are emerging as novel biological targets for medicinal chemists to develop chemical tools for intracellular regulation. In this context, the discovery of small-molecule drugs targeting specific miRNAs and modulating their production or function represents a very promising approach that could be further developed for targeted therapy in miRNA-related pathologies. Here, we describe the design of multimodal small molecules as RNA ligands targeting DICER-mediated miRNA maturation. The synthesis and the biochemical evaluation as ligands of stem-loop-structured precursor microRNAs (pre-miRNAs) are reported.

**Key words** microRNAs, Ligands, Inhibitors, DICER cleavage, Synthetic small molecules

## 1 Introduction

In recent years, the interest about ribonucleic acid (RNA) targeting using small molecules strongly increased together with the need of new synthetic and theoretical methods for the preparation of strong and selective RNA ligands [1]. In fact, RNA represents a particularly relevant biological target since both coding and noncoding RNAs are involved in a large number of biological processes essential for cell survival and homeostasis. Recently, a particular type of noncoding RNAs, i.e., microRNAs, retained large attention for its intrinsic therapeutic potential [2]. microRNAs (miRNAs or miRs) are single-stranded RNAs of 18–25 nucleotides that act as posttranscriptional regulators of gene expression upon binding to the 3′ untranslated regions (3′-UTR) of specific target messenger RNAs (mRNAs). The recognition of the mRNA target usually leads to gene silencing by repression of mRNA translation and acceleration of mRNA degradation [3]. The miRNAs biogenesis process starts with the transcription of a long RNA of several kilobases, so-called primary microRNA (pri-miRNA), which is processed in the nucleus by the enzyme Drosha into the

Marco F. Schmidt (ed.), *Drug Target miRNA: Methods and Protocols*, Methods in Molecular Biology, vol. 1517,
DOI 10.1007/978-1-4939-6563-2_10, 

shorter (ca. 70 nucleotides) stem-loop-structured precursor microRNA (pre-miRNA) [4]. This latter is exported to the cytoplasm, where it becomes a substrate for the DICER nuclease. Processing by DICER produces the mature miRNA, which is loaded onto the microRNA-induced silencing complex (miRISC) and subsequently targets complementary sequences on mRNA [5]. The pivotal role that miRNAs play in the regulation of a wide range of biological processes, including cell cycle progression and proliferation, differentiation, cell survival, and development, has become increasingly evident in recent years. Furthermore, tremendous observations have been made in linking the aberrant expression levels of miRNAs to the initiation and development of human diseases such as cancers, genetic disorders, and altered immune system function [6]. Based on these findings, it is now clear that miRNAs represent a particularly interesting target for the discovery of new therapeutic strategies for a number of diseases.

In this context, two strategies have been developed in order to interfere with miRNAs biogenesis/function: (1) direct strategies based on the use of oligonucleotides to supply for an underexpressed miRNA or to inhibit an overexpressed miRNA and (2) indirect strategies based on the use of small molecules. While oligonucleotides are very efficient and extremely specific, their use in therapy remains limited because of their poor bioavailability and unfavorable pharmacological properties. Therefore, the research of small molecules capable of tuning miRNAs production or function emerged as a promising route to restore physiological miRNAs amounts. To date, only few examples of small-molecule drugs have been reported to modulate miRNA expression by targeting their transcription and/or their processing [7–10]. These have been discovered after the screening of large chemical libraries or after the study of established RNA ligands. In parallel to these studies, we contributed to the field with the design of new RNA ligands inhibitors of oncogenic miRNA-372 and -373 production [11]. These two miRNAs are implicated, for instance, in the development and progression of gastric cancer [12]. The new ligands (Fig. 1) are composed of two different RNA-binding motives: (1) an aminoglycoside (neomycin) known to strongly interact with stem-loop RNAs with high affinity [13] and (2) natural and artificial nucleobases designed to specifically recognize a RNA base of the single-stranded region or a RNA base pair of the double-stranded region of the pre-miRNA [14–19].

The conjugation of nucleobases to aminoglycosides allowed the obtention of ligands that bind with high affinity to stem-loop-structured pre-miRNAs, thus leading to the inhibition of the production of the corresponding miRNA. In particular, some of these compounds showed an antiproliferative effect which is highly specific for gastric cancer cells overexpressing the targeted miRNA-372 and miRNA-373, while no effect is observed in

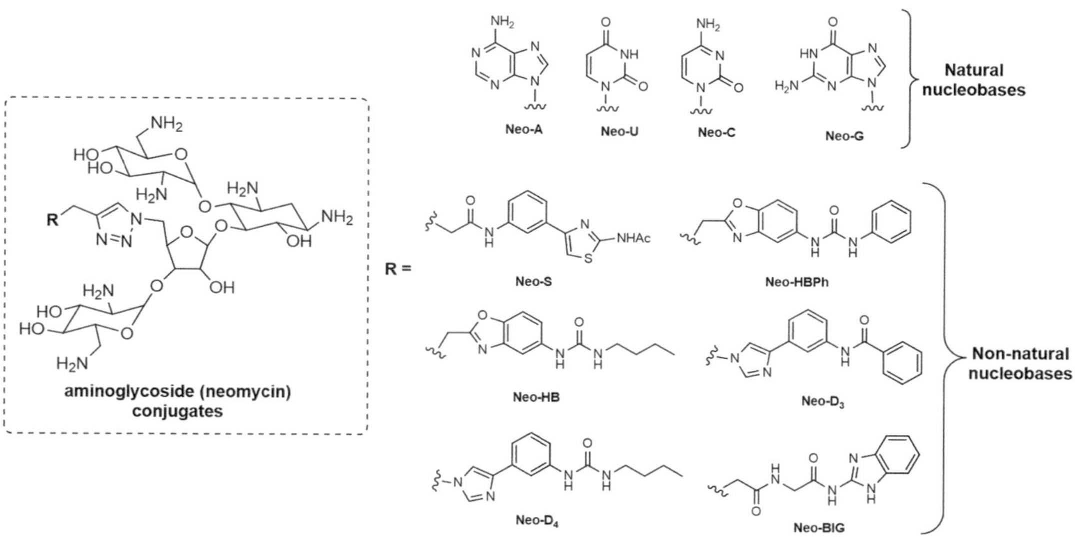


**Fig. 1** Neomycin–nucleobase conjugates that can be synthesized using the methodology described as follows

other gastric epithelial cell lines that do not express these miRNAs. Our experiments demonstrated that the biological activity is directly correlated to the inhibition of the production of these oncogenic miRNAs, thus leading to the restoration of normal mRNA translation in the target protein LArge Tumor Suppressor 2 (LATS2) [11]. This approach, based on the conjugation of different RNA-binding domains, demonstrated to be successful for the targeting of oncogenic miRNAs and opens the way for the rational design of pre-miRNAs ligands. Here, we report the methodology that has been employed for the design and the synthesis of these conjugates as well as for their in vitro screening in order to select the most promising compounds for intracellular assays. The synthesis of aminoglycoside–nucleobase conjugates relies on 1,3-dipolar cycloaddition reaction between an azido-derivative of the aminoglycoside neomycin and an alkyne derivative of the nucleobase moiety. The same synthetic pathway can be applied to other RNA-binding moieties in order to prepare various multimodal conjugates. After the synthesis of these compounds, we will describe the cell-free assay based on the fluorescence resonance energy transfer (FRET) technique that we applied in order to screen the RNA ligands for their ability to inhibit DICER cleavage of a particular pre-miRNA. Finally, the fluorescence-based assay allowing the measurement of dissociation constants ($K_D$) illustrating their affinity toward the pre-miRNAs will be reported. These cell-free assays demonstrated to be reliable for the selection of most active compounds and their activity for intracellular assays.

## 2 Materials

### *2.1 Reagents and Solvents for Chemical Synthesis*

1. Solvents (pyridine, dimethylformamide, dichloromethane, methanol, diethyl ether, toluene and acetonitrile, deuterated methanol, and deuterated water) (Sigma Aldrich) can be used without further purification. Dimethylformamide and pyridine need to be in their anhydrous form.
2. Neomycin, di-*tert*-butyldicarbonate ($Boc_2O$), triisopropylbenzenesulfonyl chloride (TIPBSCl), sodium azide, 4-pentynoic acid, triethylamine ($Et_3N$), copper iodide, *N,N*-diisopropylethylamine (DIPEA), trifluoroacetic acid (TFA), acetic acid, ninhydrin, tetrabutylammonium fluoride (TBAF), triphenylphosphine, diisopropylazodicarboxylate (DIAD), adenine (A), uracil (U), cytosine (C), guanine (G), and ninhydrin (Sigma Aldrich) can be used without further purification.
3. Sodium bicarbonate, potassium carbonate, propargyl bromide, chloromethylpyridium iodide, 1-hydroxybenzotriazole (HOBt), and *N,N'*-diisopropylcarbodiimide (DIC) (Alpha Æsar, Heysham, UK) can be used without further purification.
4. All aqueous solutions must be prepared using distilled water. This latter is necessary also for the workup of all reactions.
5. Column chromatography needs to be performed using silica gel 60 Å (40–63 μm, Merck, Darmstadt, Germany) in a 50-fold excess with respect to the amount of product that has to be purified.
6. Thin layer chromatography (TLC) needs to be conducted on precoated silica gel 60F254 (Macherey Nagel, Düren, Germany) and compounds can be visualized by UV irradiation (aromatic systems) and/or by staining with ninhydrin (primary amines). For the preparation of ninhydrin staining solution, dissolve 1.5 g of ninhydrin in 100 mL of ethanol and add 3 mL of acetic acid.
7. All synthesized compounds are analyzed by NMR spectrometry. All intermediates that do not contain the aminoglycoside moiety can be analyzed using a 200 MHz spectrometer, while compounds containing the aminoglycoside moiety need at least a 500 MHz spectrometer.
8. The purity of final compounds needs to be checked by HPLC on a $C_{18}$ reversed phase column. Toward this aim we employed a 250×4.6 mm (5 μm) by Thermo Scientific and a gradient from 5 to 100% over 20 min of acetonitrile in water both containing 0.1% of trifluoroacetic acid. The flow rate is 1 mL/min.
9. High-resolution mass spectrometry (HRMS) can be finally used in order to characterize each compound. Toward this aim we used a LTQ Orbitrap hybrid mass spectrometer with an electrospray ionization probe (Thermo Scientific).

### 2.2 Cell-Free Assays Components

1. Milli-Q® water (Millipore) should be used for all biochemical manipulations.
2. Oligonucleotides for FRET assays are double labeled with fluorescein at the 5′ position and with dabcyl at the 3′ position. Oligonucleotides for $K_D$ measurements are labeled at the 5′ position with fluorescein. All oligonucleotides were purified by HPLC (IBA GmbH, Göttingen, Germany). For the analysis of oligonucleotides, we employed a Discovery® BIO Wide Pore $C_8$, 5 μm, 15 cm × 4.6 mm HPLC column (Supelco, Sigma Aldrich) and a gradient from 0 to 40% of acetonitrile over 40 min in 0.5 M of triethylammonium acetate (TEAA) buffer.
3. Filter all solutions and buffers using Stericup® Filter Units of 0.2 μm (Millipore).
4. Prepare Tris(hydroxymethyl)aminomethane hydrochloride (Tris–HCl) buffer using preset Trizma® Pre-set crystal pH 7.4 (Sigma Aldrich).
5. Magnesium chloride and sodium chloride (Calbiochem) need to be purchased as molecular biology grade reagents.
6. Dithiothreitol (DTT, Applichem, Darmstadt, Germany) needs to be purchased as molecular biology grade reagent.
7. Human recombinant DICER (Genlantis, San Diego, CA, USA) was purchased by Biocat (Heidelberg, Germany) as a 0.5 U/μL solution.
8. All cell-free assays can be performed in black 384-well flat bottom plates (Greiner Bio-one). Black 96-well flat bottom plates (Nunc) can be used for the preparation of compounds' dilutions as described in Subheading 3.2.1, **step 7**.
9. Gloves and all materials used during RNA manipulations need to be cleaned with RNase away™ spray (Molecular BioProducts, San Diego, CA, USA).

## 3 Methods

In the first part of this Subheading 3.1, the synthetic methods used for the preparation of multimodal RNA ligands illustrated in Fig. 1 will be outlined. This description includes (1) the preparation of the azido-substituted derivative of aminoglycosides (Fig. 2), (2) the propargyl-substituted nucleobases (Fig. 3, 4, and 5), and (3) the conjugation of these two chemical entities using 1,3-dipolar cycloaddition reaction (Fig. 6). In the second part of this Subheading 3.2, the methodology employed for the cell-free assay of synthesized compounds as DICER cleavage inhibitors and RNA binders will be reported.

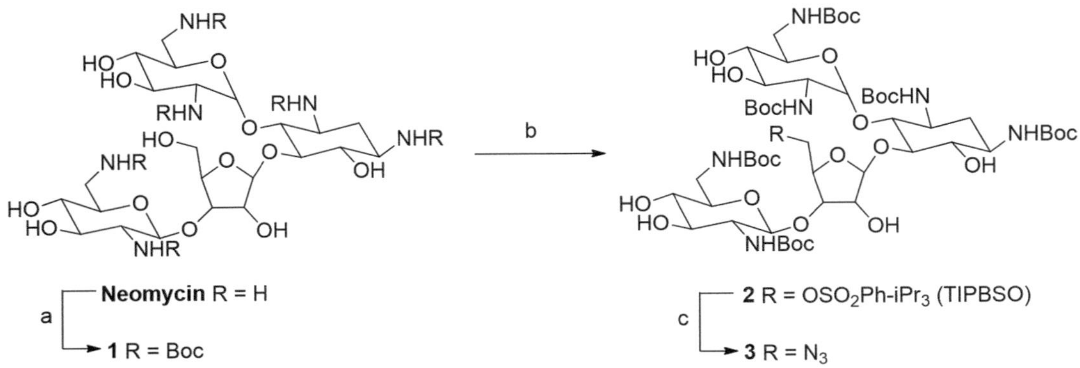


**Fig. 2** Synthesis of azide-substituted neomycin derivative **3**. Reagents: (**a**) $Boc_2O$, MeOH, $H_2O$, $Et_3N$, 60 °C, overnight; (**b**) TIPBSCl, pyr, overnight; (**c**) $NaN_3$, DMF, 100 °C, overnight

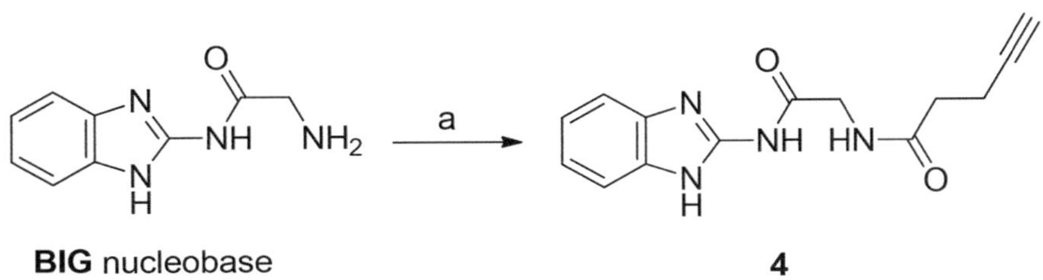


**Fig. 3** Synthesis of alkyne-substituted **BIG** nucleobase **4**. Reagents: (*a*) 4-pentynoic acid, HOBt, DIC, DMF, r.t., overnight

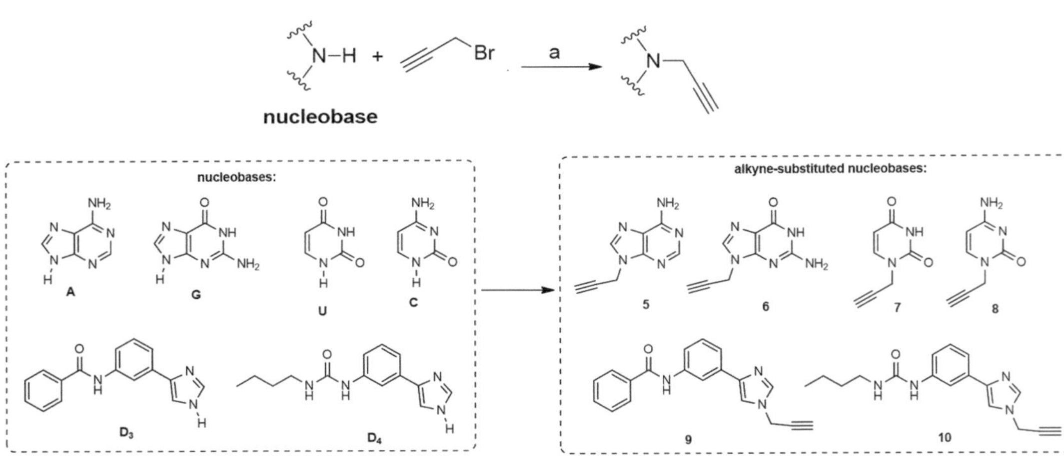


**Fig. 4** Synthesis of alkyne-substituted nucleobases 5–10. Reagents: (*a*) propargyl bromide, $K_2CO_3$, toluene, 60 °C, overnight

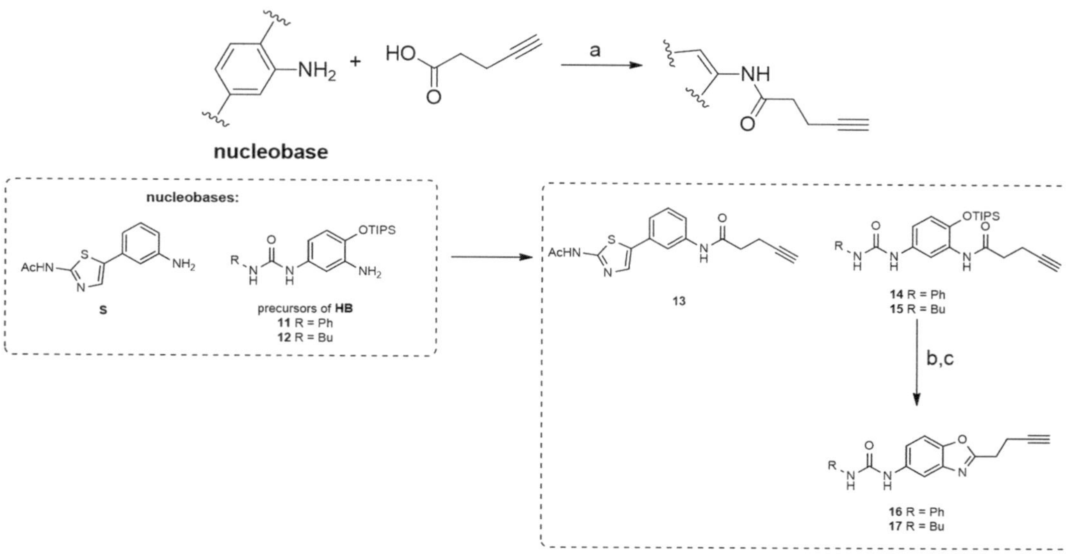


**Fig. 5** Synthesis of alkyne-substituted nucleobases **13**, **16**, and **17**. Reagents: (*a*) chloromethylpyridinium iodide, $Et_3N$, $CH_2Cl_2$, 1 h; (*b*) TBAF, THF, r.t., 1 h; (*c*) DIAD, $PPh_3$, r.t., overnight

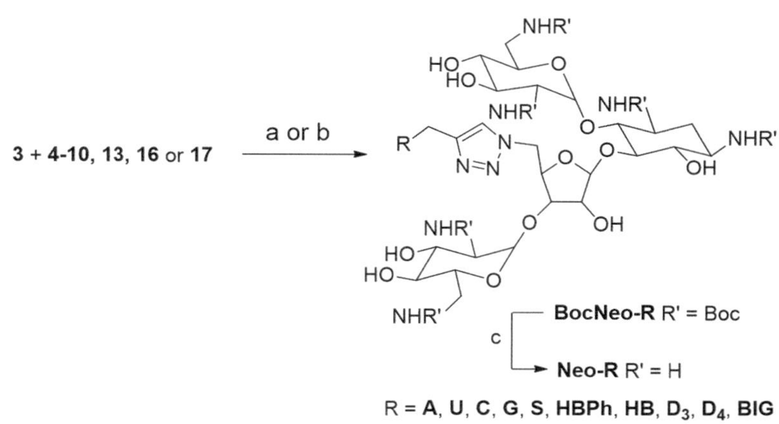


**Fig. 6** Synthesis of final conjugates **Neo-A**, **Neo-U**, **Neo-C**, **Neo-G**, **Neo-S**, **Neo-HBPh**, **Neo-HB**, **Neo-D3**, **Neo-D4**, and **Neo-BIG**. Reagents: (*a*) CuI, DIPEA, $CH_3CN$, r.t., overnight; (*b*) CuI, DIPEA, toluene, Δ, overnight; (*c*) TFA, $CH_2Cl_2$, r.t., overnight

## 3.1 Synthetic Methods

### 3.1.1 Aminoglycosides Protection/Activation/Substitution Strategy

1. Dissolve 1.5 g of neomycin sulfate (1.65 mmol) in 15 mL of a mixture $MeOH/H_2O$ 1:1 in the presence of 5.73 mL of $Et_3N$ (41.2 mmol, 25 eq.).
2. Add 3.6 g of di-*tert*-butyldicarbonate ($Boc_2O$, 16.5 mmol, 10 eq.) and stir the mixture at 60 °C overnight (*see* **Note 1**).
3. Remove methanol by evaporation and partition the residue between 300 mL of ethyl acetate and 150 mL of distilled water.

Finally, extract the aqueous layer with ethyl acetate (2 × 75 mL), combine organic layers, dry them with anhydrous $Na_2SO_4$ and remove the solvent under reduced pressure.

4. Purify the crude product by flash chromatography on a silica gel column using a mixture $CH_2Cl_2$/acetone 3:2. This affords Boc-protected aminoglycoside **1** as a white solid in 1.5 g yield (75%).
5. Dissolve 1.5 g of compound **1** (1.24 mmol) in 25 mL of dry pyridine (*see* **Note 2**).
6. Add 11.9 g of triisopropylbenzenesulfonyl chloride (TIPBSCl, 39.5 mmol, 32 eq.) and leave the reaction mixture stirring overnight at room temperature.
7. Quench the reaction with a saturated solution of sodium bicarbonate and remove the pyridine under reduced pressure. After dissolving the mixture in 300 mL of water, extract it twice with ethyl acetate (2 × 300 mL). Combine organic layers, dry them with anhydrous $Na_2SO_4$ and remove the solvent under reduced pressure.
8. Purify the crude product by flash chromatography on a silica gel column using a mixture $CH_2Cl_2$/MeOH 97:3. This leads to compound **2** as a white solid in 1.02 g yield (56%) (*see* **Note 3**).
9. Dissolve 1.02 g of compound **2** (0.689 mmol) in 10 mL of dry DMF.
10. Add 449 mg of sodium azide (6.89 mmol, 10 eq.).
11. Stir the reaction mixture at 100 °C overnight and then evaporate the solvent under reduced pressure.
12. Dissolve the crude product in 150 mL of ethylacetate and extract it twice with water (2 × 150 mL) and once with a saturated solution of NaCl (100 mL). Combine organic layers, dry them with anhydrous $Na_2SO_4$, and remove the solvent under reduced pressure.
13. Purify the crude product by flash chromatography on a silica gel column using a mixture $CH_2Cl_2$/MeOH 9:1. This leads to compound **3** as a white solid in 820 mg yield (96%) (*see* **Note 4**).

#### *3.1.2 Alkyne Introduction in Artificial Nucleobases Containing a Primary Amine (See Note 5)*

1. Dissolve 123.6 mg of 4-pentynoic acid (1.26 mmol, 1.2 eq.) in 5 mL of DMF.
2. Add 172.9 mg of *N,N'*-diisopropylcarbodiimide (DIC, 1.37 mmol, 1.3 eq.), 185.1 mg of 1-hydroxybenzotriazole hydrate (HOBt, 1.37 mmol, 1.3 eq.), and 379 μL of triethylamine (2.52 mmol, 2.5 eq.).
3. Stir this reaction mixture for 1 h.
4. Dissolve 200 mg of benzaminoimidazol-glycyl (**BIG**) nucleobase (1.05 mmol) in 5 mL of DMF and add this solution to the previously prepared reaction mixture.

5. Stir the reaction mixture at room temperature overnight and then evaporate the solvent under reduced pressure.
6. Add 50 mL of $CH_2Cl_2$ and extract it twice with water (2 × 50 mL) and once with a saturated solution of NaCl (50 mL). Combine organic layers, dry them with anhydrous $Na_2SO_4$ and remove the solvent under reduced pressure.
7. Purify the crude product by flash column chromatography using a mixture $CH_2Cl_2$/MeOH 95:5. This leads to desired compound **4** as a white solid in 150 mg yield (53%).

*3.1.3 Alkyne Introduction in Nucleobase Moiety Containing a Secondary Amine*

1. Dissolve 500 mg of secondary amine (3.70 mmol of adenine, 3.31 mmol of guanine, 4.50 mmol of cytosine, 4.46 mmol of uracil, 1.90 and 1.94 mmol of 4-(3-substituted-amidophenyl) imidazole ($D_3$ or $D_4$)) in 20 mL of DMF.
2. Add 0.5 equivalents of $K_2CO_3$ and 1.0 eq. of propargyl bromide (80% weight solution in toluene) and then stir the reaction mixture at 60 °C overnight.
3. Purify the crude product by flash chromatography on a silica gel column using a mixture $CH_2Cl_2$/MeOH 95:5. This leads to propargyl-nucleobases as white solids in 294.9 mg (**5**, 46%), 175.3 mg (**6**, 28%), 408.4 mg (**7**, 61%), 651.5 (**8**, 97%), 286.1 mg (**9**, 50%), and 286.9 mg (**10**, 50%) yields (*see* **Notes 6** and 7).

*3.1.4 Alkyne Introduction in Nucleobase Moiety Containing an Aromatic Amine*

1. Dissolve 140 mg of 4-pentynoic acid (1.43 mmol) in 30 mL of dry dichloromethane.
2. Add 731 mg of chloromethylpyridinium iodide (2.86 mmol, 2 eq.) and 0.4 mL of triethylamine (2.86 mmol, 2 eq.).
3. Add 1.2 equivalents of the appropriate amine (399 mg of nucleobase **S**, 870 mg of 1-(1-*O*-Triisopropylsilyloxy-2-aminophenyl)-4-phenylurea or 836 mg 1-(1-*O*-Triisopropylsilyloxy-2-aminophenyl)-4-butylurea) (1.71 mmol, 1.2 eq.).
4. Stir the reaction mixture under reflux for 1 h and then evaporate the solvent under reduced pressure.
5. Purify the crude products by flash chromatography on a silica gel column using a mixture 1:1 cyclohexane-EtOAc. Desired compounds **13–15** are obtained as slightly yellow solids in 374 mg (70%), 615 mg (61%), and 593 mg (61%), respectively (*see* **Note 8**).
6. Dissolve 615 mg of compounds **14** or 593 mg of compound **15** (1.28 mmol) in 5 mL of THF.
7. Add 2.50 mL of a 1 M solution of tetrabutylammonium fluoride (TBAF) in THF (2.50 mmol, 1.2 eq.) (*see* **Note 9**).

8. Stir the solution 1 h at room temperature and then evaporate the solvent under reduced pressure.
9. Dissolve the crude product in 20 mL of EtOAc and extract it twice with water (2 × 15 mL) and once with a saturated solution of NaCl (15 mL). Combine organic layers, dry them with anhydrous $Na_2SO_4$, and remove the solvent under reduced pressure.
10. Dissolve the crude product in 15 mL of THF (*see* **Note 10**).
11. Add 1.29 g of diisopropyl azodicarboxylate (DIAD, 6.40 mmol, 5 eq.) and 1.68 g of triphenylphosphine (6.40 mmol, 5 eq.)
12. Stir the reaction mixture under an argon atmosphere overnight at room temperature and then remove the solvent under reduced pressure.
13. Purify the crude products by flash column chromatography using a mixture 6:4 cyclohexane/ethyl acetate. This leads to final compounds **16** in 250 mg yield and **17** in 234 mg yield (79 %) as slightly yellow solids.

### 3.1.5 1,3-Dipolar Cycloaddition and Deprotection Reactions

1,3-Dipolar cycloaddition allows for the coupling of neomycin azide **3** with the appropriately modified nucleobases **4–10** and **13–15** in order to obtain the conjugates illustrated in Fig. 1. $CH_3CN$ was used when performing the reaction at room temperature while toluene was used when performing the reaction under heating.

1. Dissolve 50 mg of neomycin azide **3** (0.0403 mmol) in 4 mL of acetonitrile or toluene.
2. Add 1.1 equivalents (0.0443 mmol) of the appropriate alkyne previously dissolved in 4 mL of acetonitrile (**5**, **7–10**, **13**) or toluene (**4**, **6**, **14–15**) (*see* **Note 11**).
3. Add 3.2 mg of copper iodide (0.0161 mmol, 0.4 eq.) and 42 μL of *N*,*N*′-diisopropylethylamine (0.242 mmol, 6 eq.).
4. Stir the reaction mixture at room temperature or under reflux, overnight.
5. Remove the solvent under reduced pressure.
6. Purify the crude residue by flash chromatography on a silica gel column using a mixture $CH_2Cl_2$/MeOH 95:5. Desired 1,4-disubstited-1,2,3-triazole compounds containing Boc group on amine substituents are obtained as white solids in 50.1 mg (**BocNeo-A**, 87 %), 34.5 mg (**BocNeo-U**, 61 %), 44.0 mg (**BocNeo-C**, 78 %), 20.9 mg (**BocNeo-G**, 36 %), 53.8 mg (**BocNeo-S**, 86 %), 41.7 mg (**BocNeo-HBPh**, 67 %), 36.9 mg (**BocNeo-HB**, 60 %), 47.6 mg (**BocNeo-D3**, 76 %), 49.4 mg (**BocNeo-D4**, 79 %), and 34.7 mg (**BocNeo-BIG**, 57 %) yields.
7. Dissolve Boc-protected compounds in 5 mL of dichloromethane.

8. Add 3 mL of trifluoroacetic acid (TFA, large excess).
9. Stir the reaction mixture at room temperature overnight.
10. Remove the solvent and the residues of TFA under reduced pressure (*see* **Note 12**).
11. Final precipitation in a mixture $Et_2O$/MeOH 49:1 leads to pure final compounds as white solids (TFA salts) in 49.2 mg (**Neo-A**, 93%), 21.6 mg (**Neo-U**, 59%), 43.9 mg (**Neo-C**, 94%), 20.4 mg (**Neo-G**, 92%), 51.1 mg (**Neo-S**, 90%), 33.4 mg (**Neo-HBPh**, 76%), 30.0 mg (**Neo-HB**, 77%), 46.6 mg (**Neo-D3**, 93%), 49.4 mg (**Neo-D4**, 95%), and 33.7 mg (**Neo-BIG**, 92%) yields (*see* **Note 13**).

### 3.2 Cell-Free Biological Assays

This section describes the methodologies that can be used in order to evaluate (1) $IC_{50}$ values for compounds able to inhibit DICER cleavage of a pre-miRNA (Subheading 3.2.1) and (2) $K_D$ (dissociation constants) values for compounds able to bind the target pre-miRNA (Subheading 3.2.2).

In all assays that need RNA manipulation, it is necessary to work under a PCR hood using gloves cleaned with RNase away solution and to use sterilized and safe-lock tubes as well as sterilized and filtered tips for micropipettes.

#### 3.2.1 FRET DICER Assay

This section describes the cell-free assay based on the FRET technique that allows obtaining $IC_{50}$ values related to the inhibition of DICER cleavage reaction of the pre-miRNA beacon. In this assay, inspired by a previously reported test [20], targeted pre-miRNAs have been double labeled with a fluorophore (fluorescein) and a quencher (4-([4-(dimethylamino)phenyl]azo)benzoic acid; dabcyl) at 3′ and 5′ ends, respectively. The FRET-based assay is planned for 384-well plates and it is performed in a final volume of 40 μL. This assay is perfectly suited for an automated pipetting system (we used the 5070 epMotion® by Eppendorf). Each well contains 50 nM of RNA beacon, 0.25 U of recombinant DICER, and the appropriate concentration of ligand. Each compound is tested in duplicate (8 compounds/plate each one occupying two rows) and in 12 different concentrations, typically going from 125 μM to 15.26 nM (each one occupying a column of the plate). The 13th column of the plate is reserved to negative controls that are buffer alone and RNA beacon alone (0% fluorescence). Positions 14A and 14B of the plate are reserved to the positive control containing the RNA beacon and DICER enzyme in the absence of ligand (100% fluorescence).

In the presence of recombinant DICER enzyme, this latter cleaves the RNA and appearance of fluorescence is observed (positions 14A–14B, positive controls). If an RNA ligand is able to strongly bind to the structured pre-miRNA and inhibit the cleavage by DICER no fluorescence is detected. The variation of fluorescence as a function of the 12 different concentrations of each ligand allows obtaining $IC_{50}$ values (Fig. 7).

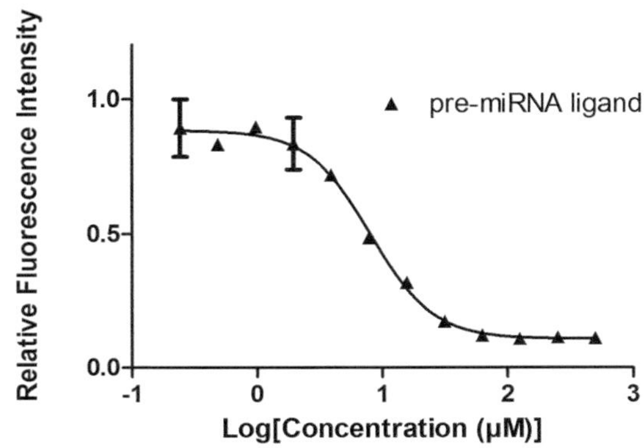


**Fig. 7** Typical example of sigmoidal curve obtained measuring fluorescence variation as a function of pre-miRNA ligand concentration

1. Prepare Tris–HCl buffer pH 7.4 at 100 mM concentration.
2. Dilute 200 mL of Tris–HCl buffer to 1 L with Milli-Q water (final concentration 20 mM) and add 238 mg of $MgCl_2$ (final concentration 2.5 mM) and 701 mg of NaCl (final concentration 12 mM).
3. Add 200 µL of dithiothreitol (DTT) to this buffer solution and filter using Stericup® Filter Units of 0.2 µm (Millipore).
4. Dissolve 4.8 nmol of double-labeled RNA beacon (*see* **Note 14**) in 1 mL of the buffer solution obtained at **step 3** in a sterilized tube of 1.5 mL. Heat the tube 2 min at 90 °C, then put it immediately at 4 °C during 10 min, and finally allow it to return to 25 °C. Add 3.8 mL of buffer to have a final volume of 4.8 mL and a final concentration of 100 nM.
5. Put the RNA solution prepared in step 4 in a reservoir. If performing the assay using an automated pipetting system, use the appropriate Eppendorf 30 mL reservoir (*see* **Note 15**).
6. Prepare a second reservoir containing 10 mL of buffer.
7. Prepare 125 µL of a solution of each one of the eight compounds to be tested. The concentration of this solution must be eight times greater than the first desired concentration in the 384-well plate. Typically, prepare 125 µL of a 1 mM solution of each compound in order to start measurements at 125 µM in the plate. Put each one of the 8 solutions in 1.5 mL tubes.
8. Dilute each compound's solution twice 12 times in a 96-well plate using a multichannel micropipette or an automated pipetting system. For this, add 100 µL of buffer in the 96 wells of the plate and then add 100 µL of each compound's solution in the 8 wells of column 1 (row A for compound 1, row B for compound 2, etc., until row H for compound 8). Mix each well of column 1, take 100 µL from each well of column 1, and put

them in column 2A-H. Repeat this procedure 12 times until the last column of the plate. Take 100 μL from each well of column 12 and throw them away. At the end, each row contains 100 μL of the 12 dilutions of each one of the eight compounds.

9. Prepare a 384-well plate containing each compound dilution mixed with RNA. For this, put 10 μL of each compound dilution contained in the 96-well plate prepared in **step 7**, in the 384-well plate rows in duplicate (rows A–B for compound 1, C–D for compound 2, etc., until N–P for the 8th compound). This will fill all rows from column 1 to column 12 with 10 μL of each compound' solutions.
10. Add 40 μL of buffer in column 13, rows A, C, E, G, J, I, M, O. These will be negative controls containing buffer alone.
11. Add 20 μL of buffer in column 13, rows B, D, F, H, K, L, N, P. These will be negative controls containing RNA alone.
12. Add 20 μL of the RNA solution in each well from column 1–12 as well as in column 13, lines B, D, F, H, K, L, N, P. At this point each well from column 1–12 contains 30 μL while each well of column 13 contains 40 μL.
13. Incubate the plate 30 min at 25 °C.
14. Dilute the solution of recombinant DICER (0.5 U/μL) 20 times in order to obtain 2.5 mL of a solution at 0.25 U/10 μL. For this, add 2375–125 μL of recombinant DICER.
15. Add 10 μL of diluted recombinant DICER obtained in step 13 to each well from column 1 to 12 (*see* **Note 16**).
16. Finally, put 10 μL of buffer in positions 14A–B, add 20 μL of the RNA solution and 10 μL of diluted recombinant DICER.
17. Incubate the plate 4 h at 37 °C (*see* **Note 17**) and then measure fluorescence signals using a plate reader with an excitation filter of 485 ± 10 nm and an emission filter of 535 ± 15 nm (*see* **Note 18**).

#### *3.2.2 Binding Experiments and $K_D$ Determination*

This section describes the fluorescence-based assay that allows measuring dissociation constants ($K_D$) related to the binding of ligands to the targeted pre-miRNAs. In this assay, the pre-miRNA is labeled with fluorescein at its 5′ end. Binding experiments are planned for 384-well plates and they are performed in a final volume of 60 μL. This assay is perfectly suited for an automated pipetting system (we used the 5070 epMotion® by Eppendorf). Each well contains 10 nM of RNA beacon and the appropriate concentration of ligand. Each compound is tested in duplicate (tight compounds/plate each one occupying two rows) and in 15 different concentrations, typically going from 500 μM to 30.52 nM (each one occupying a column of the plate). The 16th column of the plate is reserved to negative controls that are buffer alone and RNA beacon alone (100% fluorescence).

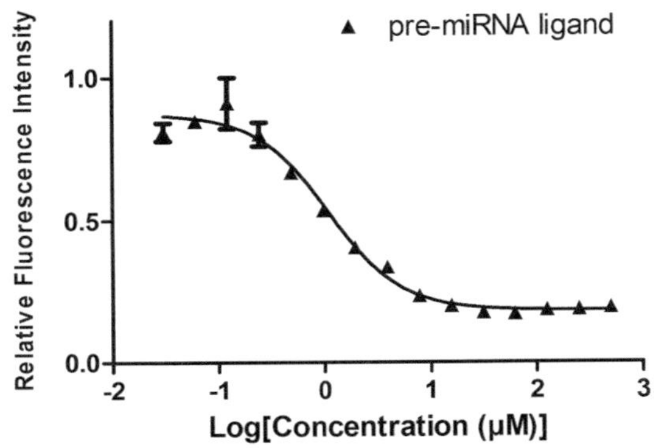


**Fig. 8** Typical example of sigmoidal curve obtained measuring fluorescence variation as a function of pre-miRNA ligand concentration

In the presence of increasing concentrations of each ligand, a decrease in fluorescence is observed. The variation of fluorescence as a function of the 15 different concentrations of each ligand allows obtaining $K_D$ values (Fig. 8).

1. Prepare Tris–HCl buffer as described in Subheading 3.2.2, **steps 1–3**.
2. Dissolve 0.1 nmol of RNA beacon 5′-labeled with fluorescein in 1 mL of Tris · HCl buffer in a sterilized tube of 1.5 mL (*see* **Note 19**). Heat the tube 2 min at 90 °C, then put it immediately at 4 °C for 10 min, and finally allow it to return to 25 °C. Add 9 mL of buffer to have a final volume of 10 mL and a final concentration of 20 nM.
3. Put the RNA solution prepared in **step 2** in a reservoir. If performing the assay using an automated pipetting system, use the appropriate Eppendorf 30 mL reservoir (*see* **Note 15**).
4. Prepare a second reservoir containing 10 mL of buffer.
5. Prepare 125 μL of a solution of each one of the eight compounds to be tested. The concentration of this solution must be four times greater than the first desired concentration in the plate. Typically, prepare 125 μL of a 2 mM solution of each compound in order to start measurements at 500 μM in the plate. Put each one of the eight solutions in 1.5 mL tubes.
6. In a 384-well plate, add 30 μl of buffer in all wells from column 1 to 16.
7. Add 30 μL of buffer in column 16 A, C, E, G, J, I, M, O. These will be negative controls containing buffer alone.
8. Add 30 μL of each compound's solution contained in the eight tubes of 1.5 mL prepared in **step 5**, in column 1 of the 384-well plate in duplicate (rows A–B for compound 1, C–D for compound 2, etc., until N–P for compound 8).

9. Mix all wells of column 1, take 30 μL of each solution in column 1, and put it in the following wells (column 2). Mix all wells of column 2, take 30 μL of each solution in column 2, and put it in the following wells (column 3). Repeat this procedure until column 15.
10. Take 30 μL of each solution in column 15 and throw them away. At this point each well from column 1 to 15 contains 30 μL.
11. Add 30 μL of the RNA solution in all positions from column 1 to 15.
12. Add 30 μL of the RNA solution in column 16, rows B, D, F, H, K, L, N, P. These will be negative controls containing RNA alone.
13. Incubate the plate overnight at 4 °C (*see* **Note 20**) and then measure fluorescence signals after incubation 30 min at 37 °C (*see* **Note 21**) using a plate reader with an excitation filter of 485 ± 10 nm and an emission filter of 535 ± 15 nm (*see* **Note 22**).

## 4 Notes

1. In all reactions that need to be heated to succeed, a reflux of glycol ethylene automatically chilled at 5 °C must be used.
2. All anhydrous reactions have been performed under an Argon atmosphere. Flask and stirring bars have been dried at 80 °C overnight before use.
3. The yield of this reaction varies and can be lower than described especially when scaling up the reaction. 1.5 g of starting material seems to be the ideal amount in order to have the best yield. Increasing this amount over 2 g leads to a strong decrease of the amount of final compound.
4. The same protection–activation–substitution procedure can be applied to any aminoglycoside containing a primary alcohol that can be selectively activated by triisopropylbenzenesulfonyl chloride before its substitution with $NaN_3$. For example, we applied this procedure to apramycin (unpublished results, Fig. 4). When a primary alcohol is not present in the aminoglycoside derivative, such as in the case of neamine and 2-deoxystreptamine (2-DOS) other protection strategies can be employed in order to isolate a free hydroxyl group that can be selectively substituted (Fig. 9, unpublished results).
5. The methodology employed in order to introduce the propargyl chain on various heteroaromatic nucleobases varies since the nature of the amine as well as the desired compound change. In fact, in the case of secondary amines, we wanted to synthesize the alkylated compound and substitution with propargyl bromide was the most appropriate procedure.

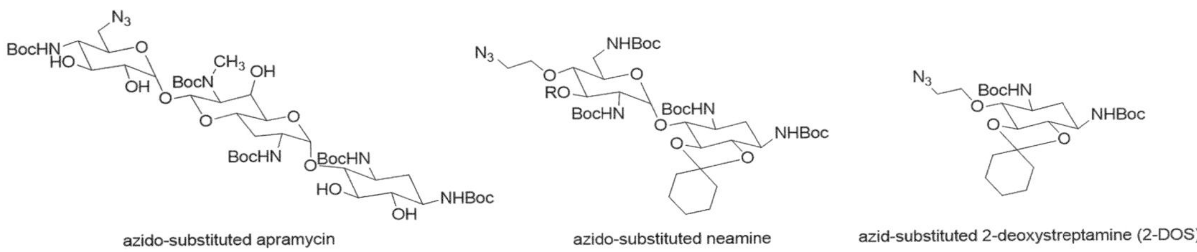


**Fig. 9** Examples of aminoglycosides and derivatives containing the azide group necessary for 1,3-dipolar cycloaddition reaction during the preparation of conjugates for pre-miRNAs binding

However, in other cases we desired to maintain the NH group in an amide bond in order to have the NH free to form hydrogen bonding with the RNA target. It was thus more convenient to perform an amide coupling in this case (primary and aromatic amines).

6. Substitution of secondary amines with propargyl bromide is a straightforward reaction with excellent yields. However, some natural and modified nucleobases as the ones described here are only partially soluble in most solvents. This render the reaction more difficult and lower the yields and explains why in some cases we obtained yields of about 50% as it was the case for alkynes **5** and **10**.
7. In some cases concomitant protection of other amine groups present in the starting material is necessary in order to obtain the desired product in good yields. This is the case for A, C, and G that have been protected using acetyl protecting group [21, 22].
8. The starting material of this reaction comes from the deprotection of a Boc group on the amine suing TFA in $CH_2Cl_2$. This leaves the compound as a TFA salt. The residual TFA leads, during this step, to the trifluoroacetamide secondary product and explains the lower yield of the coupling.
9. TBAF has been used as a 1.0 M solution in dry THF.
10. The intermediate compound with a free OH group is rapidly engaged in the following reaction without purification because this is a very unstable compound that sticks to the silica gel.
11. The use of toluene associated with heating to 110 °C is necessary for compounds that are hardly soluble in other solvents at room temperature.
12. Efficient removal of TFA is obtained by coevaporation in the presence of toluene. Add 2 mL of toluene and dry under vacuo three times allows the elimination of TFA excess.
13. Final conjugates need to be checked for their purity by HPLC and HRMS using the instruments and methodology described

in Subheading 2, **steps 8** and **9**. Stability of final conjugates can also be checked by HPLC after incubating each compound at room temperature in Tris–HCl buffer that will be employed during biochemical assays. Analytical HPLC performed after 1 h, 24 h, 48 h, and 1 week allows for the evaluation of the stability of each conjugate.

14. Previous to DICER assays, prepare aliquots of RNA beacon containing 4.8 nmol each, lyophilize and store them dry at −20 °C.

15. The reservoirs containing the RNA solutions need to be coated before use since adsorption of RNA is probable on most plastic material used. For this, we suggest to prepare a 1 g/L solution of BSA in milli-Q water, fill the reservoir with this solution, and store it at 4 °C overnight. Removal of the BSA solution allows obtaining the coated reservoir that is ready to be used for the RNA solution.

16. The FRET-based assay can also be performed using cell lysates. In this case, use a concentration of 250 μg/mL and add the same volume.

17. In order to determine the time of incubation at 37 °C after adding recombinant DICER enzyme, we checked the kinetic of DICER in our system. After a 4-h incubation fluorescence signal reaches a maximum and do not change anymore. Evaluation of fluorescence variation over time allows for the evaluation of the kinetic of the cleavage reaction and of its inhibition.

18. The fluorescence was measured on a GeniosPro (Tecan) plate reader. Each point was measured ten times with a 500 μs integration time and averaged. Inhibition data were analyzed using Graphpad Prism 5 software using nonlinear regression following the equation: $Y = \text{Bottom} + (\text{Top} - \text{Bottom})/1 + 10^{[(\text{LogIC50-X})\times \text{Hills Slope}]})$.

19. Previous to binding assays, prepare aliquots of RNA beacon containing 0.1 nmol each, lyophilize and store them dry at −20 °C.

20. The 384-well plates were incubated at 4 °C overnight in order to facilitate the binding of each ligand to the RNA target. After this incubation, the plate can be read at the desired temperature after incubating at least 30 min at this temperature.

21. $K_D$ values are measured and reported at 37 °C. However, it can be extremely useful to measure $K_D$ values at different temperatures (typically 5, 10, 15, 20, 25, 30, and 35 °C) in order to use the obtained values for the calculation of thermodynamic parameters of the interaction ($\Delta G°$, $\Delta H°$, $T\Delta S°$, and $\Delta Cp°$).

22. Binding data were analyzed using Graphpad Prism 5 software. Unless otherwise stated, binding profiles were well modeled using a simple model assuming the one-to-one stoichiometry.

## Acknowledgement

This work was supported by ANR (Agence Nationale de la Recherche, France) grant (ANR JS07-011-1).

### References

1. Guan L, Disney MD (2012) Recent advances in developing small molecules targeting RNA. ACS Chem Biol 7:73–86
2. Li Z, Rana TM (2014) Therapeutic targeting of microRNAs: current status and future challenges. Nat Rev Drug Discov 13:622–638
3. Ambros V (2008) The evolution of our thinking about microRNAs. Nat Med 14:1036–1040
4. Park JE, Heo I, Tian Y, Simanshu DK, Chang H, Jee D, Patel DJ, Kim VN (2011) Dicer recognizes the 5′ end of RNA for efficient and accurate processing. Nature 475:201–205
5. Kim VN, Han J, Siomi MC (2009) Biogenesis of small RNAs in animals. Nat Rev Mol Cell Biol 10:126–139
6. Calin GA, Croce CM (2006) MicroRNA signatures in human cancers. Nat Rev Cancer 6:857–866
7. Disney MD, Yildirim I, Childs-Disney JL (2014) Methods to enable the design of bioactive small molecules targeting RNA. Org Biomol Chem 12:1029–1039
8. Monroig P, Chen L, Zhang S, Calin GA (2015) Small molecule compounds targeting miRNAs for cancer therapy. Adv Drug Deliv Rev 81:104–116
9. Velagapudi SP, Vummidi BR, Disney MD (2015) Small molecule chemical probes of microRNA function. Curr Opin Chem Biol 24:97–103
10. Jayaraj GG, Nahar S, Maiti S (2015) Nonconventional chemical inhibitors of microRNA: therapeutic scope. Chem Commun 51:820–831
11. Vo DD, Staedel C, Zehnacker L, Benhida R, Darfeuille F, Duca M (2014) Targeting the production of oncogenic microRNAs with multimodal synthetic small molecules. ACS Chem Biol 9:711–721
12. Cho WJ, Shin JM, Kim JS, Lee MR, Hong KS, Lee JH, Koo KH, Park JW, Kim KS (2009) miR-372 regulates cell cycle and apoptosis of ags human gastric cancer cell line through direct regulation of LATS2. Mol Cells 28:521–527
13. Magnet S, Blanchard JS (2005) Molecular insights into aminoglycoside action and resistance. Chem Rev 105:477–498
14. Malnuit V, Duca M, Benhida R (2011) Targeting DNA base pair mismatch with artificial nucleobases. Advances and perspectives in triple helix strategy. Org Biomol Chem 9:326–336
15. Guianvarc'h D, Benhida R, Fourrey JL, Maurisse R, Sun JS (2001) Incorporation of a novel nucleobase allows stable oligonucleotide-directed triple helix formation at the target sequence containing a purine.pyrimidine interruption. Chem Commun 18:1814–1815
16. Lecubin F, Benhida R, Fourrey JL, Sun JS (1999) NMR recognition studies of C•G base pairs by new easily accessible heterobicyclic systems. Tetrahedron Lett 40:8085–8088
17. Wang W, Purwanto MG, Weisz K (2004) CG base pair recognition by substituted phenylimidazole nucleosides. Org Biomol Chem 2:1194–1198
18. Sasaki S, Nakashima S, Nagatsugi F, Tanaka Y, Hisatome M, Maeda M (1995) Design of a novel artificial nucleobase for the selective formation of a triple-complex with a cytosine-guanine base pair. Tetrahedron Lett 36:9521–9524
19. Griffin LC, Kiessling LL, Beal PA, Gillespie P, Dervan PB (1992) Recognition of all four base pairs of double-helical DNA by triple-helix formation: design of nonnatural deoxyribonucleosides for pyrimidine.cntdot.purine base pair binding. J Am Chem Soc 114:7976–7982
20. Davies BP, Arenz C (2006) A homogenous assay for micro RNA maturation. Angew Chem Int Ed 45:5550–5552
21. Krim J, Sillahi B, Taourirte M, Rakib EM, Engels JW (2009) Microwave-assisted click chemistry: synthesis of mono and bis-1,2,3-triazole acyclonucleoside analogues of Acyclovir via copper(I)-catalyzed cycloaddition. ARKIVOC 8:142–152
22. Lindsell EW, Murray C, Preston PN, Woodman TAJ (2000) Synthesis of 1,3-diynes in the purine, pyrimidine, 1,3,5-triazine and acridine series. Tetrahedron 56:1233–1245

# Chapter 11

# Machine Learning Approaches Toward Building Predictive Models for Small Molecule Modulators of miRNA and Its Utility in Virtual Screening of Molecular Databases

**Vinita Periwal and Vinod Scaria**

## Abstract

The ubiquitous role of microRNAs (miRNAs) in a number of pathological processes has suggested that they could act as potential drug targets. RNA-binding small molecules offer an attractive means for modulating miRNA function. The availability of bioassay data sets for a variety of biological assays and molecules in public domain provides a new opportunity toward utilizing them to create models and further utilize them for in silico virtual screening approaches to prioritize or assign potential functions for small molecules. Here, we describe a computational strategy based on machine learning for creation of predictive models from high-throughput biological screens for virtual screening of small molecules with the potential to inhibit microRNAs. Such models could be potentially used for computational prioritization of small molecules before performing high-throughput biological assay.

**Key words** microRNA, Machine learning, miRNA inhibitors, Molecular descriptors, Random forest, Naïve Bayes, Pubchem, ZINC database

## 1 Introduction

MicroRNAs (miRNAs) have extensively been discussed as attractive targets for therapeutic intervention [1–3]. A large number of classes of small molecules including many therapeutically active classes of molecules which have RNA-binding potential have been identified previously [4, 5]. The recent advancements in synthesis of novel and large compound libraries being made available for biological screening pose a high demand for predictive computational methods that can prioritize molecules for biological screening. A number of approaches including molecular modeling and simulation, molecular docking and virtual screening, and machine learning methods have been recently adopted for virtual screening to assign classifications in terms of molecular activities [6, 7]. A major focus of machine learning methods has been to automatically learn to recognize complex patterns of features from bioassay

Marco F. Schmidt (ed.), *Drug Target miRNA: Methods and Protocols*, Methods in Molecular Biology, vol. 1517,
DOI 10.1007/978-1-4939-6563-2_11, 

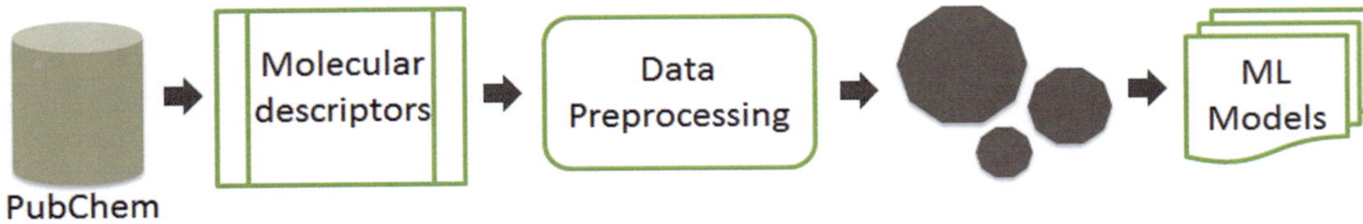


**Fig. 1** Graphical abstract depicting overview of the methodology employed to train machine learning models from small molecular modulators

datasets to make intelligent decisions or classifications. We have previously shown that machine learning-based classification models targeting tropical diseases such as Tuberculosis [8, 9], Malaria [10], Leishmaniasis [11], and Schistosomiasis [12] can be effectively used to prioritize small molecules. Similar approaches have also been employed for a variety of diseases and targets and extensively reviewed in literature [13–15].

Here, we have provided a detailed methodology of building machine learning-based predictive models of small molecules with potential to inhibit miRNAs (specifically miR-21) (Fig. 1) [16]. It has previously been shown that miRNAs are oncogenic or tumor suppressive thereby resulting in altered miRNA expression levels associated with human cancers [17, 18]. The overexpression of miR-21 has been associated with a variety of human tumors [19]. The predictive models built by using this methodology could be potentially used for computational/virtual screening of chemical compounds before performing high-throughput experimental screen as well as picking potential hits from large chemical structure databases.

Utilizing this methodology, we have trained two classification models based on Naïve Bayes and Random Forest to build predictive models for small molecule modulators of miR-21 with an average accuracy of 80% [16]. These models were used to screen approved drugs from DrugBank database [20] and resulted in short-listing of 43 drugs which could potentially target miR-21 thus suggesting a probable novel mechanism of off-target activity of these drugs (Fig. 2).

## 2 Materials

### 2.1 Hardware

1. Workstation (for large datasets, RAM 8GB and above)/PC (for small datasets, at least 4GB RAM).

### 2.2 Software

1. Java (preferably 1.5 and above, prerequisite for Weka).
2. Perl (for running scripts).
3. Microsoft .net 1.1 and above (required for PowerMv).

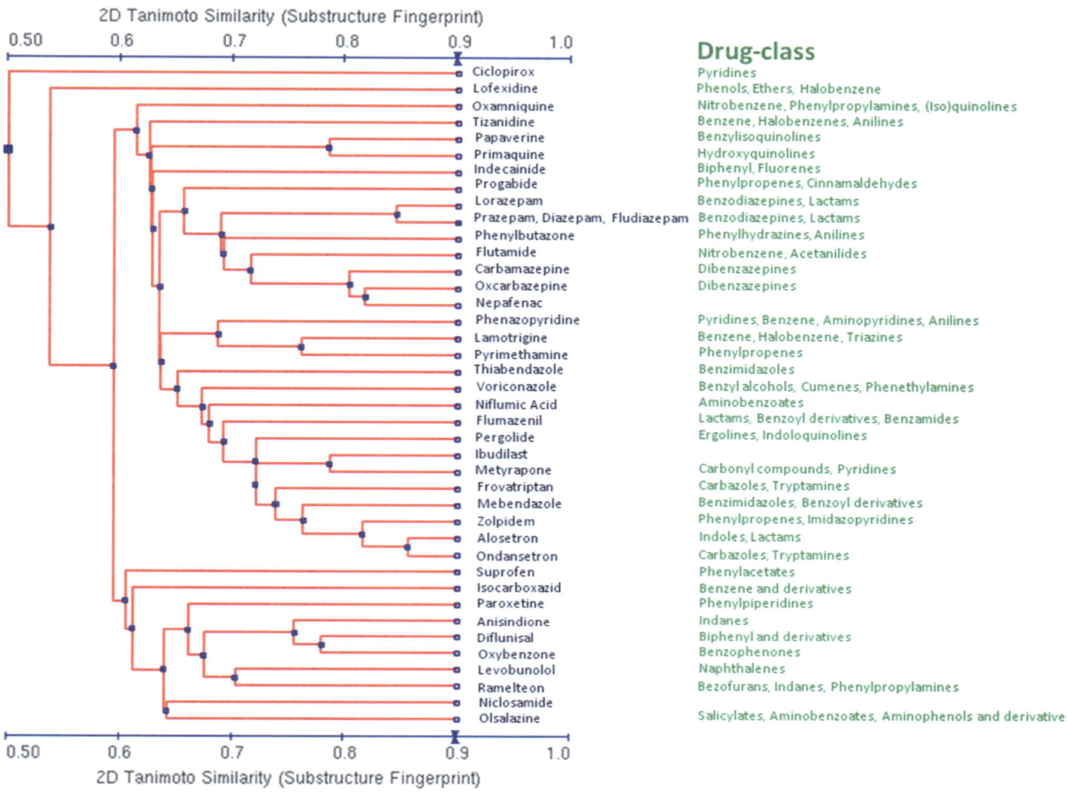


**Fig. 2** The figure shows clustering of 43 drugs from DrugBank which were predicted as actives against miR-21, based on Tanimoto similarity

4. Any text editor (Notepad++, EditPlus, Excel).
5. PowerMV (for molecular descriptor calculation, windows based).
6. Weka suite of machine learning algorithms (for various machine learning classifiers).
7. MayaChemTools (script to split large SDF files).

### 2.3 Data Source

The high-throughput dataset consists of a library of small molecule modulators of human microRNA, miR-21. The bioassay Id for the miR-21 dataset available in PubChem is: 2289.

## 3 Methods

### 3.1 Obtaining Bioassay Data from PubChem

1. Browse to PubChem (https://pubchem.ncbi.nlm.nih.gov/) (*see* **Note 1**).
2. Select BioAssay tab and type in the assay Id for miR-21 and hit go.
3. Download structures of both active and inactive compounds in SDF (structure data format) format. Similarly download data

from a counter-screen (AID: 588342) of miR-21 project from the same depositor (*see* **Note 2**).

4. Overlap actives obtained from both assays (i.e., AID 2289 and 588342) to filter out false positives and retain true positives only.

#### 3.2 Split Large SDF Files to Smaller Files (Use SplitSDFiles.pl)

1. Download and install MayaChemTools (http://www.mayachemtools.org/Download.html) (*see* **Note 3**).
2. Open command prompt (in windows)/terminal (in Ubuntu/linux).
3. Specify the path to SplitSDFiles.pl script and split the SDF data file into smaller chunks using the command "perl SplitSDFiles.pl -n number file_name.sdf." Number denotes the number of desired file subsets example: -n 20 would split the file into 20 subsets.

#### 3.3 Generate Molecular Descriptors (Use PowerMv)

1. Download and install PowerMv (http://nisla05.niss.org/PowerMV/) (*see* **Note 4**).
2. Start PowerMV by clicking on its icon.
3. Load one of the SD file obtained after splitting, right click on compound file to open a list of preferences. From there choose Generate Table.
4. In the subsequent dialog box, select the molecular descriptors pharmacophore fingerprints (147), weighted burden number (24), and properties (8) descriptors and click generate.
5. After the 179 descriptors are calculated, right click and open the file in any text editor of your choice. Append an additional column at the end and fill it with bioactivity value (i.e., Outcome either active or inactive). Save the file as .CSV (Comma Separated Values).
6. Repeat **steps 3–5** for all subsequent SD files.
7. Merge all .CSV files together to generate a single file of calculated molecular descriptors for both active and inactive datasets with their bioactivity values appended as the last column. The merged .CSV file should look like a matrix with all molecule Ids depicting row heading and the 179 molecular descriptor categories as column heads with an additional Outcome head denoting the class: active or inactive. Sort the file on last Outcome column such that all actives are enlisted first followed by inactives. As a next step, delete the Row column containing molecule Id from the file (*see* **Note 5**).

#### 3.4 Weka: Handling OutOfMemory Exception

1. Download and install Weka (http://www.cs.waikato.ac.nz/ml/weka/downloading.html) according to your system specifications and java version in use. If java is not installed then first install java (https://www.java.com/en/download/) (*see* **Note 6**).

By default Weka's maximum heap size is set to 128mb, so datasets larger than this size doesn't open in Weka and one gets an out of memory exception. Most Java virtual machines only allocate a certain maximum amount of memory to run Java programs. Usually this is much less than the amount of RAM in your computer. However, you can extend the memory available for the virtual machine by setting appropriate options.

*For windows users*

1. Go to the parent directory where Weka is installed, say: C:/Program Files/Weka-3-6/.
2. Locate RunWeka.ini file. Open the file in any text editor.
3. Scroll to line: maxheap = 128 m ('m' stands for MB).
4. Change it to: maxheap = 1500 m (i.e., 1.5GB for a 32-bit windows system with 3GB RAM, you can keep this according to your system specifications). Save file and exit.

*For Ubuntu/Linux users*

1. Go to terminal. Locate Weka.jar.
2. Start Weka with increased heap size such as:
   java -classpath /usr/local/weka.jar -Xmx4000m
   With Sun's JDK, use –Xmx option to increase heap size. The earlier example starts Weka with an increased heap of 4 GB.

### 3.5 Weka: Data Preprocessing and Perl Script: Train and Test Split

1. Start Weka (manage OutOfMemoryException as discussed in Subheading 3.4).
2. Open/Load your .CSV file in Weka. In the data preprocessing step, we remove attributes of no variation, i.e., descriptors which contain only 1's and 0's throughout their entire column.
3. In the Preprocess tab, choose unsupervised filter → attributes → RemoveUseless and then click apply.
4. Attributes of no variation are removed and then save your file as .CSV.
5. Next, we split our dataset into a training and test set (*see* **Note 7**).
6. Assuming that the Perl script (*see* **Note 8**) is present in your Perl's bin directory run the script as:
   perl split_train_test.pl
7. If the script runs without any error, you should have two new .CSV files in your directory.

### 3.6 Weka: CSV to ARFF Conversion

1. Open your .CSV file in Weka using the 'Open file' button in Weka explorer.
2. Once open you can save your file in different format using the 'Save' file button in Weka explorer. Choose .ARFF (Attribute-Relation File Format) from drop down options.

### 3.7 Weka: Classification Runs (For Windows Users)

1. At this stage you should have two files test and train both in ARFF format (*see* **Note 9**).
2. Start Weka explorer, in the Preprocess tab, open file and open training file in ARFF format.
3. Now click on classify tab in the menu bar.
4. We will first train a model using Naïve Bayes classifier; we will first apply standard classifiers and if there will be less than 20% False Positive rate than we will use cost-sensitive classifier (*see* **Notes 10** and **11**).
5. Click on Choose button to select a classifier. From Bayes folder select the algorithm Naïve Bayes (*see* **Note 12**).
6. Use fivefold cross-validations for larger datasets such as the miR-21 data in current example (*see* **Note 13**).
7. Now click on start button, model will start building. Since we have used fivefold cross-validation so it will build models for fivefolds. The output (classification results with confusion matrix (*see* **Note 14**)) is generated in the classifier output window.
8. This is the model generated by Naïve Bayes classifier by using training set. Next step is to test this model on the independent test set. Go to section test options select Supplied test set and click on set. Open the test file.
9. After reading the file close the Test instances dialog by clicking on close. Now right-click on your model in result list and choose Re-evaluate model on current test set.
10. Now, we will set cost-sensitive classifier to improve the results. For Naïve Bayes we will use Weka's CostSensitiveClassifier. Cost is gradually increased in stages starting from 2 until a 20% threshold of false positive rate is reached. So, we will set up a cost matrix by starting with a misclassification cost of 2 (*see* **Note 15**).
11. Go to choose button, select CostSensitiveClassifier from meta folder.
12. Click on the text box to open the GenericObjectEditor dialog box.
13. In the dialog box, select Naïve Bayes from choose classifier. Next, click on costMatrix to set up the misclassification cost.
14. We have two classes in our dataset, i.e., actives and inactives so we will set up a 2X2 Matrix (For TP, FP, TN, and FN) (*see* **Note 16**). In classes enter 2. Click on resize to create a 2X2 matrix. Change misclassification cost for false negatives to 2. Then close the dialog box.
15. Leave all other options default and now close GenericObjectEditor dialog by clicking OK. Click start to begin building cost-sensitive model.
16. Repeat **steps 8** and **9** as described earlier for testing.

17. Similarly, you can build models using Random Forest as classifier.

### 3.8 Weka: Classification Runs (for Ubuntu/Linux Users)

1. Commands to be used to train classifiers using command line (*see* **Note 17**):
   Example: for Random Forest
   java -classpath /usr/local/weka.jar -Xmx4000m weka.classifiers.trees.RandomForest -t $1 -x 5 -d $2 -i
   -t → specifies training file. $1 → name of training file (input.arff).
   -x → Sets number of folds for cross-validation (default: 10).
   -d → specifies model output file.
   $2 → name of model file (out.model).
   -i → Outputs detailed information-retrieval statistics for each class.
2. Example script showing use of meta-learners:
   For CostSensitiveClassifier Naïve Bayes (CSCNB)
   java -classpath /usr/local/weka.jar -Xmx4000m weka.classifiers.meta.CostSensitiveClassifier -cost-matrix "[0.0 2.0; 1.0 0.0]" -t $1 -x 5 -d $2 -W weka.classifiers.bayes.NaiveBayes -i
   Format of the cost matrices: Matlab single-line format [0.0 2.0; 1.0 0.0]
   -cost-matrix → The cost matrix in Matlab single line format
   -t → specifies training file
   $1 → name of training file (input.arff)
   -x → Sets number of folds for cross-validation (default: 10)
   -d → specifies model output file
   $2 → name of model file (out.model)
   -W → Full name of base classifier. (default: weka.classifiers.rules.ZeroR)
   -i → Outputs detailed information-retrieval statistics for each class
3. Command for testing model:
   java -classpath /usr/local/weka.jar -Xmx4000m weka.classifiers.trees.RandomForest -l $1 -T $2 - i
   -I → specifies load previously saved model
   $1=rf.model (model file)
   -T → Sets test file. If missing, a cross-validation will be performed on the training data
   $2=test.arff (test file)
   -i → Outputs detailed information-retrieval statistics for each class

*Using the models to classify molecules*

1. Obtain the molecules or chemical compounds for whose binding activity is to be tested by the machine learning models, for example, against miR-21 target.
2. Generate molecular descriptors in PowerMV as described in Subheading 3.3. In order to remove the descriptors which

were not present in the training file after data preprocessing, use the Perl script header_match.pl (*see* **Note 18**) as:
perl header_match.pl test_file.csv new_file.csv out_file.csv

3. Open Weka, load the CSV file, and then save the file in ARFF format.
4. From the filters, select the filter unsupervised attribute Add. In the dialog box that appears fill attributeName with Outcome, attributeType as nominal, and nominalLabels as active, inactive (*see* **Note 19**).
5. To add classifications labels to this new dataset, gain choose filters → supervised attribute AddClassification.
6. In the dialog box that appears, select the classifier you used to build the model, i.e., either Naïve Bayes or Random Forest.
7. Turn outputClassification to True and in serializedClassifier-File load the respective model file, i.e., either Naïve Bayes or Random Forest model.
8. Set Ok and click Apply.
9. Now you can click on Edit tab to see that new classification results have been appended to your file as the last column. This is the probable activity added to each of the molecules depending on your trained model's predictions.

## 4 Notes

1. PubChem is a database of chemical compounds which provides information on biological activity of small molecules [21]. It has three linked databases called PubChem Substance, PubChem Compound, and PubChem BioAssay.
2. The bioactivity of compounds in the miR-21 screen 2289 was measured in a cell-based Firefly Luciferase (FLuc) reporter gene assay. Since, earlier reports suggest that compounds which resemble substrates of FLuc can potentially function as competitive inhibitors of the enzyme and can give rise to counterintuitive phenomenon of signal activation. Thus, the apparent increase in luminescence could be mistakenly interpreted as an activity. Therefore, we also used the counter-screen (AID: 588342) of miR-21 project to remove this discrepancy.
3. MayaChemTools is a free software repository of useful Perl scripts. It can be downloaded on both Ubuntu/Linux and windows platforms. If using windows install it in C drive. All scripts can be found in the Bin folder of the mayachemtools directory. Most of the BioAssay datasets are large enough that they cannot be loaded for descriptor calculation in one run, thus this necessitates to split the SD file into smaller files, calculate descriptors, and then merge them back. SplitSDFiles splits large SD files into smaller subsets of desired numbers.

4. PowerMv is windows-based software only and requires Microsoft .net 1.1 and above for its functioning [22]. It can additionally be used for molecule viewing, descriptor generation, and similarity searches.
5. For merging all .CSV files together you can use concat command in Linux/Ubuntu and in windows use copy command. Don't forget to remove the extra column headers from each individual CSV files else this will lead to file reading error in Weka. Your final file shall contain only one column header. We don't use compound ids during model building, as training data is ordered by class, so compound id will appear to be a good predictor on cross-validation, but it will not work on the test data, so delete column Row containing compound Ids from the dataset.
6. If you start the java virtual machine without any parameters it takes default values for stack and heap. The stack size does not pose a problem in most cases, but the heap size does, since it limits the amount of memory a Java program can use for its data structures. In Java 1.4 it was by default 64 MB, which is quite often not enough for programs, especially in Machine Learning.
7. In every classification experiment, you divide your data points into a training set which is used to train the classifier and a test set which is used to independently predict the class of your data points thus ensuring model robustness. A train and test split can be chosen arbitrarily keeping more than half of the dataset in train file and a minor fraction in test set. Some common splits used are 80:20; 70:30; 75:25.
8. A working Perl script code is given here, which can be customized according to user needs. For nonprogrammers, copy this code in any text editor and save the file with a .pl extension such as split_train_test.pl. The datasets are randomly split into 80% training and validation set and 20% independent test set, so we should have two files for each dataset one for training the classifier and one for testing the model built by that classifier.

```
#Program to split data into 80% training and 20% test set.
#input required: sorted data file in csv format. csv is comma
separated file.
#!usr/bin/perl
use strict;
use warnings;
open(FILE,"File_name.csv");
my @file=<FILE>;
close FILE;
my $len=scalar(@file);
my $header=$file[0]; #header contains title of descriptors
my @test, my @train, my $i; #declare variables
push(@test,$header);
```

```
push(@train,$header);
for($i=1;$i<$len;$i++){
my $num=$i/5; #divide by 5 for 20% data
if($num=~ /^\d*$/){#matches nondecimal number
my $test=$file[$i];
push(@test,$test);
}elsif($num=~ /^\d*\.\d*$/){#matches decimal number
my $train=$file[$i];
push(@train,$train);
}
}
open(TRAIN,">train_set.csv");
print TRAIN "@train\n";
close TRAIN;
open(TEST,">test_set.csv");
print TEST "@test\n";
close TEST;
exit;
```

9. All datasets should be in ARFF format, otherwise Weka will complain for incompatible format during training and testing. We have two goals: to find most robust and versatile classifier for imbalanced bioassay data and to find out optimal misclassification cost setting for a classifier.
10. One of the drawbacks of virtual screening experiments is the imbalance between active and inactive compounds. A dataset is considered to be imbalanced if one of the classes is overrepresented by large number of instances as compared to other. To address this problem cost-sensitive classification is introduced. In cost-sensitive learning, misclassification of the marginal class is assigned a high cost which the training algorithm in use will then attempt to lessen.
11. Selecting FP rate less than 20% is arbitrary and usually depends on the stringency required to build or train models. The misclassification cost for False Negatives has to be set in order to achieve maximum number of True Positives with a False Positive rate less than 20%.
12. Naïve Bayes is one of the simplest probabilistic classifier. The technique is based on Bayes theorem in statistics. A Bayesian classifier considers each structural feature or descriptor independent of the other descriptors, and the probability of activity is considered to be proportional to the ratio of actives to inactives that share the descriptor value. The final probability that a compound is active is a product of all descriptor-based probabilities.
13. Cross-validation is a technique in which data is partitioned into subsets, performing the analysis on one subset (called the training set), and validating the analysis on the other subset (called the validation set or testing set).

**Table 1**
**Illustration of a confusion matrix for a two-class classifier**

| A | B | ← Classified as |
|---|---|---|
| True Positives (TP) | False Negative (FN) | a = active |
| False Positive (FP) | True Negative (TN) | b = inactive |

14. CostSensitiveClassifier is used for base classifiers Naïve Bayes and Random Forest, as it outperforms other meta-learners. For Naïve Bayes and Random Forest, all other options are kept at default.
15. A confusion matrix contains information about actual and predicted classifications done by a classification system. Performance of such systems is commonly evaluated using the data in the matrix. Table 1 presents the confusion matrix for a two-class classifier.
16. Sensitivity, Specificity, and Accuracy are expressed in terms of true positive (TP), false negative (FN), true negative (TN), false positive (FP) rates. A True Positive Rate (TPR) is the proportion of actual positives which are correctly predicted as actives (TP/TP + FN). False Positive Rate (FPR) is ratio of predicted false actives to actual number of inactives (FP/FP + TN). Accuracy indicates overall effectiveness of the classifier. It can be calculated as (TP + TN/TP + TN+ FP + FN). Sensitivity refers to proportion of actual positives which are predicted positives (TP/TP + FN). Specificity refers to proportion of actual negatives which are predicted negatives (TN/TN + FP).
17. A more comprehensive practical guide to Weka command line can be viewed at https://weka.wikispaces.com/Primer.
18. The script compares two CSV files and removes descriptor columns which are not present in training/test file. This step is important because if descriptor headers will not match between your model file and new file on which prediction has to be done Weka will generate error message of "headers don't match."

```
#Program to match two CSV files. Extract columns with same headers only.
#!usr/bin/perl
use strict;
use warnings;
my $base_file = shift;    #train/test file in which columns have been removed with RemoveUseless
```

```
my $orig_file=shift;    #name of new descriptor file for which
columns need to be matched
my $out_file=shift;
open(FILE1,$base_file) || die $!;
****open(FILE2,$orig_file) || die $!;
my @base_file=<FILE1>;
close FILE1;
my @orig_file=<FILE2>;
close FILE2;
open(OUTFILE,">>$out_file");
my $header_base=$base_file[0];    #extract header of train/
test file
my $header_orig=$orig_file[0]; #extract header of new file
my @headers_base=split_data($header_base);
my @headers_orig=split_data($header_orig);
my $i, my @matches, my $j, my @elements, my @match;
#for loop to match headers and collect matching positions of
headers in new file.
for($i=0;$i<scalar(@headers_orig);$i++){
for($j=0;$j<scalar(@headers_base);$j++){
if($headers_orig[$i]=~ /$headers_base[$j]/){
push(@matches,$i);
push(@match,$headers_orig[$i],",");
}
}
}
pop(@match);    #removes last ','
print OUTFILE @match;
#for loop to extract cells with matching header numbers only.
for($i=1;$i<scalar(@orig_file);$i++){
my @data=split_data($orig_file[$i]);
for(my $k=0;$k<scalar(@matches);$k++){
my $element=$data[$matches[$k]];
push(@elements,$element,",");
}
pop(@elements);    #removes last ','
print OUTFILE @elements;
@elements="";
}
exit;
##################################################
############
sub split_data{
my($line)=@_;
my @data=split(',',$line);
return @data;
}
exit;
```

19. Note that at this stage the file doesn't contain the last Outcome attribute as nothing is known about the activity of these molecules against the given target. The labels should match case as is given in training and test files while building the models.

## Acknowledgement

The authors acknowledge Open Source Drug Discovery (OSDD) consortium under which this work was carried out. This work was funded by the Council of Scientific and Industrial Research (CSIR), India for funding through the Open Source Drug Discovery Project (HCP001).

### References

1. Bader AG, Brown D, Winkler M (2010) The promise of microRNA replacement therapy. Cancer Res 70(18):7027–7030. doi:10.1158/0008-5472.CAN-10-2010
2. Scaria V, Hariharan M, Brahmachari SK, Maiti S, Pillai B (2007) microRNA: an emerging therapeutic. ChemMedChem 2(6):789–792. doi:10.1002/cmdc.200600278
3. Garofalo M, Croce CM (2013) MicroRNAs as therapeutic targets in chemoresistance. Drug Resist Updat 16(3-5):47–59. doi:10.1016/j.drup.2013.05.001
4. Gumireddy K, Young DD, Xiong X, Hogenesch JB, Huang Q, Deiters A (2008) Small-molecule inhibitors of microrna miR-21 function. Angew Chem Int Ed Engl 47(39):7482–7484. doi:10.1002/anie.200801555
5. Connelly CM, Deiters A (2014) Identification of inhibitors of microRNA function from small molecule screens. Methods Mol Biol 1095:147–156. doi:10.1007/978-1-62703-703-7_12
6. Vert JP, Jacob L (2008) Machine learning for in silico virtual screening and chemical genomics: new strategies. Comb Chem High Throughput Screen 11(8):677–685
7. Schierz AC (2009) Virtual screening of bioassay data. J Cheminformatics 1:21. doi:10.1186/1758-2946-1-21
8. Periwal V, Kishtapuram S, Scaria V (2012) Computational models for in-vitro anti-tubercular activity of molecules based on high-throughput chemical biology screening datasets. BMC Pharmacol 12:1. doi:10.1186/1471-2210-12-1
9. Periwal V, Rajappan JK, Jaleel AU, Scaria V (2011) Predictive models for anti-tubercular molecules using machine learning on high-throughput biological screening datasets. BMC Res Notes 4:504. doi:10.1186/1756-0500-4-504
10. Jamal S, Periwal V, Scaria V (2013) Predictive modeling of anti-malarial molecules inhibiting apicoplast formation. BMC Bioinformatics 14:55. doi:10.1186/1471-2105-14-55
11. Jamal S, Scaria V (2013) Cheminformatic models based on machine learning for pyruvate kinase inhibitors of Leishmania mexicana. BMC Bioinformatics 14:329. doi:10.1186/1471-2105-14-329
12. Gaba S, Jamal S, Open Source Drug Discovery C, Scaria V (2014) Cheminformatics models for inhibitors of Schistosoma mansoni thioredoxin glutathione reductase. SciWorldJ 2014:957107. doi:10.1155/2014/957107
13. Kourou K, Exarchos TP, Exarchos KP, Karamouzis MV, Fotiadis DI (2014) Machine learning applications in cancer prognosis and prediction. Comput Struct Biotechnol J 13:8–17. doi:10.1016/j.csbj.2014.11.005
14. Kang J, Schwartz R, Flickinger J, Beriwal S (2015) Machine learning approaches for predicting radiation therapy outcomes: a clinician's perspective. Int J Radiat Oncol Biol Phys 93(5):1127–1135. doi:10.1016/j.ijrobp.2015.07.2286
15. Mousavian Z, Masoudi-Nejad A (2014) Drug-target interaction prediction via chemogenomic space: learning-based methods. Expert Opin Drug Metab Toxicol 10(9):1273–1287. doi:10.1517/17425255.2014.950222
16. Jamal S, Periwal V, Consortium O, Scaria V (2012) Computational analysis and predictive modeling of small molecule modulators of microRNA. J Cheminformatics 4(1):16. doi:10.1186/1758-2946-4-16

17. Esquela-Kerscher A, Slack FJ (2006) Oncomirs – microRNAs with a role in cancer. Nat Rev Cancer 6(4):259–269. doi:10.1038/nrc1840

18. Ruan K, Fang X, Ouyang G (2009) MicroRNAs: novel regulators in the hallmarks of human cancer. Cancer Lett 285(2):116–126. doi:10.1016/j.canlet.2009.04.031

19. Tong AW, Nemunaitis J (2008) Modulation of miRNA activity in human cancer: a new paradigm for cancer gene therapy? Cancer Gene Ther 15(6):341–355. doi:10.1038/cgt.2008.8

20. Knox C, Law V, Jewison T, Liu P, Ly S, Frolkis A, Pon A, Banco K, Mak C, Neveu V, Djoumbou Y, Eisner R, Guo AC, Wishart DS (2011) DrugBank 3.0: a comprehensive resource for 'omics' research on drugs. Nucleic Acids Res 39(Database issue):D1035–D1041. doi:10.1093/nar/gkq1126

21. Wang Y, Xiao J, Suzek TO, Zhang J, Wang J, Zhou Z, Han L, Karapetyan K, Dracheva S, Shoemaker BA, Bolton E, Gindulyte A, Bryant SH (2012) PubChem's bioassay database. Nucleic Acids Res 40(Database issue):D400–D412. doi:10.1093/nar/gkr1132

22. Liu K, Feng J, Young SS (2005) PowerMV: a software environment for molecular viewing, descriptor generation, data analysis and hit evaluation. J Chem Inf Model 45(2):515–522. doi:10.1021/ci049847v

# Chapter 12

# Identification of Small Molecule Modulators of MicroRNA by Library Screening

Zhangang Xiao and Yangchao Chen

## Abstract

MicroRNAs (miRNAs) function as oncogenes or tumor suppressors and are dysregulated in cancer. miRNAs therefore represent promising therapeutic targets for cancer. Small molecules that could modulate the expression of miRNAs would thus have potential as anticancer agents. Library screening of small molecules targeting miRNAs is a useful technology platform for anticancer drug development. Here, we describe a hepatocellular carcinoma (HCC) cell-based luciferase reporter system which could be used to screen for small molecule modulators of tumor suppressor microRNA-34a.

**Key words** microRNA, Cancer, Library screening, Small molecule

## 1 Introduction

MicroRNAs (miRNAs) are a class of single-stranded, noncoding RNAs, which regulate the expression of target genes by translational repression [1]. It is estimated that 25–70% of human genes are regulated by miRNAs [2, 3]. miRNAs function as oncogenes or tumor suppressors in various cancer. Their roles are manifested in almost all aspects of cancer biology, such as proliferation, apoptosis, invasion, metastasis, and angiogenesis [4]. Therefore, the use of microRNAs as therapeutic drugs or the screening of compounds which target tumor-associated miRNAs are two potential applications of microRNA-based cancer therapy.

Currently, nucleic acid-based drugs still exhibit poor pharmacodynamic and pharmacokinetic properties. Small molecules are low molecular weight compounds that may demonstrate a potent biological effect. It is reported that small molecules provide significant advantages for anticancer drug development: the wide range of compounds can be synthesized in a short time; the compounds can be easily screened for specificity and capacity of binding with a target; and most importantly, small molecules are orally bioavailable and their manufacturing is cost effective [5]. These are important

Marco F. Schmidt (ed.), *Drug Target miRNA: Methods and Protocols*, Methods in Molecular Biology, vol. 1517,
DOI 10.1007/978-1-4939-6563-2_12, 

advantages for patients and healthcare systems. Many commonly used anticancer drugs are small molecules, such as Imatinib, Gefitinib, Erlotinib, and Sorafenib. In light of the intriguing roles of miRNAs in cancers and the advantages of small molecules as anticancer agents, it would be promising to identify small molecule which could modulate the expression of miRNAs implicated in caner as potential anticancer agent.

Due to unavailable effective therapeutics, hepatocellular carcinoma (HCC) is still one of the most common malignancies and is a leading cause of cancer-related deaths [6]. MicroRNA-34a (miR-34a) is one of the most well-studied tumor suppressor microRNAs

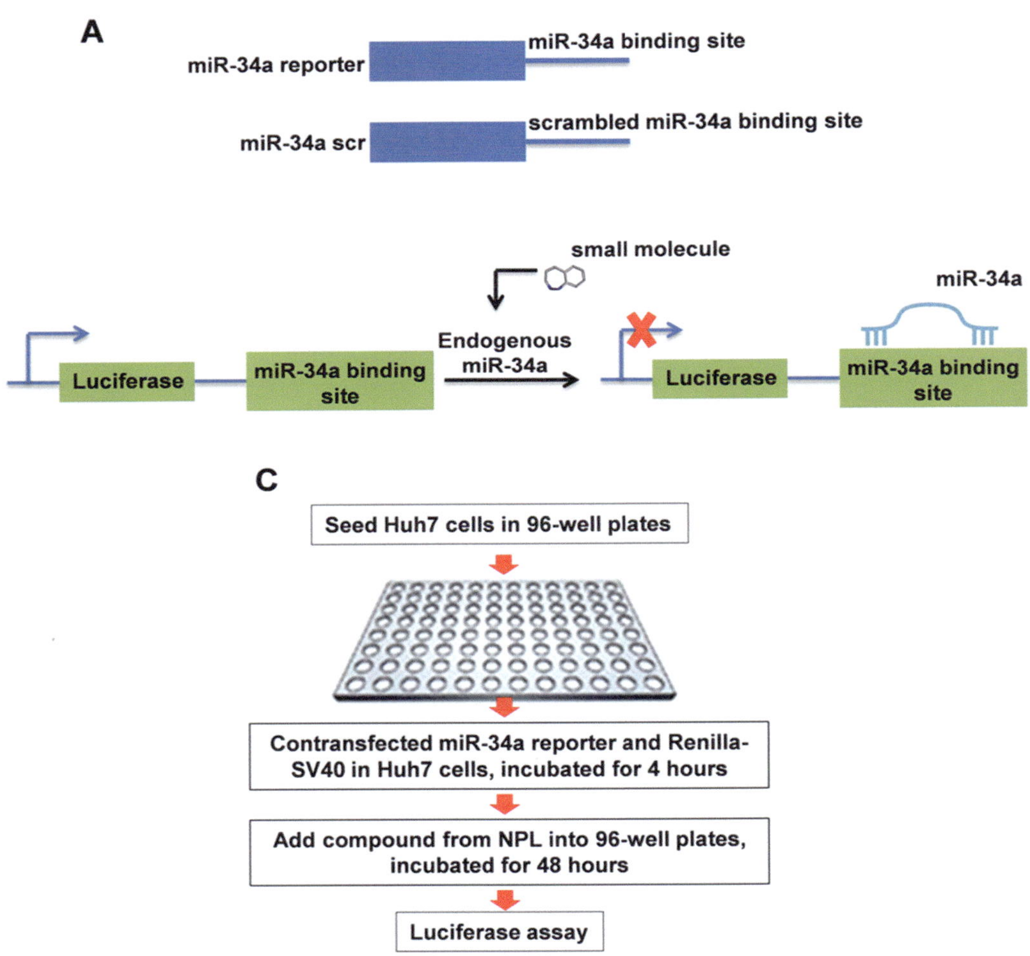


**Fig. 1** Identification of miR-34a modulator through library screening. (**a**) Schematic illustration of miR-34a reporter system. The complementary sequences including mature miR-34a and the scrambled miR-34a sequence were cloned into pMIR-REPORT™ miRNA Reporter Vector to establish miR-34a reporter and miR-34a. (**b**) Working mechanism of the miR-34a reporter. The miR-34a reporter could detect the presence of functional mature miR-34a as reflected by the rate of luciferase activity repression. (**c**) The process of library screening for the identification of miR-34a modulators

that is down-regulated or silenced in a variety of cancers including HCC [7–10]. Therefore, compounds that could selectively restore miR-34a expression in HCC cells would be potential therapeutic agents for HCC. Here, we describe a luciferase reporter system which could be used to screen miR-34a modulators in cell culture models. Using this system, we have identified a small molecule after screening a natural product library which could selectively modulate miR-34a expression in HCC cells (Fig. 1).

## 2 Materials

Prepare all solutions with Millipore water. Prepare and store all reagents at room temperature (unless indicated otherwise). Follow all waste disposal regulations when disposing waste materials.

### 2.1 Constructs and Oligonucleotides

1. pmiR-REPORT luciferase plasmid (Ambion), stored at-20 °C (*see* **Note 1**).
2. Oligonucleotides: DNA oligonucleotide containing the miR-34a-binding site (Forward: 5′-CTGGCAGTGTCTTAGCTGG TTGTA-3′; Reverse: 5′-AGCTTACAACCAGCTAAGACA CTGCCAGAGCT-3′). Scrambled miR-34a binding site (Forward: 5′-CTGTTTCGTTGGGCGTTTCGAAGA-3′; Reverse: 5′-AGCTTCTTCGAAACGCCCAACGAAACAG AGCT-3′) (TechDragon, Hong Kong), stored at-20 °C (*see* **Note 2**).
3. Renilla luciferase pRL-SV40 (Promega, USA): Stored at −20 °C.
4. Sequencing primers: Forward 5′-AGGCGATTAAGTTG GGTA-3′ (*see* **Note 3**).
5. 0.1% Diethylpyrocarbonate (DEPC) water: Dissolved in water, mix, and let sit at room temperature overnight and then autoclaved.
6. miR-34a mimics/inhibitors solution (20 μM): miR-34a mimics (sense:5′-UGGCAGUGUCUUAGCUGGUUGU-3′, anti-sense: 5′-AACCAGCUAAGACACUGCCAUU-3′), negative control for miR-34a mimices (sense: 5′-UUCUCCGA ACGUGUCACGUTT-3′,antisense: 5′-ACGUGACACGUUC GGAGAATT-3′), miR-34a inhibitors ( 5′-ACAACCAGCUAA GACACUGCCA-3′), negative control for miR-34a inhibitor (5′-CAGUACUUUUGUGUAGUACAA-3′) (Genepharma Shanghai, China). 1 OD oligonucleotides are dissolved in 125 μL DEPC water. Aliquot the solution and stored at −80 °C.

### 2.2 Cloning Components

1. Restriction enzymes: Sac I/Hind III and NEB buffer 1, 2, 3, 4 (10 units each in 50 μL reaction, NEB, UK).
2. T4 DNA ligase and T4 DNA ligase buffer (200 units in 10 μL reaction, NEB, UK).

3. 50× TAE buffer: 242 g Tris-base, 57.1 mL acetate (100% acetic acid),100 mL 0.5 M sodium ethylenediaminetetraacetic acid (EDTA); add water up tol L.
4. Agarose gel: Set 1% agarose gel by adding 1 g agarose into 100 mL 1× TAE.
5. DH5α competent cells.
6. Ampicillin (100 mg/mL): 1 g sodium ampicillin, add water up to 10 mL.
7. Lysogeny broth (LB): 10 g Bacto-tryptone, 5 g yeast extract, 10 g NaCl, add water up to 1 L. Sterilize by autoclaving. Add another 15 g agar for LB agar preparing.

### 2.3 Cell Culture

1. The human HCC cell line Huh7 was provided by Dr Nakabayashi, Hokkaido University School of Medicine, Japan. The human HCC cell line HepG2 was purchased from American Type Culture Collection.
2. Dulbecco's Modified Eagle Medium (DMEM): Invitrogen/Gibco (packs of 10×1-L packages), 3.7 g $NaCO_3$, Add water up to 1 L (Adjust the final pH to 7.4). Sterilize with 0.22 μm filter and stored at 4 °C in the dark. Compete DMEM: Add 100 mL FBS into 900 mL DMEM.

### 2.4 Library Screening Components

1. Lipofectamin 2000 (Invitrogen, USA).
2. DharmaFECT siRNA transfection reagent (Thermo Scientific, USA).
3. Dual-Luciferase® Reporter assay system (Promega, USA).
4. Natural products library (NPL): NPL contains 640 compounds including natural products and their derivatives (TimTec, USA).
5. Phosphate-buffered saline (PBS): 8 g NaCl, 0.2 g KCl, 1.42 g $Na_2HPO_4$, 0.24 g $KH_2PO_4$, add water up to 1 L (adjust the final pH to7.4).
6. Dimethyl sulfoxide (DMSO) (Promega, USA).
7. Wallac VICTOR$^3$V luminometer (PerkinElmer, USA).

## 3 Methods

All procedures are carried out at room temperature unless otherwise specified.

### 3.1 Construction of miR-34a Luciferase Reporter

1. Assemble the annealing mixture in a nuclease-free tube as follows: 2 μL sense oligonucleotide, 2 μL antisense oligonucleotide (the oligonucleotides containing the miR-34a binding site or scrambled miR-34a binding site), 46 μL 1× T4 ligase buffer.

2. Heat the annealing mixture to 95 °C for 5 min and then place in a 37 °C incubator in 1 h.
3. The annealed inserts can be ligated into pMIR-report luciferase vector immediately or stored at −20 °C for 6 months.
4. Digest pmiR-REPORT™ luciferase plasmid with restriction enzyme Sac I and Hind III following NEB user manual.
5. Loading the digested pmiR-REPORT™ luciferase plasmid and running on agarose gel.
6. Purify the digested pmiR-REPORT™ luciferase plasmid after gel electrophoresis.
7. The inserts from **step 3** are ligated into Sac I and Hind III double digested pmiR-REPORTTM luciferase plasmid according to routine subcloning procedures (*see* **Note 4**).
8. Transform DH5α competent cells with the ligation products (*see* **Note 5**).
9. Spread the transformed DH5α competent cells on LB agar containing 50 μg/mL ampicillin. Place in a 37 °C incubator overnight.
10. Pick clones, isolate plasmid DNA, and perform DNA sequencing using the plasmid DNA (*see* **Note 6**).
11. Purify plasmids for transfection after identifying the right plasmids with inserts. The plasmid containing the miR-34a binding site is termed miR-34a reporter. The plasmid containing scrambled miR-34a binding site is termed miR-34a scr.

### 3.2 Validation of miR-34a Reporter

1. Seed Huh7 and HepG2 cells into 96-well plate, respectively ($2 \times 10^3$cells/well), incubate at 37 °C overnight.
2. MiR-34a report and miR-34a scr (100 ng/well) are transfected into Huh7 and HepG2 cells, respectively, using Lipofectamin 2000 according to the manufacturer's protocol. Renilla luciferase pRL-SV40 is cotransfected with miR-34a report or miR-34a scr at a ratio of 1:100. Incubate at 37 °C for 4 h and then change with fresh complete DMEM (*see* **Note 7**).
3. Incubate at 37 °C for 48 h.
4. Wash the cells with PBS twice, harvest the cells, and prepare cell lysis according to the protocol of Dual Luciferase Reporter Assay kit.
5. The cell lysis is used to measure luciferase activities with a Wallac VICTOR$^3$V luminometer.
6. Calculate the ratio of firefly luciferase to Renilla expression to calculate the luciferase activity of each well after treatment (*see* **Note 8**).
7. As start from **step 2**, miR-34a mimics (2 μM) are transfected into Huh7, miR-34a inhibitor (2 μM) are transfected into

HepG2 cells, respectively (*see* **Note 9**) using DharmaFECT siRNA transfection reagent (*see* **Note 10**).

8. Follow **steps 3–6**.
9. Analysis the luciferase activities data from above treatments, confirm whether miR-34a reporter is responsive to the endogenous miR-34a.

   In this study, the data supports that miR-34a reporter is responsive to the endogenous miR-34a level (Fig. 2) (*see* **Note 11**).

### 3.3 Identification of Small Molecule Modulators of miR-34aby Library Screening in HCC Cells

1. Seed Huh7 cells into 96-well plates ($2 \times 10^3$ cells/well) and incubate at 37 °C overnight.
2. miR-34a report and miR-34a scr (100 ng/well) are, respectively, transfected into Huh7 cells using Lipofectamin 2000. Renilla luciferase pRL-SV40 is cotransfected with miR-34a report or miR-34a scramble at a ratio of 1:100.
3. Incubate at 37 °C for 4 h.
4. Add 640 small molecules from the library into 96-well plates, respectively, at a final concentration of 10 μM (one small molecule/well), the complete DMEM containing 0.1% DMSO was used as a control (*see* **Note 12**).
5. Incubate at 37 °C for 48 h (*see* **Note 13**).
6. Wash the cells twice with PBS, harvest the cells, and prepare cell lysis according to the protocol of Dual Luciferase Reporter Assay kit.

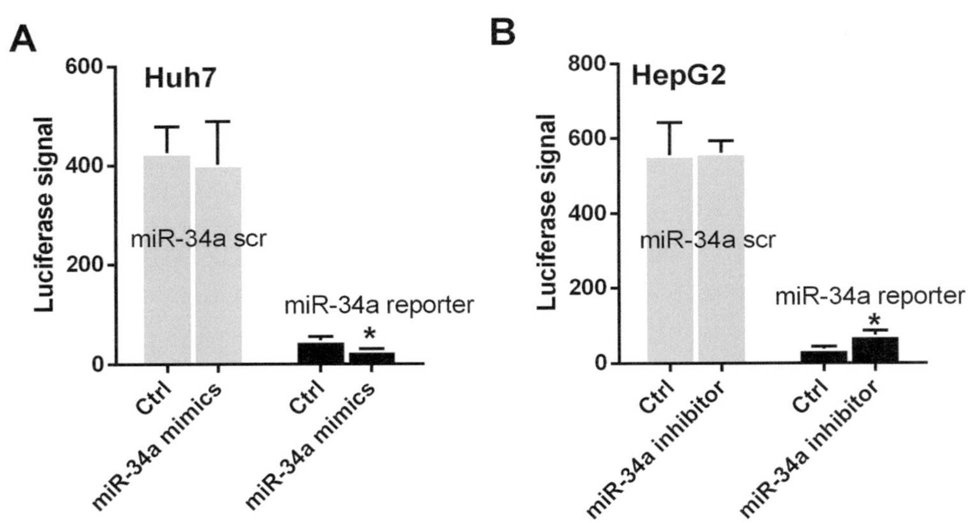


**Fig. 2** The established miR-34a reporter was responsive to the endogenous miR-34a level. (**a**, **b**) Cotransfection of miR-34a mimics and miR-34a reporter decreased the luciferase signal in Huh7 cells. Cotransfection of miR-34a inhibitor and miR-34a reporter increased the luciferase signal in HepG2 cells. No luciferase signal was changed in control group where miR-34a reporter was replaced with miR-34a scr. Error bars represent means ± SD of three independent experiments. *$p$ Values less than 0.05 were considered statistically significant

7. The cell lysis is used to measure luciferase activities with a Wallac VICTOR$^3$V luminometer.
8. Calculate the ratio of firefly luciferase to renilla expression to calculate the luciferase activity of each well after small molecule treatment.
9. Choose the small molecules which down-regulate the luciferase activity in Huh7 cells (*see* **Note 14**).
10. Repeat **steps 1–3**.
11. Add the chosen small molecules from **step 9** into 96-well plates at a final concentration of 10 μM (one small molecule/3 wells, $n=3$), the complete DMEM containing 0.1% DMSO was used as a control.
12. Follow **steps 5–8** to further confirm whether these small molecules could decrease luciferase activities (*see* **Note 15**). Two small molecules are validated.
13. Repeat **steps 1–3**.
14. Add small molecules from **step 12** into 96-well plates at a final concentration of 1, 2, 5, and 10 μM, respectively, the complete DMEM containing 0.1% DMSO was used as a control (*see* **Note 16**).
15. Following **steps 5–8** to confirm whether compounds can decrease luciferase activities in a dose-dependent manner. In our study, we finally found that a small molecule named Compound 3 significantly inhibited the luciferase activity of miR-34a reporter at a dose-dependent manner (Fig. 3). Compound 3 is a

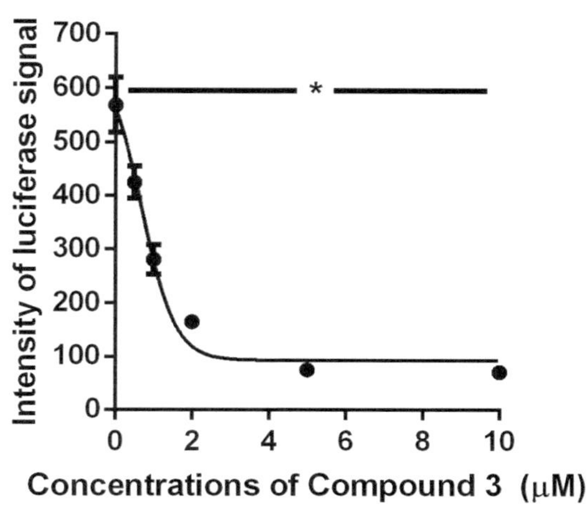


**Fig. 3** A small molecule named Compound 3 significantly inhibited the luciferase activity of miR-34a reporter at a dose-dependent manner. Huh7 cells were transfected with miR-34a reporter and then treated with indicated concentrations of Compound 3 for 48 h. Cell lysates were subjected to luciferase assay. Results are expressed as luciferase activity values. Error bars represent means ± SD of three independent experiments. *$p$ Values less than 0.05 were considered statistically significant

chemically synthesized plant chalcone derivative with a molecular weight of 374.

## 4 Notes

1. pmiR-REPORT luciferase plasmid can be used to analyze the effects of 3′-UTR sequences on gene expression. 3′-UTR regulatory sequences have shown to be important for mRNA stability, translation, and transport. miRNA-binding sites can be inserted into 3′-UTR of pmiR-REPORT luciferase plasmid. And the luciferase signal can be directly affected by dysregulated miRNA expression level. Therefore, the luciferase signals can be measured to screen small molecules which can modulate miRNA expression.
2. DNA oligonucleotides containing the miR-34a binding sites completely reverse complement of mature miR-34a. Make sure that scrambled miR-34a binding site does not contain complement-reverse bases of mature miR-34a. The cohesive end of Sac I/Hind III must be included in miR-34a-binding site or scrambled miR-34a-binding site. Thereafter, anneal synthetic oligonucleotides containing the miR-34a-binding site or scrambled miR-34a-binding site can be directly ligated into Sac I/Hind III double digested pmiR-REPORTTM luciferase plasmid.
3. This primer locates at the downstream of 3′-UTR of pmiR-REPORT luciferase. By sequencing, it is easy to confirm whether the ligation is correct.
4. Ligating a threefold molar of insert into prepared pmiR-REPORT luciferase plasmid.
5. The total ligation volume should be less than 10 μL when use 50 μL DH5α competent cells.
6. To avoid the salt, proteins, and other contaminates for efficient transfection, the commercial plasmid purification kit should be used.
7. The transfection media could be replaced 4–6 h to reduce cytotoxicity after transfection. According to our experience, we found most transfection reagents exhibited high transfection efficiency after 4–6 h transfection, including DharmaFECT siRNA transfection reagent and lipofectamin 2000. To avoid the potential cytotoxicity, we tended to change the medium after 4–6 h transfection.
8. By the end of this step, according to the luciferase activity in Huh7 and HepG2 cells, we can confirm whether miR-34a reporter responses to the endogenous miR-34a level.

9. miR-34a expression is higher in HepG2 than that in Huh7, so we up-regulate miR-34a expression with miR-34a mimics in Huh7 cells and down-regulate miR-34a expression with miR-34a inhibitor in HepG2 cells.
10. According to our experience, during miRNA mimics or inhibitor transfection, DharmaFECT siRNA transfection reagent shows higher transfection efficiency than that of lipfectamin.
11. The luciferase activities in Huh7 cells were significantly higher than that in HepG2 cells. The endogenous miR-34a level in HepG2 cells is significantly higher than that in Huh7 cells as measured by qRT-PCR [11]. These results indicate that miR-34a reporter is responsive to the endogenous miR-34a. The luciferase activities are decreased in miR-34a mimics treated Huh7 cells while increased in miR-34a inhibitors treated HepG2 cells. No luciferase signal changed in control group where miR-34a reporter was replaced with miR-34a scr (Fig. 2a, b). Further confirms that miR-34a reporter is responsive to the endogenous miR-34a specifically.
12. The concentration of small molecule stock is 10 mM in DMSO, dilute the small molecule with DMSO first, then dilute the small molecule with PBS, make sure that the complete DMEM must contain 0.1% DMSO in each treatment. Taking this strategy can prevent the precipitation of some small molecules with poor solubility.
13. We examined the luciferase activities 48 h after treatment with small molecule. The process of miRNAs including producing primary miRNAs, precursor miRNAs, and mature miRNAs, there is no study reporting the actual time period for this process. Typical time points for detecting targets are 24–48 h for mRNA and 48–96 h for protein. In other reports, the luciferase assay for miRNAs was usually performed 48 h after inducible treatment [12, 13]. So, we performed luciferase assay 48 h after small molecule treatment.
14. The decreased luciferase signal means that the expression of miR-34a is up-regulated due to the small molecule treatment.
15. Due to the instability of luciferase signal, the candidate small molecule must be repeated with miR-34a reporter. In our study, we also further validate potential miR-34a modulators three times after the primary screening.
16. Dose-dependent assay is necessary; in our study, we also excluded one small molecule which did not show any dose-dependent inhibition on luciferase signal.

## Acknowledgment

The work described in this paper was supported by grants from the Research Grants Council-General Research Fund of Hong Kong Special Administrative Region, China (CUHK462211, CUHK462713, and 14102714), National Natural Science Foundation of China (81101888 and 8142730), Shenzhen Basic Research Program (JC201105201092A), and Direct Grant from CUHK to Y.C.


## References


1. Carthew RW (2006) Gene regulation by microRNAs. Curr Opin Genet Dev 16:203–208
2. Lewis BP, Burge CB, Bartel DP (2005) Conserved seed pairing, often flanked by adenosines, indicates that thousands of human genes are microRNA targets. Cell 120:15–20
3. Selbach M, Schwanhausser B, Thierfelder N, Fang Z, Khanin R, Rajewsky N (2008) Widespread changes in protein synthesis induced by microRNAs. Nature 455:58–63
4. Hwang HW, Mendell JT (2007) MicroRNAs in cell proliferation, cell death, and tumorigenesis. Br J Cancer 96(Suppl):40–44
5. Kuentz MT, Arnold Y (2009) Influence of molecular properties on oral bioavailability of lipophilic drugs – mapping of bulkiness and different measures of polarity. Pharm Dev Technol 14:312–320
6. Kim HY, Park JW (2014) Clinical trials of combined molecular targeted therapy and locoregional therapy in hepatocellular carcinoma: past, present, and future. Liver Cancer 3:9–17
7. Welch C, Chen Y, Stallings RL (2007) MicroRNA-34a functions as a potential tumor suppressor by inducing apoptosis in neuroblastoma cells. Oncogene 26:5017–5022
8. Bommer GT, Gerin I, Feng Y, Kaczorowski AJ, Kuick R, Love RE, Zhai Y, Giordano TJ, Qin ZS, Moore BB, MacDougald OA, Cho KR, Fearon ER (2007) p53-mediated activation of miRNA34 candidate tumor-suppressor genes. Curr Biol 17:1298–1307
9. Yamakuchi M, Ferlito M, Lowenstein CJ (2008) miR-34a repression of SIRT1 regulates apoptosis. Proc Natl Acad Sci U S A105:13421–13426
10. Tarasov V, Jung P, Verdoodt B, Lodygin D, Epanchintsev A, Menssen A, Meister G, Hermeking H (2007) Differential regulation of microRNAs by p53 revealed by massively parallel sequencing: miR-34a is a p53 target that induces apoptosis and G1-arrest. Cell Cycle 6:1586–1593
11. Xiao Z, Li CH, Chan SL, Xu F, Feng L, Wang Y, Jiang JD, Sung JJ, Cheng CH, Chen Y (2014) A small-molecule modulator of the tumor-suppressor miR34a inhibits the growth of hepatocellular carcinoma. Cancer Res 74:6236–6247
12. Gumireddy K, Young DD, Xiong X, Hogenesch JB, Huang Q, Deiters A (2008) Small-molecule inhibitors of microrna miR-21 function. Angew Chem Int Ed Engl 47:7482–7484
13. Young DD, Connelly CM, Grohmann C, Deiters A (2010) Small molecule modifiers of microRNA miR-122 function for the treatment of hepatitis C virus infection and hepatocellular carcinoma. J Am Chem Soc 132:7976–7981

# Chapter 13

# Rapid Generation of miRNA Inhibitor Leads by Bioinformatics and Efficient High-Throughput Screening Methods

**Christopher L. Haga, Sai Pradeep Velagapudi, Jessica L. Childs-Disney, Jacqueline Strivelli, Matthew D. Disney, and Donald G. Phinney**

## Abstract

The discovery of microRNAs (miRNAs) has opened an entire new avenue for drug development. These short (15–22 nucleotides) noncoding RNAs, which function in RNA silencing and posttranscriptional regulation of gene expression, have been shown to critically affect numerous pathways in both development and disease progression. Current miRNA drug development focuses on either reintroducing the miRNA into cells through the use of a miRNA mimic or inhibiting its function via use of a synthetic antagomir. Although these methods have shown some success as therapeutics, they face challenges particularly with regard to cellular uptake and for use as systemic reagents. We recently presented a novel mechanism of inhibiting miR-544 by directed inhibition of miRNA biogenesis. We found that inhibition of DICER processing of miR-544 through the use of a small molecule abolished miR-544 function in regulating adaptation of breast cancer cells to hypoxic stress. Herein, we describe a protocol that utilizes bioinformatics to first identify lead small molecules that bind to DICER cleavage sites in pre-miRNAs and then employ an efficient, high-throughput fluorescent-based screening system to determine the inhibitory potential of the lead compounds and their derivatives.

**Key words** MicroRNA, miRNA, Therapeutics, Small molecule, DICER, High-throughput screening

## 1 Introduction

microRNAs (miRNAs) were first described in 1993 by Victor Ambros in *C. elegans* when it was revealed that the *lin-4* gene was capable of repressing the *lin-14* gene through a novel mechanism of producing a short, noncoding RNA that bound to the 3′ UTR region of the *lin-14* mRNA [1]. Shortly thereafter, numerous miRNAs were discovered in mouse and humans that regulate up to 60% of all genes. Many of these miRNAs were found to play an important role in disease pathophysiology, prompting widespread efforts to exploit miRNAs for their therapeutic potential.

Marco F. Schmidt (ed.), *Drug Target miRNA: Methods and Protocols*, Methods in Molecular Biology, vol. 1517, DOI 10.1007/978-1-4939-6563-2_13, 

Typically, miRNAs that are repressed in the disease state can be restored using miRNA mimics which are short RNA sequences that associate with the RISC complex and restore the function of the endogenous miRNA. Similarly, miRNAs that are overexpressed in disease can be inhibited by use of an antagomir, which is a small inhibitory RNA (siRNA) against the native miRNA. However, both of these approaches have limitations that are largely inherent to the use of RNA as a treatment option. For therapeutic purposes, RNA oligonucleotides do not readily permeate the cell membrane and often require a carrier molecule such as a lipid in order to increase cellular entry potential [2]. Additionally, RNA oligonucleotides have poor penetration throughout the human body, often being filtered out before they can achieve their therapeutic benefits [3]. These poor pharmacokinetic properties of oligonucleotides in general limit their usefulness as therapeutics and have served as a driving factor in the development of novel methods to modulate miRNA function in cells.

Instead of focusing our research efforts on developing carrier systems for inhibitory RNA-based oligonucleotides, we developed a system for identifying small molecule inhibitors of miRNA biogenesis or maturation. miRNA maturation is a coordinated multistep process and it should be noted that any step in the process can be targeted to inhibit the function of a particular miRNA. Generation of a mature miRNA begins by RNA transcription of the appropriate gene by either RNA polymerase II or III, which results in the formation of a hairpin loop structure commonly known as a primary microRNA (pri-miRNA) [4]. This pri-miRNA is then cleaved by the ribonuclease Drosha to form a shortened hairpin loop structure known as a pre-miRNA, which is then exported from the nucleus by Exportin-5. Once in the cytoplasm, the endoribonuclease DICER cleaves the precursor microRNA (pre-miRNA) hairpin to form a miRNA duplex that unwinds to yield one or two mature miRNAs. The mature miRNAs then associates with the microRNA-induced silencing complex (miRISC) wherein they suppress translation of target genes by binding to their 3′ untranslated regions.

Identifying molecules that are capable of inhibiting miRNAs is done through large-scale drug screens utilizing a reporter system. A miRNA and its target are introduced into a cell line, compounds are added, and a reporter gene is used to determine whether or not a particular compound has an inhibitory effect on the miRNA–target interaction. There are two limitations with this approach. First and foremost is the fact that screening thousands of compounds may not lead to a single hit. Second, even if a hit is identified, there is no data given about the mechanism of inhibition. Therefore, significant time and effort must be spent ruling out false positives or identifying the underlying mechanism of inhibition. Alternatively, methods outlined herein (Fig. 1) to identify inhibitors of miRNA biogenesis combine a rational design-based approach to identify lead small molecules that are capable of binding to the DICER and

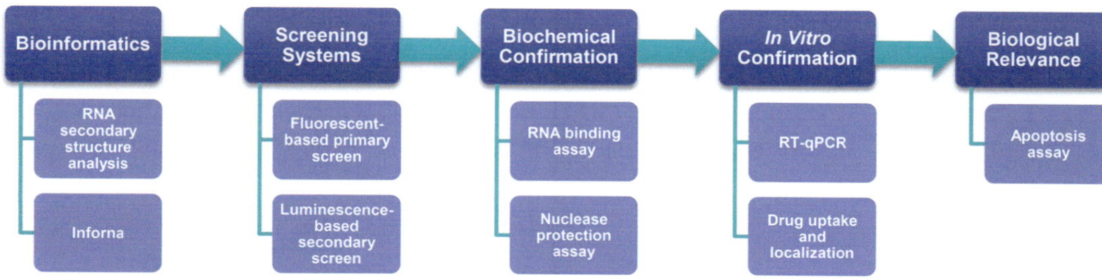


**Fig. 1** Schematic overview of identification of miRNA inhibitory small molecule compounds

Drosha sites within the pre-miRNA hairpin secondary structure and a novel fluorescent-based screening platform to confirm the activity of the leads. By targeting the DICER or Drosha binding site, the small molecules prevent cleavage of the pri- or pre-miRNA thereby blocking formation of the mature miRNA. Leads are identified using an algorithm referred to as *Inforna* [5], which parses the pri/pre-miRNA secondary structure for matching composite motifs and compares them to a database of RNA–small molecule interactions. The chapter describes, as an example, the identification of small molecule inhibitors of miR-544 biogenesis [6], which has a $1 \times 1$ nucleotide UU internal loop in both the DICER and Drosha binding sites. miR-544 was identified as playing an important role in regulating cellular proliferation in tumorigenesis and was shown to be upregulated under hypoxic conditions [6, 7]. Query of the *Inforna* database allowed us to identify several molecules that were capable of binding these sites. From there, we evaluated the inhibitory potential of lead compounds using a fluorescent-based screening platform that is amenable to high throughput. After secondary screening confirmation, RNA binding and RNAse protection assays confirmed the selectivity of lead compounds for the target sequence and cell-based assays revealed the effect of miRNA inhibition on apoptosis of hypoxic breast cancer cells.

## 2 Materials

### 2.1 Identification of Potential Lead Compounds

1. Access to *Inforna* database (*see* **Note 1**).

### 2.2 Fluorescence- and Luciferase-Based Drug Screening

1. Human embryonic kidney (HEK-293) cell line (ATCC CRL-1573).
2. Dulbecco's Minimum Essential Media (DMEM) with glutamine and high glucose (Gibco).
3. Fetal bovine serum (FBS) (Atlanta Biologicals).

4. Penicillin–Streptomycin (100×) (Gibco).
5. Trypsin–Ethylenediaminetetraacetic acid (EDTA) (0.25%) (Gibco).
6. Complete culture media: DMEM, 10% FBS, 1× penicillin–streptomycin.
7. RNAiMax Transfection Reagent (Life Technologies).
8. Lipofectamine 2000 (Life Technologies) (*see* **Note 2**).
9. Vector pGRB-miR.
10. Vector pmiR-GLO (Promega).
11. miR-544 antagomir (Qiagen).
12. Plate reader with fluorescent and luminescent capabilities (*see* **Note 3**).

### 2.3 RNA-Binding Assay

1. Short hairpin construct of miR-544 mimic (or other RNA of interest).
2. 1× RNA binding buffer (8 mM $Na_2HPO_4$, pH 7.0, 185 mM NaCl, and 1 mM EDTA).
3. Bovine serum albumin (BSA).
4. Small molecule of interest.
5. Black 96-well or 384-well plates (Corning Costar # 3686).
6. Fluorescent plate reader (BioTek FLx800) (*see* **Note 4**).

### 2.4 Nuclease Protection Assay

1. pre-miR-544 DNA template (5′-ATTTTCATCACCTAGGGA TCTTGTTAAAAAGCAGATTCTGATTCAGGGACC AAGATTCTGCATTTTTAGCAAGTTCTCAAGTG ATGCTAA-3′).
2. 1× PCR Buffer (10 mM Tris, pH 9.0, 50 mM KCl, and 0.1% (v/v) Triton X-100).
3. Forward DNA primer (5′-GGCCGAATTCTAATACGACT CACTATAGGATCTTGTTAAA AAGCA-3′).
4. Reverse DNA primer (5′-GAGAACTTGCTAAAAATGCA-3′).
5. 4.25 mM $MgCl_2$ working solution.
6. 330 μM deoxynucleotide triphosphate (dNTPs) working solution.
7. Taq DNA polymerase (NEB).
8. 1× Folding reaction buffer (Genlantis).
9. 1 mM ATP working solution.
10. Recombinant human DICER (Genlantis).
11. 1× RNA hydrolysis buffer (50 mM $NaHCO_3$, 1 mM EDTA, pH 9.4).
12. Denaturing polyacrylamide gel (15% acrylamide).
13. Molecular Dynamics Typhoon phosphorimager.

**2.5 Gene Expression Analysis**

1. Mammary adenocarcinoma (MDA-MB-231) cell line (ATCC HTB-26).
2. Roswell Park Memorial Institute media (RPMI 1640) with glutamine (Lonza).
3. Fetal bovine sera (Atlanta Biologicals).
4. Penicillin–Streptomycin (100×) (Gibco).
5. Trypsin–EDTA (0.25 %) (Gibco).
6. Complete culture media: RPMI 1640, 10% FBS, 1× penicillin–streptomycin.
7. miR-544 antagomir (Qiagen).
8. RNAiMax transfection reagent (Life Technologies).
9. Zymo Quick-RNA miniprep (Zymo Research).
10. miScript II RT Kit (Qiagen #218161).
11. Power SYBR Green Master Mix (Life Technologies).
12. ABI Prism 7900HT Sequence Detection System.
13. Thermocycler.

**2.6 Drug Uptake and Cellular Localization**

1. Mammary adenocarcinoma (MDA-MB-231) cell line (ATCC HTB-26).
2. miR-544 antagomir-FITC (Ambion).
3. RNAiMax transfection reagent (Life Technologies).
4. LSRII flow cytometer (BD Biosciences).
5. CyTRAK Orange nuclear counterstain (eBiosciences).
6. SYTO RNASelect Green Fluorescent cell stain (Life Technologies).
7. Leica DMI3000 B upright fluorescent microscope.

**2.7 Apoptosis Assay**

1. Mammary adenocarcinoma (MDA-MB-231) cell line (ATCC HTB-26).
2. miR-544 antagomir (Qiagen).
3. Annexin V APC Apoptosis Detection Kit (eBiosciences).
4. Propidium iodide (1 μg/mL).
5. LSRII flow cytometer (BD Biosciences).

## 3 Methods

**3.1 Identification of Potential Lead Compounds**

1. The Disney laboratory has developed a bottom-up approach, named *Inforna*, to identify lead small molecules for an RNA target of interest [5]. Briefly, *Inforna* compares motifs that comprise an RNA's secondary structure to a database of annotated RNA motif–small molecule interactions (Fig. 2). Overlap indi-

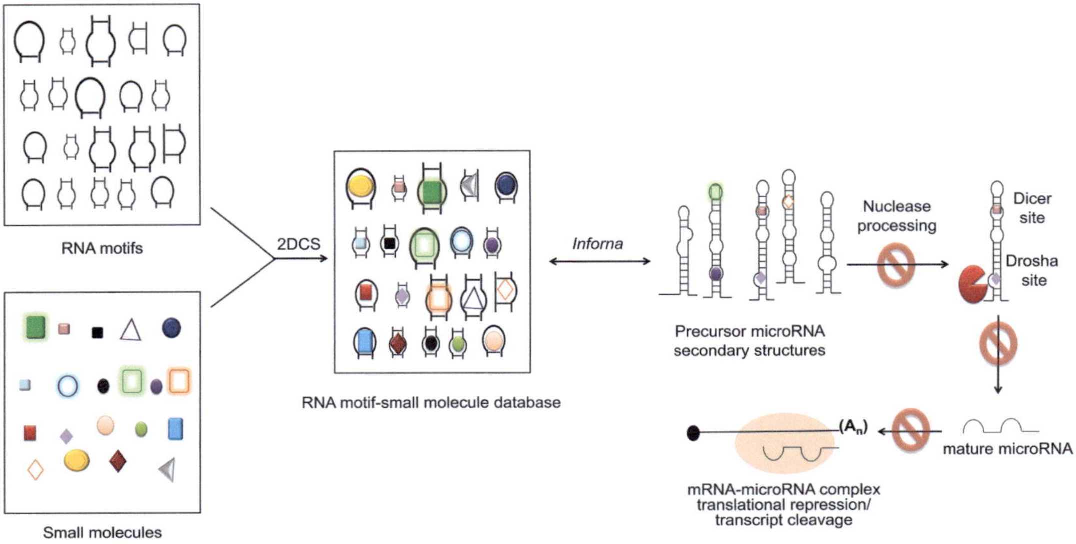


**Fig. 2** Schematic overview of *Inforna* demonstrating the use of RNA motifs to identify small molecule compounds capable of binding to DICER or Drosha sites in miRNAs

cates a targetable motif and *Inforna* outputs the motif, the small molecule that binds it, and related metadata. The most important metadata are Fitness Scores, which are a metric of affinity and selectivity and are derived from measured affinities and statistical analysis. Optimal interactions are defined as a Fitness Score of 100. Lead compounds are then evaluated in vitro or in cellular assays as described in the sections following.

2. Generate a connectivity table (.ct) file that describes the RNA's secondary structure. Various databases have .ct files for RNAs of known structure available for download. If they are not available, .CT files can be generated using software such as RNAstructure (http://rna.urmc.rochester.edu/RNAstructure.html), mFOLD (http://unafold.rna.albany.edu/?q=mfold/download-mfold), or ViennaFold (http://rna.tbi.univie.ac.at/) [8–11] (*see* **Note 5**). For detailed protocols for RNA secondary structure prediction, please *see* refs. 12, 13. The structures of miRNA precursors are available in miRBase [14].

3. Search the database for targetable motifs in the RNA of interest: Login to the *Inforna* server and upload the .ct file (*see* **Note 1**). Specify the stringency of the search by selecting (a) including the closing base pairs (most stringent); (b) search only loop nucleotides without the closing base pairs; or (c) search for variable nucleotides using 'N' to indicate any nucleotide (least stringent) (*see* **Note 6**).

4. View lead compounds: After the search is complete, *Inforna* outputs the targetable motif in the RNA of interest, the structure

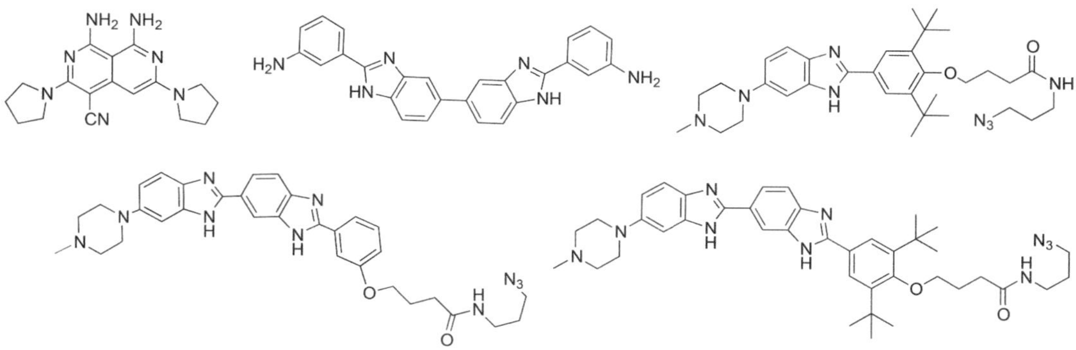

**Fig. 3** Lead compounds identified via *Inforna*. Reprinted after modification with permission from [6]

of the lead compound, and related meta data including affinity (if measured), Fitness Score, and PMID that report the RNA motif–small molecule interaction. The results can be viewed directly or exported as an .xlsx file. The structures of small molecule leads are exported as a simplified molecular input line entry system (SMILES) notation, which can easily be converted back into the chemical structure by using ChemDraw (CambridgeSoft; "Paste Special" fun4ction) or with PubChem Sketcher V2.4 (https://pubchem.ncbi.nlm.nih.gov/edit2/index.html). For miR-544, the molecules identified by *Inforna* as potential DICER and Drosha inhibitors are shown in Fig. 3.

### 3.2 Binding Assay

1. After lead small molecules have been generated by *Inforna*, their affinities and selectivities for the RNA of interest can be measured. Such parameters are often informative in downstream assays whether in vitro or in cells. RNAs can either be purchased commercially or can be produced by in vitro transcription [15]. There are a variety of methods to measure affinity, including competition dialysis [16], electrophoretic mobility shift assays, dye displacement assays [17], or fluorescence-based assays. Following we describe a fluorescence-based assay (*see* **Note 7**).
2. It is important that the RNA is properly folded prior to measurement of affinity. To fold, dilute the RNA to the desired concentration (up to 50 μM depending on the expect $K_d$) in 1× Binding Assay Buffer supplemented with 40 μg/mL bovine serum albumin in a total volume of 400 μL (96-well plate) or 100 μL (384-well plate). Heat the RNA for 5 min at 60–70 °C for 5 min and then slowly cool to room temperature on the bench top. After folding is complete, add the small molecule to the RNA solution to a final concentration of 50–1000 nM (or the concentration of small molecule that generates signal/noise ratio >3 in the absence of RNA) (*see* **Note 8**).

3. Complete a 12-point 1:2 serial dilution. Prepare a solution containing the small molecule of interest (at the same concentration in **step 2**) in 1× Binding Assay Buffer supplemented with 40 μg/mL bovine serum albumin (2250 μL for 96-well-plate and 600 μL for 384-well plate). Aliquot the small molecule into 11 microcentrifuge tubes (180 μL for 96-well plate and 40 μL for 384-well plate). Complete 1:2 serial dilutions in tubes 1–10; the remaining tube should contain no RNA. Incubate the solutions at room temperature for 30–60 min to allow for equilibration.
4. Aliquot each dilution prepared in **step 3** into three wells of a micro-well plate (50 μL for a 96-well plate; 10 μL for a 384-well plate) (*see* **Note 9**). Measure the fluorescence intensity or polarization using the appropriate excitation and emission wavelengths.
5. Calculate the change in fluorescence intensity as compared to samples containing no RNA. Plot the change in fluorescence intensity as a function of RNA concentration and fit the curve to the following equation if appropriate (1:1 binding stoichiometry):

$$I = I_0 + 0.5\Delta\varepsilon\left(\left([FL]_0 + RNA_0 + K_t\right) - \left(\left([FL]_0 + RNA_0 + K_t\right)^2 - 4[FL]_0\, RNA_0\right)^{0.5}\right)$$

where $I$ and $I_0$ are the observed fluorescence intensity in the presence and absence of RNA, respectively, $\Delta\varepsilon$ is the difference between the fluorescence intensity in the absence of RNA and in the presence of infinite RNA concentration, $[FL]_0$ and $[RNA]_0$ are the concentrations of small molecule and RNA, respectively, and $K_t$ is the dissociation constant (*see* **Note 10**).

### 3.3 Nuclease Protection Assays

1. After confirming that the small molecule binds with high affinity and selectivity to the miRNA of interest, it is important to determine if binding is sufficient to inhibit processing by Drosha or DICER. The assay requires labeling of the RNA, commonly by using [$\gamma$-$^{32}$P] ATP and T4 polynucleotide kinase. Alternatively, the RNA can be internally labeled during in vitro transcription using [$\alpha$-$^{32}$P] ATP or fluorescently labeled posttranscription.
2. Generate the DNA template for generation of pre-miRNAs via in vitro transcription: Genomic DNA or a synthetic DNA template is PCR amplified with 2 μM each of forward primer (containing a T7 promoter; 5′-GGCCGAATTCTAATACGAC TCACTATA) and reverse primer to generate a double-stranded DNA. RNAs are transcribed in 1× Transcription Buffer (40 mM Tris–HCl, pH 8.1, 1 mM spermidine, 0.001 % (v/v)

Triton X-100 and 10 mM DTT), 2.25 mM of each ribonucleoside triphosphate (rNTP), 5 mM $MgCl_2$, and T7 RNA polymerase by incubation at 37 °C overnight [15]. Transcribed RNAs are purified on a denaturing polyacrylamide gel and isolated. Concentrations are determined by absorbance at 260 nm and the corresponding extinction coefficient [18].

3. Preparation of RNA substrates: Briefly, prepare $^{32}P$-labeled RNA (~10,000 cpm) in 1× Reaction Buffer in a total volume of 100 mL. For DICER protection assays, 10× Reaction Buffer is provided by the manufacturer (Genlantis). Fold the RNA by incubating at 60 °C for 5 min and slowly cooling to room temperature (*see* **Note 11**). For Dicer protection assays, samples are supplemented with ATP to a final concentration of 1 mM. For Drosha protection assays, samples are supplemented with $MgCl_2$ to a final concentration of 6.4 mM. RNA is dispensed into 1×20 and 6×10 mL aliquots. Small molecule is added to final concentration between 10 and 50 mM into the 20 mL aliquot. Serial dilutions are then completed with five of the 10 mL aliquots. The remaining tube contains only RNA (no compound). The samples are then incubated at room temperature for 15 min.
4. Preparation of enzymes. Recombinant DICER is commercially available (Genlantis). Inhibition of Drosha activity can be assessed using cell lysates. Briefly, HEK 293T cells are cultured in a 100 mm dish transfected with a plasmid containing Drosha-c-Myc using lipofectamine-2000 according to manufacturer's protocol. Cells are collected by scraping into 1 mL of ice-cold 1× DPBS and centrifuged at 3300×*g* for 5 min at 4 °C. Cells are suspended in 500 μL 1× Lysis Buffer (20 mM Tris–HCl, pH 8.0, 100 mM KCl, and 0.2 mM EDTA) and sonicated for 30 s. Cellular debris is removed by centrifugation at 13,400×*g* for 15 min at 4 °C. The lysate is transferred to a new tube.
5. DICER Protection Assay: After the 15 min incubation of RNA and small molecule, 0.001 units/μL of recombinant human Dicer are added and the samples are incubated at 37 °C overnight. Reactions are stopped by adding an equal volume of Stop Buffer (Genlantis). The reaction products are resolved on a denaturing 10% polyacrylamide gel.
6. Drosha protection assay: After the 15 min incubation of RNA and small molecule, 1 μL of cell lysate in which Drosha was overexpressed is added, and the samples are incubated at 37 °C for 3 h. The reactions are quenched by phenol–chloroform extraction followed by ethanol precipitation. The pellet is then dissolved in 10 μL 1× Loading Buffer (4 M urea, 25 mM EDTA, 0.05% (w/v) bromophenol blue and 0.05% xylene cyanol). The reaction products are resolved on a denaturing 10% polyacrylamide gel (*see* **Note 12**).

### *3.4 Fluorescence- and Luciferase-Based Preliminary Drug Screening*

1. A fresh vial of HEK-293 cells is thawed for 5 min at 37 °C and then plated in a 100 mm culture dish in complete culture medium. After 16 h, the medium is changed. Cells are passaged every 3 days for a minimum of three times before transfection (*see* **Note 13**).
2. pGRB-miR is a tricolor (green, red, blue) fluorescent vector that allows for rapid screening of lead compounds with minimal handling (Fig. 4a). A pre-miR of interest is cloned downstream of the GFP reporter and a complementary 3′ untranslated region (UTR) is cloned downstream of the RFP reporter. The miRNA suppresses RFP expression by binding to the 3′ UTR. To clone a pre-miRNA fragment into pGRB-miR, the fragment can either be amplified from genomic DNA via polymerase chain reaction (PCR) or obtained from a commercial source. PCR primers for the pre-miRNA should be designed such that the forward primer includes either a 5′ XhoI or SalI restriction digest site and a 3′ HindII, EcoRV, or EcoRI restriction site (Fig. 4b). The 3′ UTR fragment can be isolated from either genomic DNA or obtained through a commercial source. PCR primers for subcloning the 3′ UTR into pGRB-miR should include a 5′ XmaI, SmaI, or BamHI restriction site and a 3′ XbaI or NotI restriction site (Fig. 4c). Several orthologous control vectors should be constructed including ones lacking the pre-miRNA and one lacking the 3′ UTR in addition to vectors where either the pre-miRNA or the 3′ UTR complementary sequence are mutated (*see* **Note 14**).

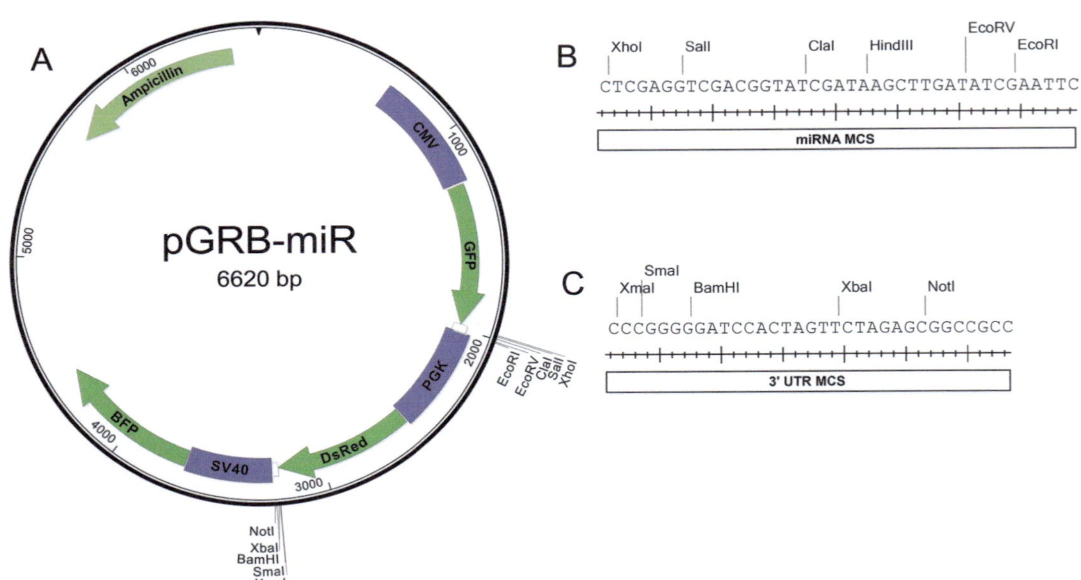


**Fig. 4** (**a**) pGRB-miR. (**b**) MiRNA multiple cloning site. (**c**) 3′ UTR multiple cloning site

3. The pGRB-miR vector is transfected into HEK-293 cells using Lipofectamine 2000. One day prior to transfection, HEK-293 cells are plated such that they obtain 80% confluence at the time of transfection. PGRB-miR vector (4 μg) and Lipofectamine 2000 (4 μL) are added to separate tubes containing 250 μL of DMEM without FBS and antibiotics. The tubes are then combined, vortexed for 1 min, incubated at room temperature for 20 min, and then added to the HEK-293 cells. The following day, cells are washed 3× with PBS and fed with fresh complete culture media (2 mL). At 48 h posttransfection cells are visualized by fluorescent microscopy for expression of green fluorescent protein, red fluorescent protein, and blue fluorescent protein (GFP, RFP, and BFP, respectively) (*see* **Note 15**). Cells are then harvested using trypsin, diluted to $1 \times 10^5$ cells/mL, and cell aliquots (100 μL) are plated into 96-well plates. RFP is read at 563 nm excitation/595 nm emission, GFP at 480 nm excitation/525 nm emission, and BFP at 325 nm excitation/450 nm emission (*see* **Note 16**).
4. The lead compounds are added to the wells in triplicate at dilutions ranging from 1 nM to 1 μM. Cells are then incubated at 37 °C for 48 h. After the incubation period, cells are analyzed again using the fluorescent plate reader with the settings previously described. The ratio of RFP, an indicator of 3′ UTR activity, to BFP, an internal transfection control, is used to ascertain the inhibitory or stabilizing potential of lead compounds (*see* **Note 17**). Molecules that show inhibitory potential will be utilized in secondary luciferase screening to determine whether the inhibitory potential is related to inhibition of miRNA biogenesis.
5. The pmiR-Glo vector system serves as a secondary screening system to determine the mechanism of miRNA inhibition. The system will use a vector containing the pre-miRNA in addition to miRNA mimics. If biogenesis of the miRNA is inhibited, only the pre-miRNA vector should be inhibited by the lead compounds.
6. In order to generate the screening vector, the 3′ UTR target of the miRNA is first cloned into the restriction sites downstream of the luciferase gene in the pmiR-Glo vector and confirmed by DNA sequencing. Orthologous control vectors are also generated including a vector wherein the 3′ UTR is mutated to eliminate the miRNA seed sequence and a vector that lacks the 3′ UTR.
7. Additionally, a pre-miRNA expression vector must be either purchased or generated. Generating a pre-miRNA expression vector can be accomplished by cloning GFP into the multiple cloning site of pcDNA3.1 and then adding the pre-miRNA sequence, obtained from genomic DNA, downstream of the GFP stop codon. Expression vectors including a scrambled

pre-miRNA vector and a vector lacking the pre-miRNA sequence can be generated in a similar manner. miRNA mimics may be obtained from commercial sources.

8. HEK-293 cells (~70% confluent) are transfected with either the pmiR-Glo vector (250 ng) containing the 3′ UTR target sequence or orthologous control vectors in 6-well plates using Lipofectamine 2000 as described earlier. At 24 h posttransfection, cells are harvested by addition of trypsin (100 μL) and diluted in 5 mL of fresh complete culture media. An aliquot (100 μL) of the cell suspension is plated in triplicate in 96 well black walled plates. At 24 h after plating, the pre-miRNA expression vector (100 ng) or miRNA mimic (100 nM) is transfected using either Lipofectamine 2000 or Lipofectamine RNAiMax, respectively (*see* **Note 18**). Cells are incubated overnight and then fed with 75 μL of fresh complete culture media. Lead compounds are then added at their predetermined concentrations obtained from the fluorescence assay. Plates are incubated for at least 24 h at 37 °C before performing the luciferase expression assay.
9. The luciferase expression assay is carried out using the Dual-Glo Luciferase Assay System. Dual-Glo reagent (75 μL) is added to each well and incubated for 15 min at room temperature. Firefly luminescence (the control reporter) is then measured using a plate reader with luminometer capabilities. Dual-Glo Stop & Glo reagent (75 μL) is then added to each well and the plate is incubated for 15 min at room temperature. Renilla luminescence (the experimental reporter) is then measured using the plate reader. The readout is calculated as the ratio of renilla luciferase luminescence over firefly luciferase luminescence (*see* **Note 19**).
10. Lead compounds that are found to inhibit pre-miRNA biogenesis may be used in subsequent assays.

### 3.5 Gene Expression Analysis

1. Although there are several systems available to analyze gene expression, we find that real-time quantitative polymerase chain reaction (RT-qPCR) is the most cost effective and efficient way of gauging changes in miRNA and gene expression levels in cells treated with lead compounds. Because we are measuring pre-miRNA, mature miRNA, and gene expression levels the miScript II RT Kit is well suited toward generating cDNA for SYBR Green RT-qPCR analysis with minimal manipulation. miR-544 is upregulated in hypoxic breast cancer cells; therefore, for this protocol, the cells will be cultured under hypoxic conditions prior to analysis.
2. MDA-MB-231 cells are cultured in 100 mm cell culture dishes under normoxic conditions (21% $O_2$) in complete culture media. Cells are passaged every 3–4 days for a minimum of three times before exposure to hypoxic conditions (*see* **Note 20**).

3. For this assay, it is important to compare the changes in miRNA expression as well as gene expression relative to untreated samples and also to samples treated with a miRNA antagomir that ablates the miRNA activity (*See* **Note 21**). The antagomir is introduced into cells by reverse transfection using RNAiMax Lipofectamine. Briefly, antagomir (500 nmol) is added to 200 μL of DMEM then RNAiMax (1 μL) is added to the solution, which is mixed rapidly by vortexing for 1 min. The resulting solution is incubated at room temperature for 25 min. During this incubation period, confluent MDA-MB-231 cells are harvested as described previously and diluted 1:20 in complete culture media. After the incubation period is finished, the transfection solution is added directly to one well of a 6-well plate followed by an aliquot (2 mL) of the diluted MDA-MB-231 cells. An aliquot (2 mL) of cells is also added to other wells of the 6-well plate, which serve as controls. The cells are incubated overnight under normoxic conditions. This experiment should be repeated using biological triplicates.
4. The following day, all wells of the 6-well plate are washed twice with 1× PBS and replaced with fresh complete culture media. Lead compounds are added in the appropriate concentrations to non-antagomir-treated wells just prior to culturing cells under hypoxic conditions using a Billups-Rothenberg chamber (*see* **Note 22**). Cells are exposed to hypoxia for a period of 5 days (*see* **Note 23**).
5. After the specified amount of time in hypoxia, cells are removed from the hypoxic chamber and are immediately lysed with RNA lysis buffer (*see* **Note 24**). Isolation of RNA is carried out using the Zymo Research Quick-RNA Miniprep protocol including the optional DNAse I treatment step as described by the manufacturer (*see* **Note 25**). The purified RNA is then analyzed using a NanoDrop Spectrophotometer to determine concentration and assess purity.
6. The isolated RNA is used to generate cDNA using the Qiagen miScript II RT Kit. The Qiagen miScript II RT Kit comes supplied with two buffers: a HiSpec and a HiFlex buffer. For analysis of mature miRNA, the HiSpec buffer is used. In these studies, the pre-miRNA, mature miRNA, and downstream target genes are to be analyzed. Therefore, the HiFlex buffer is appropriate. To generate cDNA the reaction mixture consists of HiFlex Buffer (4 μL), 10× DNTPs (2 μL), reverse transcriptase mix (2 μL), purified RNA (1 μg), and PCR grade water to bring the reaction to 20 μL. The reaction is incubated at 37 °C for 60 min, 95 °C for 5 min, and then placed on ice until qPCR analysis.
7. Quantitative reverse transcription polymerase chain reaction (RT-qPCR) analysis is carried out using a SYBR Green qPCR

system. For this application, we used the Power SYBR Green Master Mix. Due to the large number of genes that can potentially be affected by each miRNA, we generally carry out analyses using 10 μL reactions consisting of 0.5 μL of forward and reverse primers (10 μM) (*see* **Note 26**), 2.5 μL of PCR grade water, 2 μL of cDNA (5 ng/μL), and 5 μL of master mix in 384-well qPCR plates. The reaction is run in an Applied Biosystems 7900HT Fast Real-Time PCR System set for reading SYBR Green. The number of cycles should be set to 40 in order to detect genes that may have low expression levels.

8. Data analysis is straightforward and involves quantifying expression levels of each individual gene transcript relative to the appropriate housekeeping gene(s). Small RNAs (pre-miRNA and miRNA) are compared relative to the small RNA RNU6 housekeeping gene while mRNAs are compared relative to GAPDH in our analysis. The expected result is an upregulation of the miRNA target gene(s) if miRNA biogenesis is blocked by the lead compound or inhibited by the miRNA antagomir when compared to untreated samples. Additionally, if miRNA biogenesis is inhibited, mature miRNA expression level should decrease and pre-miRNA levels should increase in lead compound-treated cells in comparison to untreated cells.

### 3.6 Drug Uptake and Cellular Localization

1. Many of small RNA-binding lead compounds have fluorescent properties that can be exploited in order to easily determine cellular drug uptake and subcellular localization by flow cytometric analysis and microscopy, respectively. It should be noted that only lead compounds with fluorescent properties will be able to be analyzed with the methods described in this section. The first method describes cellular uptake of the lead compounds by flow cytometry and compares the uptake against a fluorescently labeled antagomir (*see* **Note 27**). The second method utilizes microscopy to visualize lead compound cellular localization.
2. MDA-MB-231 cells are passaged a minimum of 3 times before transfection and should be 90% confluent the day prior to transfection. The day of transfection cells are harvested with trypsin as described earlier and diluted 1:10 in complete culture medium. Cells are then transfected with the fluorescently labeled antagomir using RNAiMax Lipofectamine using the reverse transfection method. Briefly, fluorescently labeled antagomir (500 nanomoles) is added to 200 μL of DMEM without serum, then RNAiMax Lipofectamine (2 μL) is added to this mixture, which is mixed by vortexing for 1 min. After a 25 min incubation at room temperature, the reaction mixture is added to one well of a 6-well plate, then an aliquot (2 mL) of MDA-MB-231 cells is added on top of the reaction mixture. Cell aliquots (2 mL) are also added to other wells of the 6-well plates for testing of lead compounds and for use as nontreated controls.

3. The following day all wells are fed with complete culture media. Then, lead compounds are added to nontransfected wells and incubated for a minimum of 30 min. After incubation, cells are lifted from the plate with trypsin (100 μL) and suspended in 1 mL of complete culture media. Cells are collected by centrifugation at 700 × *g* for 5 min, washed twice with 1× PBS, and suspended in an appropriate volume of FACS analysis buffer.
4. Flow cytometric analysis is carried out on a LSRII flow cytometer (*see* **Note 28**). The miR-544 inhibitor lead compound fluoresces at approximately 460 nm ("blue channel"). Therefore, both the blue channel emission and the side scatter are collected at acquisition. Similarly, the fluorescent antagomir emission channel is collected and compared to side scatter.
5. The overall percent of cells taking up the lead compound or antagomir are compared to untreated cells in order to determine the uptake efficiency of the two treatments. Generally, the efficiency of lipofectamine-based transfection is not 100%, whereas uptake of the lead compound should be nearly 100% (*see* **Note 29**).
6. Fluorescent microscopy can be used to analyze the subcellular localization of fluorescent lead compounds. Small RNA-binding compounds have the potential to also bind DNA causing unwanted effects whereas compounds that are excluded from the nucleus may be more beneficial for clinical use. Using an RNA staining dye, a nuclear staining dye, and the fluorescent lead compound, it is possible to determine nuclear exclusion.
7. MDA-MB-231 cells are cultured on Lab-Tek chamber slides until 50% confluent. Lead compounds are then added to each well and incubated at 37 °C for a period of 48 h (*see* **Note 30**). Cells are then stained with a mixture of CyTRAK Orange nuclear counterstain (5 μM) and SYTO RNASelect RNA stain (500 nM) for 30 min at 37 °C (*see* **Note 31**). Cells are then washed 3× for 5 min each with warm 1× PBS. The chamber portion of the slide is then carefully removed and a glass coverslip is secured over the slide with an appropriate adhesive.
8. Cells are imaged using a Leica DMI3000 B upright fluorescent microscope attached to a DFC295 digital camera. Blue, red, and green wavelength channel images are acquired in addition to phase contrast. After acquisition, image overlays are created using appropriate imaging software package.
9. If the lead compound being tested is excluded from the nucleus, there should be no overlap between the nuclear counterstain and the lead compound fluorescence. Lead compound should be localized to the cytoplasm with the RNA as visualized using the RNASelect dye.

### 3.7 Apoptosis Assay

1. The last section of this protocol will focus on measuring a biological effect of cancer cells treated with the lead compound, in this case, apoptosis of breast cancer cells in which miR-544 biogenesis is inhibited. In this assay, MDA-MB-231 cells are treated with either miR-544 antagomir or lead compound and then are cultured under hypoxic conditions. Cells are then analyzed for apoptosis and necrosis by flow cytometry after staining with Annexin V and propidium iodide.
2. MDA-MB-231 cells passaged a minimum of three times are transfected with miR-544 antagomir by reverse transfection in a 6-well plate as described earlier. At 24 h posttransfection, a well of nontransfected cells is treated with the lead compound at an appropriate concentration and all cells are immediately placed under hypoxic conditions as described earlier for a period of 5 days.
3. After cells are removed from hypoxia the culture supernatant is collected and centrifuged at 700 × *g* for 5 min. Accutase Cell Detachment Solution (200 μL) is then added to the plate to detach the adherent cells, which are collected in 500 μL of 1× PBS. The adherent cells are added to the tube with the previously collected cells and again centrifuged at 700 × *g* for 5 min after which the supernatant is discarded (*see* **Note 32**).
4. Cells are stained by suspending in 1× Annexin V binding buffer (300 μL) together with an APC-conjugated Annexin V antibody (10 μL) (*see* **Note 33**). Cells are incubated at room temperature for 10–15 min, washed once with 1× and suspended in 200 μL of binding buffer. Propidium iodide (5 μL) is added to the suspension, which is then kept at 4 °C in the dark until the cells can be analyzed by flow cytometry.
5. Cells are analyzed on an LSRII flow cytometer for Annexin V/APC and PI staining. In our experimentation, miR-544 inhibition by either miR-544 antagomir or our lead compound under hypoxic conditions leads to an increase in Annexin V+ and Annexin V+/PI+ cells indicative of an increase in apoptotic activity compared to untreated cells.

## 4 Notes

1. Access to the *Inforna* server can be found at http://www.scripps.edu/disney/software.html.
2. Although other transfection reagents such as PEI-based reagents can be used in this assay, we have found that Lipofectamine-based reagents tend to transfect HEK-293 cells at the highest efficiency while maintaining low toxicity making them ideal for use in these screening assays.

3. For the pGRB-miR vector drug screening vector system, a plate reader capable of exciting at 325, 480, and 563 nm and reading emissions at 450, 525, and 595 is required.
4. The required fluorescent capabilities of the plate reader will depend on the excitation and emission spectrum of the lead compounds.
5. Experimental constraints can be used to restrain folding and to ensure the known structure of the RNA is output.
6. The hits obtained by searching motifs including the closing base pairs (most stringent) give most reliable hits.
7. Small molecules that are not inherently fluorescent can be appended with a fluorophore. However, one must be certain that the appended fluorophore does not mask the surface involved in target recognition.
8. The concentration of the compound for fluorescence assay is determined for each compound, such that the fluorescence signal of the compound in assay buffer is at least three times above background.
9. The experiment is performed in technical triplicates and biological replicates should also be prepared. We found that using this replication scheme gives the most reliable results when dealing with small changes in fluorescence.
10. For most compounds which are strong binders we see at least a 50% increase in fluorescence upon binding RNA.
11. We recommend folding the RNA in 50 mM NaCl for the Drosha protection assay.
12. Usually the site protection is about 50%, if you increase concentration of compound to see 100% protection, there is some nonspecific protection from nuclease cleavage.
13. Cells are harvested when confluent by washing the monolayer once with 1× PBS, incubating with trypsin (1 mL) to detach the cells from the plate, and then adding fresh complete culture media (10 mL) to inactivate the trypsin. The cell suspension is then diluted 1:10 by transferring an aliquot (1 mL) to a new 100 mm cell culture dish and adding 9 mL of complete culture medium.
14. For the mutated pre-miRNA, a nonbinding miRNA sequence can be introduced into the vector by mutating the miRNA seed sequence through any number of commercially available targeted mutation kits.
15. It is important for the transfection efficiency to exceed 90% for this experiment in order for reliable results to be obtained. In general, Lipofectamine 2000 gives greater than 90% transfection efficiency with this system when used with HEK-293 cells. Should less than 90% transfection efficiency be seen, the vector should be repurified using an endotoxin-free plasmid isolation kit.

16. Certain compounds have fluorescent properties; therefore, it is necessary to obtain a fluorescent reading from the plate reader prior to addition of the compounds.
17. miRNA inhibiting molecules are expected to increase the ratio of RFP to BFP, whereas stabilizing molecules are expected to decrease the ratio of RFP to BFP. As expected, the orthologous controls should show no change in fluorescent readout compared to untreated samples.
18. RNAiMax is specifically formulated for the transfection of small RNAs and therefore is appropriately used to transfect the miRNA mimic but not the pre-miRNA vector, which can be transfected using Lipofectamine 2000.
19. In this secondary screening system, if the lead compound inhibits miRNA biogenesis treated wells expressing both the pre-miRNA and the target 3′ UTR are expected to have an increased ratio of renilla to firefly luciferase when compared to untreated wells. Treated wells that are transfected with the miRNA mimic and the 3′ UTR are expected to exhibit the same luciferase expression ratio as untreated wells. Orthologous controls should all exhibit increased renilla to firefly luciferase ratios relative to untreated pre-miRNA and miRNA mimic wells.
20. MDA-MB-231 cells are passaged by washing the monolayer twice with 1× PBS, detaching cells using 1 mL of trypsin, and then adding 10 mL of fresh complete culture media to the plate to inactivate the trypsin. The cell suspension is then diluted 1:10 by transferring an aliquot (1 mL) to a new 100 mm cell culture dish and adding 9 mL of complete culture medium.
21. For these studies we used a commercially available miR-544 antagomir purchased from Qiagen.
22. Culture dishes containing the appropriate cells are placed in the chamber along with a 100 mm culture dish containing deionized water. The chamber is flushed with $N_2$ gas for a period of 7 min using a flow rate of 25 l/min. To prevent oxygenation of the chamber, the outlet lines are clamped first followed by the intake line clamps before the $N_2$ gas flow is shut off.
23. The period of hypoxia will largely be dependent on the biological system being examined. In the case of miR-544, changes in target gene expression due to hypoxia-induced upregulation of this miRNA are best observed at 5 days postexposure. Other miRNAs may be induced by hypoxia with faster or slower kinetics and therefore require more or less time to induce downstream changes on gene expression.
24. The immediate addition of lysis buffer is crucial to the success of the experiment as cells react quickly to oxygen reexposure by upregulating molecules for DNA damage and repair.

25. For miRNA analysis, it is important to select an RNA isolation kit that is capable of isolating total cellular RNA including both large and small RNAs. We recommend using the Zymo Research Quick-RNA Miniprep kit, which has worked well in our experience.
26. The miScript II RT Kit adds a universal reverse primer tag to small RNAs which can be amplified using the Qiagen universal reverse RT-qPCR primer. Forward primers for RT-qPCR can be designed from the pre-miRNA and mature miRNA sequences. Additionally, primer sets for housekeeping control genes also need to be designed. For small RNAs, RNU6 is generally a stable housekeeping gene to use for relative qPCR analysis. For mRNA analysis, several housekeeping genes should be run for experiments involving hypoxic conditions as housekeeping genes can vary by cell type when exposed to low oxygen. For the MDA-MB-231 cell line cultured under hypoxic conditions, we found that GAPDH is generally stable.
27. The drug uptake assay is a straightforward approach to determine the cellular permeability of the lead compounds in target cells of interest. In this case MDA-MB-231 cells are incubated with lead compounds and then analyzed by flow cytometry. Fluorescent-labeled antagomirs are also transfected into cells to compare the uptake efficiency between the lead compound and the antagomir. Fluorescently labeled antagomirs can be obtained from any number of commercial sources.
28. Any flow cytometer that is equipped with the appropriate lasers to detect the fluorescent excitation and emission wavelengths of the lead compound(s) and fluorescent-labeled antagomir may be used for these analyses.
29. In the event that any cell populations excludes the lead compound of interest, those populations can be further analyzed for expression of multidrug efflux pumps, which may pump the molecule out of the cell and as such reduce its potency and as such its potential as a therapeutic agent.
30. A 48 h incubation period allows the compounds to penetrate into cells and ensures that cells have undergone at least one round of cell division, which also enables the compounds to diffuse passively into the nucleus and bind to DNA.
31. The selection of stains used for nuclear counterstaining and RNA staining will largely depend on the fluorescent emission of the lead compound being tested. The miR-544 lead compound emits in the blue channel, therefore, DAPI cannot be used as a traditional nuclear counterstain. Instead, CyTRAK Orange, which emits in the 615 nm, is used to counterstain the nucleus.
32. Because MDA-MB-231 4cells are adherent it is important to collect the supernatant, which may contain dead cells, as well as the cells still adhered to the tissue culture plate.

33. When performing Annexin V/PI staining on cells treated with lead compounds, it is imperative to account for the fluorescent properties of the compound. Annexin V is available in a wide range of fluorescently labeled conjugates. We found using APC-conjugated Annexin V allowed for the greatest emission spectrum separation and minimized fluorescent overlap with our compound.

## Acknowledgement

This work was supported by Department of Defense CDMRP Grant W81XWH-16-1-0029 to D.G.P. and M.D.D.

### References

1. Lee RC, Feinbaum RL, Ambros V (1993) The C. elegans heterochronic gene lin-4 encodes small RNAs with antisense complementarity to lin-14. Cell 75(5):843–854
2. Wang J, Lu Z, Wientjes MG, Au JLS (2010) Delivery of siRNA therapeutics: barriers and carriers. AAPS J 12(4):492–503
3. Burnett John C, Rossi John J (2012) RNA-based therapeutics: current progress and future prospects. Chem Biol 19(1):60–71
4. Cullen BR (2004) Transcription and processing of human microRNA precursors. Mol Cell 16(6):861–865
5. Velagapudi SP, Gallo SM, Disney MD (2014) Sequence-based design of bioactive small molecules that target precursor microRNAs. Nat Chem Biol 10(4):291–297
6. Haga CL et al (2015) Small molecule inhibition of miR-544 biogenesis disrupts adaptive responses to hypoxia by modulating ATM-mTOR signaling. ACS Chem Biol 10(10):2267–2276
7. Haga CL, Phinney DG (2012) MicroRNAs in the imprinted DLK1-DIO3 region repress the epithelial-to-mesenchymal transition by targeting the TWIST1 protein signaling network. J Biol Chem 287(51):42695–42707
8. Eddy SR (2004) How do RNA folding algorithms work? Nat Biotechnol 22(11):1457–1458
9. Lorenz R et al (2011) ViennaRNA Package 2.0. Algorithms Mol Biol 6:26
10. Mathews DH (2014) RNA secondary structure analysis using RNAstructure. Curr Protoc Bioinformatics Chapter 12:Unit 12.6
11. Zuker M (2003) Mfold web server for nucleic acid folding and hybridization prediction. Nucleic Acids Res 31(13):3406–3415
12. Seetin MG, Mathews DH (2012) RNA structure prediction: an overview of methods. Methods Mol Biol 905:99–122
13. Bernhart SH (2011) RNA structure prediction. Methods Mol Biol 760:307–323
14. Griffiths-Jones S, Saini HK, van Dongen S, Enright AJ (2008) miRBase: tools for microRNA genomics. Nucleic Acids Res 36(Database issue):D154–D158
15. Milligan JF, Uhlenbeck OC (1989) Synthesis of small RNAs using T7 RNA polymerase. Methods Enzymol 180:51–62
16. Chaires JB (2003) A competition dialysis assay for the study of structure-selective ligand binding to nucleic acids. Curr Protoc Nucleic Acid Chem Chapter 8:Unit 8.3
17. Tse WC, Boger DL (2005) A fluorescent intercalator displacement assay for establishing DNA binding selectivity and affinity. Curr Protoc Nucleic Acid Chem 8:85
18. Puglisi JD, Tinoco I Jr (1989) Absorbance melting curves of RNA. Methods Enzymol 180:304–325

# Chapter 14

# Peptide-Based Inhibition of miRNA-Guided Gene Silencing

**Johannes Danner, Balagopal Pai, Ludwig Wankerl, and Gunter Meister**

## Abstract

MicroRNAs (miRNAs) are a large class of small noncoding RNAs that regulate the expression of distinct target mRNAs. miRNAs are incorporated into Argonaute (AGO) proteins and guide them to their target mRNAs. Subsequently, AGO proteins recruit a member of the glycine-tryptophan-rich (GW) protein family by direct protein-protein interaction. GW proteins coordinate all downstream processes leading to robust and efficient gene silencing. A short peptide of GW proteins comprising the AGO interaction motif can be used to biochemically isolate endogenous AGO protein complexes. Furthermore, within a cell such a peptide competes with endogenous GW proteins for AGO binding and thus can be used as potent inhibitor of the miRNA pathway. Here, we describe a method that utilizes a GW-based polypeptide (T6B-assay) to validate miRNA-mRNA interactions in tissue culture systems.

**Key words** miRNA, GW proteins, Argonaute, TNRC6 proteins

## 1 Introduction

microRNAs (miRNAs) belong to a class of small noncoding RNAs (19–25 nucleotides) that are involved in posttranscriptional gene silencing in plants and animals [1]. Depending on the genomic organization, RNA polymerase II transcribes miRNA genes from individual genes or as clusters of several miRNAs. Many miRNAs, however, originate form introns and are processed from their host pre-mRNA transcript [2]. Nuclear RNase III Drosha along with the double-stranded RNA-binding protein (dsRBP) DGCR8 processes primary miRNAs (pri-miRNA) into pre-miRNA. After transport to the cytoplasm, pre-miRNAs undergo additional processing by a second RNase III enzyme, Dicer, resulting in a ~22–23 nucleotide double-stranded (ds) miRNA/miRNA* duplex. One strand of the miRNA duplex is loaded into the RNA-induced silencing complex (RISC), where it directly binds to a member of the AGO protein family whereas the other strand is often degraded [3].

AGO proteins possess an N-terminal domain, a characteristic PAZ domain, a PIWI domain, and a middle (MID) domain located

Marco F. Schmidt (ed.), *Drug Target miRNA: Methods and Protocols*, Methods in Molecular Biology, vol. 1517,
DOI 10.1007/978-1-4939-6563-2_14, © Springer Science+Business Media New York 2017

between PAZ and PIWI [4, 5]. The function of the N-terminal domain is only poorly understood, and a contribution to RISC loading has been reported [6]. The PAZ domain binds the 3′ end of the small RNA [7–10], and the MID domain anchors the 5′ end in a very specific binding pocket [11, 12]. The PIWI domain is structurally similar to RNase H, and some AGO proteins indeed possess endonucleolytic activity [13–15]. Among the four mammalian AGO proteins, only AGO2 has an active, "slicing," competent RNAse-H-like PIWI domain [16–19]. In case of full complementarity of the loaded RNA strand (miRNA or siRNA), the target is cleaved and degraded [20–22].

In animals, miRNA typically associates with partially complementary target sequences located in the 3′ untranslated region (UTR) of mRNAs. Partial complementarity prevents RNAi-like direct cleavage by AGO2 [23]. Instead, once a mature miRNA is loaded onto an AGO protein, it associates with several other proteins to form the effector miRNP or the miRNA-induced silencing complex (miRISC). In mammalian cells, AGO proteins associate with the members of the GW protein family, which coordinate all downstream silencing steps [24–26]. GW proteins are also components of cytoplasmic processing bodies (P-bodies), and these structures might be associated with miRNA-guided gene silencing [26–29].

GW proteins are a highly conserved family of proteins in vertebrates. In humans, three paralogs referred to as TNRC6A–C are found [30]. TNRC6 proteins are viewed as central cellular hubs that facilitate and coordinate all individual silencing steps. TNRC6 proteins are known to interact with poly-A-binding proteins, recruit deadenylases such as the CCR4-NOT complex, and thus initiate a cascade of gene-silencing process. The deadenylases initiate removal of poly-A tail of the target mRNA; this in turn triggers recruitment of repressor DDX6 and initiates decapping and degradation by 5′–3′ exoribonucleases like Xrn1 [31–33].

As the name indicates, the N-terminal region of GW proteins contains a high amount of glycine-tryptophan repeats that interact directly with the tryptophan-binding pockets of mammalian AGO proteins [19, 34]. The C-terminal region, which is highly unstructured, is also called the "silencing" domain, since it can induce silencing independent of AGO proteins when tethered artificially to a target mRNA [30].

Since their discovery as mediators of posttranscriptional gene regulation, miRNAs have been implicated in the pathophysiology of many human diseases. miRNAs assure a smooth balancing of cellular homeostasis by regulating gene expression, which is often dysregulated in various diseases including cancer [35, 36]. A single miRNA could target multiple mRNAs, and a single mRNA could harbor several miRNA-binding sites. Targeting even a single miRNA could thus have dramatic effects on cellular physiology. Hence, knowing the true miRNA candidate and its specificity for a particular target at a particular physiological condition is of utmost importance. Although there are several bioinformatics algorithms that predict target specificity [37], they are not capable of considering the spatiotemporal aspect of miRNA-mediated regulation. In addition, the interaction of a miRNA to its target is through the "seed region" [38], which is only 7–8 nucleotides additionally constraining the accuracy of predictions. This emphasizes the need for an assay to validate specificity of miRNA-mRNA interactions in its physiological context. For example, a luciferase-based reporter gene assay is a simple and efficient method to study miRNA-mediated regulation through the 3′-UTRs of target mRNAs.

Recently, it was shown that a short region of TNRC6B efficiently interacts with all four AGO proteins [34, 39]. Since then the TNRC6B-derived peptide (T6B-peptide) has been used to efficiently purify all four endogenous AGO proteins from different primary tissues [40]. The T6B-peptide (amino acid position 599–683 in TNRC6B) competes with endogenous TNRC6 proteins for the interaction to AGO and thus can efficiently block miRNA-mediated silencing of target mRNAs (Fig. 1) [40]. Coupled

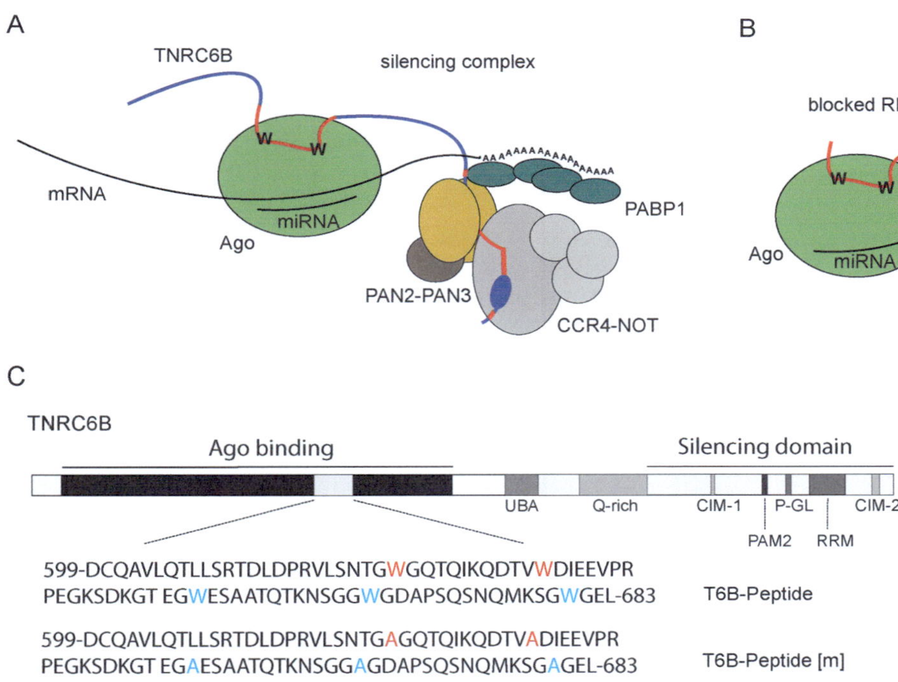


**Fig. 1** Model of small RNA-mediated gene silencing. (**a**) AGO proteins interact with small noncoding RNAs, which guide them to target mRNAs to mediate gene silencing. A functional miRNA-mediated gene-silencing complex requires at least one AGO protein, one TNRC6 protein, Poly-A-binding proteins (PABP1) bound to mRNA, the PAN2–PAN3, and CCR4-NOT deadenylase complexes. Translational repression and destabilization of the target mRNA target leads to 5′–3′ decay through exonucleases. (**b**) The silencing mechanism is blocked by a competing TNRC6B-peptide interacting with the tryptophan-binding pockets in AGO proteins. (**c**) Schematic representation of TNRC6B domain organization and its AGO-interacting region. The amino acid sequence depicts the T6B-peptide with the interacting tryptophans in *red* and the control peptide (T6B-peptide [m]) (Adapted from [40])

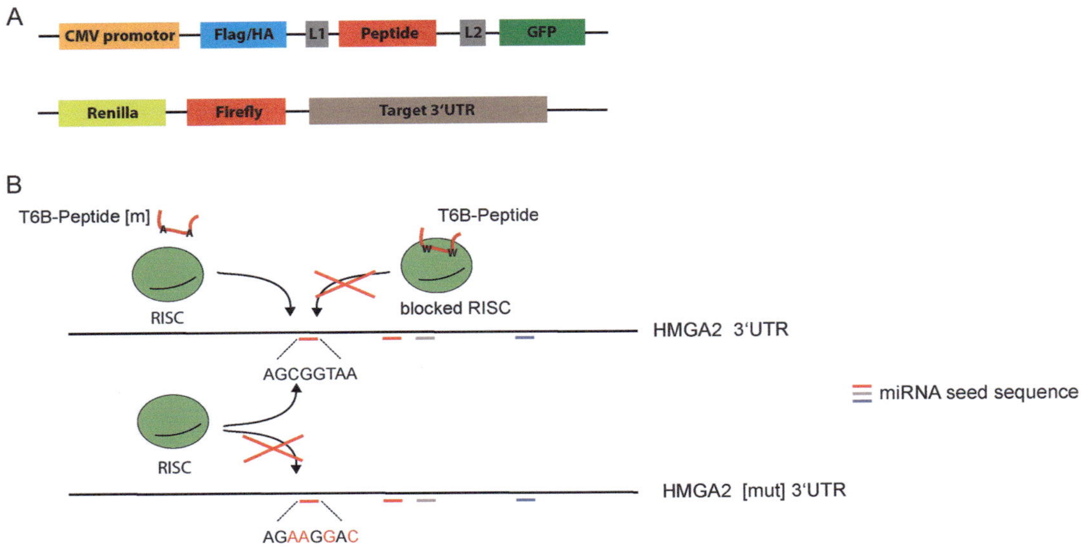


**Fig. 2** Schematic representation of vector constructs used for "T6B derepression assay." (**a**) Scheme of vectors for expression of Flag/HA-T6B-peptide-EYFP and *Renilla*/firefly target 3′-UTR. (**b**) Depiction of T6B-peptide-mediated derepression of miRNA-mediated silencing of mRNA targets while luciferase assays

with luciferase reporter transfection, the T6B-peptide can be used as an efficient readout for miRNA-mediated gene silencing in any cell type (Fig. 2). Here, we describe the "T6B-assay" that can be adapted for various cell types to analyze whether a specific target mRNA is under control of the miRNA pathway. Our assay validates specificity or miRNA-mRNA target interactions and is useful for miRNA-based drug development as well as its various validation approaches.

## 2 Materials

### 2.1 Cell Culture

1. Dulbecco's Modified Eagle's Medium (DMEM) (Sigma-Aldrich). Supplemented with 10% fetal bovine serum (FBS) (Gibco) and 1% penicillin-streptomycin (Sigma-Aldrich).
2. Phosphate-buffered saline pH 7.5 (1× PBS).
3. Trypsin-EDTA (ethylenediaminetetraacetic acid) (Sigma-Aldrich).

### 2.2 Transfection

1. Opti-MEM serum-free medium (Gibco, Life Technologies).
2. Lipofectamine 2000 (Life Technologies).
3. Multi-well cell culture plates (96 wells or 48 wells) (Nunc).

### 2.3 Lysis and Luciferase Assay

1. Passive Lysis Buffer, 5× (Promega).
2. Luciferase assay buffers:

(a) Firefly luciferase buffer (pH 8.0): 0.1 mM ethylenediaminetetraacetic acid (EDTA), 5.34 mM $MgSO_4.7H_20$, 20 mM tricine, 530 µM ATP, 270 µM coenzyme A, 470 µM d-luciferin, 33.3 mM dithiothreitol (DTT).

(b) *Renilla* luciferase buffer (pH 5.1): 2.2 mM $Na_2EDTA$, 220 mM $K_3PO_4$, 0.44 mg/mL BSA, 1.1 M NaCl, 1.3 mM $NaN_3$, 1.43 mM colenterazine.

3. Mithras LB 940 luminometer (Berthold Technologies) (or any other luminometer).
4. Luciferase plates: multi-well plates with high reflective surface pureGrade™ (brand).
5. Methanol (Sigma-Aldrich).

### 2.4 Western Blot

1. Sodium dodecyl sulfate (SDS) polyacrylamide gels (10%).
2. SDS running buffer (10×): 250 mM Tris (pH-8.5), 1.92 M glycine, 10% SDS.
3. SDS loading buffer (5× Lämmli): 300 mM Tris/HCl pH 6.8, 10% SDS, 62.5% glycerin (87%), 1 mg/mL bromphenolblue, 10% mercaptoethanol.
4. Towbin transfer buffer (1×): 25 mM Tris (pH 8.5), 192 mM glycine, 20% methanol.
5. Hybond protein nitrocellulose membrane (GE Healthcare).
6. Tris-buffered saline-Tween (TBS-T (1×)): 150 mM NaCl, 10 mM Tris pH 8.0, 1% Tween.
7. Anti-Flag, anti-HA, or anti-EYFP (Sigma-Aldrich) antibodies can be used for detection of the peptide expression levels. All antibodies were used 1:1000 diluted in 5% milk powder dissolved in 1× TBS-T.
8. Secondary antibody against anti-Mouse-IgG-IRDyeR-800C W/-680.

### 2.5 Plasmids

1. Reporter gene construct for luciferase assays:
   For identifying physiologically relevant miRNAs that target the mRNA of interest, in vivo validation in the specific cell type of interest is required. Reporter assays based on firefly luciferase are a widely used tool for empirical identification of miRNAs that target the mRNA. One major advantage of using luciferase reporter genes is the lack of endogenous background especially in mammalian cells. For the T6B-assay described here, use any custom-made or commercial luciferase gene reporter construct. Firefly and *Renilla* dual luciferase reporter constructs are a preferred combination of reporter constructs. The emission spectra of luminescence for these genes are separable, and the luminescence measurements can be performed sequentially. Clone the target gene 3′-UTR downstream to one of the

luciferase genes, into the available multiple cloning site. In addition, the second luciferase gene serves as the transfection control and normalizer.

A wild-type reporter construct should contain the 3′-UTR with intact miRNA-binding sites. A mutation in the miRNA seed site of the original 3′-UTR construct should be used as a negative control. Another negative control is an empty reporter gene construct without any target 3′-UTR (Fig. 2).

2. The T6B-peptide construct:

   The T6B peptide is expressed from a Flag/HA-T6B-EYFP vector construct based on pIRESneo [40].

   The T6B mutant vector that serves as a negative control consists of a peptide lacking all the tryptophan residues important for AGO interaction. Additional negative control is an empty Flag/HA-EYFP vector lacking the peptide-coding insert.

## 3 Methods

### *3.1 Cell Culture and Transfection*

1. Seed 50,000 HEK293T/HeLa cells per well in a 48-well cell culture plate at least 24 h before transfection. Seeding density ought to be standardized for different cell types to have ~60% confluence during transfection. Make sure that the cells attain their typical morphology before transfection (*see* **Note 1**).
2. For transfection, determine the ratio of the target 3′-UTR to the miRNA construct or miRNA mimic to achieve a significant readout. For T6B-assay we use in total 240 ng of constructs per well for a 48-well plate (80 ng of each vector) (*see* **Note 2**).
3. Just before transfection remove the medium and replace with a complete medium but without the antibiotics. This reduces the stress on the cells caused during transfection.
4. Mix the various plasmid constructs as required to have proper controls for the experiment (*see* **Notes 4** and **15**). Some of the suggested combinations are:
   (a) T6B-peptide wild type, luciferase reporter construct wild-type target 3′-UTR.
   (b) T6B-peptide wild type, luciferase reporter construct mutated target 3′-UTR.
   (c) T6B-peptide mutated, luciferase reporter construct wild-type target 3′-UTR.
   (d) T6B-peptide mutated, luciferase reporter construct mutated target 3′-UTR.
   (e) T6B-peptide wild type, luciferase reporter construct wild-type positive control target 3′-UTR.

(f) T6B-peptide wild type, luciferase reporter construct mutated positive control target 3′-UTR.

(g) T6B-peptide mutated, luciferase reporter construct wild-type positive control target 3′-UTR.

(h) T6B-peptide mutated, luciferase reporter construct mutated positive control target 3′-UTR.

5. Mix each combination of plasmids with 100 μL of Opti-MEM medium. In another tube, mix 100 μL of Opti-MEM and 1 μL Lipofectamine 2000 (*see* **Note 3**). Add the Lipofectamine 2000/Opti-MEM mix to the plasmid/Opti-MEM mix and incubate at room temperature for 20–30 min. Mix properly at each step to have a uniform suspension. Prepare all the reactions in triplicates.
6. One day after transfection, change the transfection medium with complete growth medium with antibiotics.

### 3.2 Luciferase Assay

1. *Renilla* luciferase buffer:

   (a) Prepare the *Renilla* luciferase buffer without *Renilla* substrate coelenterazine and adjust the pH to 5.0 with KOH. The buffer can be prepared as required, filter sterilized, and stored at −20 °C for months (see Note 6).

   (b) Dissolve coelenterazine in methanol (absolute) to give a 1000× stock solution. Prepare 50 μL aliquots of this and store at −80 °C in the dark.

   (c) Just before the assay, thaw the Renilla luciferase buffer on ice, add coelenterazine, and store on ice (10 μL of stock to 10 mL of the buffer).

2. Firefly luciferase buffer:

   (a) Prepare the firefly luciferase buffer without the firefly substrate d-luciferin and DTT and adjust the pH to 8.0. Cool the buffer on ice and add the d-luciferin. Once the d-luciferin has dissolved, the buffer should be stored as smaller aliquots at −80 °C for months.

   (b) Just before the assay, thaw the firefly buffer (in the dark) and add DTT to a final concentration of 33.3 mM. Mix properly and store on ice (*see* **Note 5**).

3. Dilute the 5× Passive Lysis Buffer to 1× concentration with sterile water (*see* **Notes 10** and **13**).
4. After 48 h (post-transfection), aspirate the medium as much as possible. Add 100 μL (for 48-well plate) of Passive Lysis Buffer per well or enough to cover the cell layer uniformly. Incubate the plate at room temperature for 15–20 min on a rocking platform or an orbital shaker with gentle shaking to ensure proper lysis (*see* **Notes 11** and **12**).

5. Pipette out 20 μL of the lysate to white plates (96 wells) specially designed for efficient measurement of luminescence by luciferase. Dilute the lysate as required depending on the signal intensity. We suggest performing a pilot experiment for each luciferase vector construct to find a proper dilution when necessary (*see* **Notes 9** and **14**).
6. At this point, a small aliquot of the lysate could be removed for confirming the uniform expression of the T6B-peptide that can be easily detected by a Flag antibody or a GFP-antibody by Western blot (*see* Subheading 3.3).
7. Before loading the plate on to the luminometer with injectors, for instance, Mithras LB 940 Multimode Microplate Reader, wash the injectors as suggested by the manufacturer and adjust the read settings (*see* **Notes 7** and **8**).

(See Fig. 3 for an example of validating miRNA-guided gene regulation of a specific 3′-UTR.)

### 3.3 Western Blot Analysis for Peptide Expression

1. Any standard Western blotting protocol could be used to confirm successful transfection of Flag/HA-T6B-EYFP-peptide expression levels. It is described here in brief.
2. For Western blot analysis, add SDS sample loading buffer directly to a lysate after centrifugation at 15,000 × *g* for 10 min and suspend them well by flicking or tapping the tubes gently.

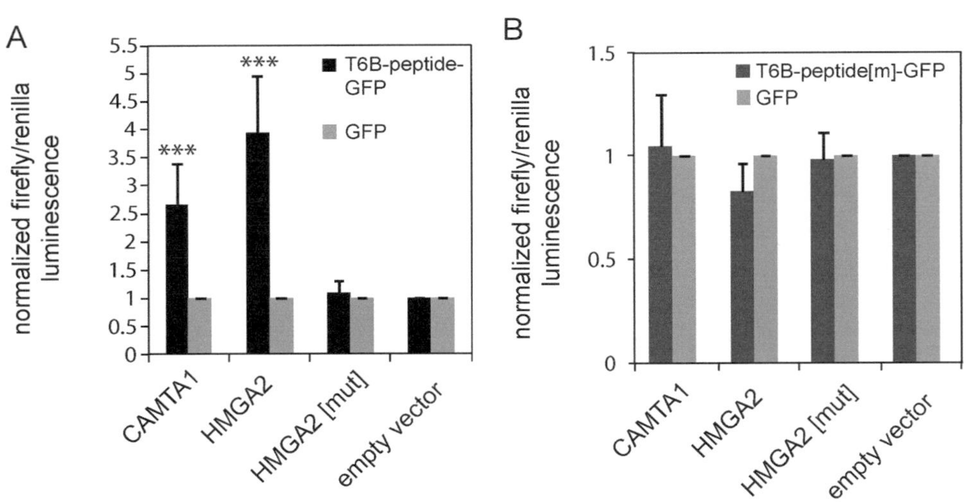


**Fig. 3** T6B-luciferase derepression assay. (**a**) Overexpression of T6B-peptide leads to a significant derepression of the CAMTA1-3′-UTR and the HMGA2-3′-UTR (target of let-7 miRNA family). Mutated HMGA2-3′-UTR and empty vector served as negative controls. (**b**) Overexpression of mutated T6B-peptide shows repression of HMGA2-3′-UTR instead of derepression

Boil the samples at 95 °C for 5 min and centrifuge them before loading the supernatant to a 10% SDS-PAGE.

3. After the transfer to a nitrocellulose membrane (semidry or wet-blot chambers can be used), block the membrane 1 h at room temperature or overnight at 4 °C using 5% milk in 0.1% TBS-T.
4. For protein detection incubate the membrane with the anti-Flag, anti-HA, or anti-EYFP antibody at 4 °C overnight or 1 h at room temperature with gentle rocking.
5. Wash the membrane and incubate for 1 h at room temperature with a secondary antibody (anti-rat-HRP or anti-Mouse-IgG-IRDyeR-800CW/-680). Follow then the standard protocols for the detection of Flag/HA-T6B-EYFP-peptide on the Western blot nitrocellulose membrane.

## 4 Notes

1. Adapt the transfection protocol according to the cell type and the transfection reagent. Make sure that the cells are only 60–65% confluent during transfection. Overly crowded cells are prone to more stress during transfection.
2. The amount of plasmid and ratios of various plasmids to be co-transfected might differ depending on the luciferase reporter system used and the target mRNA 3′-UTR. This depends on the expression levels of the miRNAs that target the 3′-UTR during the particular growth condition tested.
3. Choose a transfection reagent according to the cell type. Several cell-type-specific transfection reagents are commercially available.
4. A plasmid harboring a known miRNA target or a plasmid harboring a miRNA seed sequence downstream to luciferase could serve as a positive control. This construct can be used to standardize the luciferase assays.
5. Always prepare the luciferase reagents just before use. Coelenterazine and d-luciferin are light sensitive and temperature sensitive and once added to the respective buffers should be stored on ice. Pipette the coelenterazine carefully as it is prepared in methanol and has very low viscosity. Add the DTT to the firefly buffer just before use.
6. Sodiumazide ($NaN_3$) added to the *Renilla* buffer is toxic; handle it with care and necessary precautions.
7. When using a manual luminometer, measure the reaction as fast as possible since the luciferase-catalyzed reactions are very short. In such cases, measure few wells or individual tubes one each after adding the substrate. Using automated luminome-

ters with injectors adds the substrate and immediately measures the luminescence sequentially for both the firefly and *Renilla* luciferases, which reduces variability.

8. When using single injectors or manual luminometers, divide the lysate for measuring each luciferase activity into two different plates after lysis.
9. Determine the luminescence for each reporter construct in a pilot experiment before the actual experiment, as this varies depending on the promoters of the constructs and the expression levels in various cell types.
10. Passive Lysis Buffer (Promega) is recommended for lysing cells as it is specially formulated for luciferase assays with minimal background autoluminescence. The lysates prepared using the Passive Lysis Buffer can be used to determine total protein concentrations when necessary.
11. Cells should be no more than 95 % confluent during lysis. Add 20–50 μL of lysis buffer if using a 96-well plate or 65–100 μL for a 48-well plate. The lysis conditions can be adapted according to cell types.
12. Clarification of lysates is not usually necessary, but when necessary transfer the lysates to micro-centrifuge tubes and spin for 30 s at maximum speed.
13. Dilute the lysate where necessary to avoid saturation levels during measurement of luciferase activity. For dilution use 1× PBS or a buffer without detergents or sterile water for dilution of lysates. Make a dilution curve to determine the right amount of lysate required when necessary.
14. Determine background luminescence by including proper controls while measuring on a luminometer like non-transfected cell lysates or measuring buffer reagents without cells.
15. The amount of T6B-peptide might vary depending on cell type, growth conditions, and the targets tested. Optimize and determine the right amount of all vector construct combinations in cell types used.

## Acknowledgments

Our research is supported by grants from the Deutsche Forschungsgemeinschaft (SFB 960, FOR2127), the European Research Council (ERC grant 242792 “sRNAs,” ITN RNATrain), the Bavarian Genome Research Network (BayGene), the German Cancer Aid, and the Bavarian Systems-Biology Network (BioSysNet).

## References


1. Bartel DP (2009) MicroRNAs: target recognition and regulatory functions. Cell 136:215–233
2. Carthew RW, Sontheimer EJ (2009) Origins and mechanisms of miRNAs and siRNAs. Cell 136:642–655
3. Dueck A, Meister G (2014) Assembly and function of small RNA – argonaute protein complexes. Biol Chem 395:611–629
4. Ipsaro JJ, Joshua-Tor L (2015) From guide to target: molecular insights into eukaryotic RNA-interference machinery. Nat Struct Mol Biol 22:20–28
5. Jinek M, Doudna JA (2009) A three-dimensional view of the molecular machinery of RNA interference. Nature 457:405–412
6. Kwak PB, Tomari Y (2012) The N domain of argonaute drives duplex unwinding during RISC assembly. Nat Struct Mol Biol 19:145–151
7. Song JJ, Liu J, Tolia NH, Schneiderman J, Smith SK, Martienssen RA, Hannon GJ, Joshua-Tor L (2003) The crystal structure of the Argonaute2 PAZ domain reveals an RNA binding motif in RNAi effector complexes. Nat Struct Biol 10:1026–1032
8. Ma JB, Ye K, Patel DJ (2004) Structural basis for overhang-specific small interfering RNA recognition by the PAZ domain. Nature 429:318–322
9. Lingel A, Simon B, Izaurralde E, Sattler M (2003) Structure and nucleic-acid binding of the Drosophila argonaute 2 PAZ domain. Nature 426:465–469
10. Yan KS, Yan S, Farooq A, Han A, Zeng L, Zhou MM (2003) Structure and conserved RNA binding of the PAZ domain. Nature 426:468–474
11. Ma JB, Yuan YR, Meister G, Pei Y, Tuschl T, Patel DJ (2005) Structural basis for 5′-end-specific recognition of guide RNA by the A. fulgidus Piwi protein. Nature 434:666–670
12. Parker JS, Roe SM, Barford D (2005) Structural insights into mRNA recognition from a PIWI domain-siRNA guide complex. Nature 434:663–666
13. Song JJ, Smith SK, Hannon GJ, Joshua-Tor L (2004) Crystal structure of argonaute and its implications for RISC slicer activity. Science 305:1434–1437
14. Yuan YR, Pei Y, Ma JB, Kuryavyi V, Zhadina M, Meister G, Chen HY, Dauter Z, Tuschl T, Patel DJ (2005) Crystal structure of A. aeolicus argonaute, a site-specific DNA-guided endoribonuclease, provides insights into RISC-mediated mRNA cleavage. Mol Cell 19:405–419
15. Wang B, Li S, Qi HH, Chowdhury D, Shi Y, Novina CD (2009) Distinct passenger strand and mRNA cleavage activities of human argonaute proteins. Nat Struct Mol Biol 16:1259–1266
16. Meister G, Landthaler M, Patkaniowska A, Dorsett Y, Teng G, Tuschl T (2004) Human argonaute2 mediates RNA cleavage targeted by miRNAs and siRNAs. Mol Cell 15:185–197
17. Liu J, Carmell MA, Rivas FV, Marsden CG, Thomson JM, Song JJ, Hammond SM, Joshua-Tor L, Hannon GJ (2004) Argonaute2 is the catalytic engine of mammalian RNAi. Science 305:1437–1441
18. Elkayam E, Kuhn CD, Tocilj A, Haase AD, Greene EM, Hannon GJ, Joshua-Tor L (2012) The structure of human argonaute-2 in complex with miR-20a. Cell 150:100–110
19. Schirle NT, MacRae IJ (2012) The crystal structure of human argonaute2. Science 336:1037–1040
20. Tuschl T, Zamore PD, Lehmann R, Bartel DP, Sharp PA (1999) Targeted mRNA degradation by double-stranded RNA in vitro. Genes Dev 13:3191–3197
21. Zamore PD, Tuschl T, Sharp PA, Bartel DP (2000) RNAi: double-stranded RNA directs the ATP-dependent cleavage of mRNA at 21 to 23 nucleotide intervals. Cell 101:25–33
22. Hammond SM, Bernstein E, Beach D, Hannon GJ (2000) An RNA-directed nuclease mediates post-transcriptional gene silencing in Drosophila cells. Nature 404:293–296
23. Chen PY, Meister G (2005) microRNA-guided posttranscriptional gene regulation. Biol Chem 386:1205–1218
24. Liu J, Rivas FV, Wohlschlegel J, Yates JR 3rd, Parker R, Hannon GJ (2005) A role for the P-body component GW182 in microRNA function. Nat Cell Biol 7:1161–1166
25. Rehwinkel J, Behm-Ansmant I, Gatfield D, Izaurralde E (2005) A crucial role for GW182 and the DCP1:DCP2 decapping complex in miRNA-mediated gene silencing. RNA 11:1640–1647
26. Meister G, Landthaler M, Peters L, Chen PY, Urlaub H, Luhrmann R, Tuschl T (2005) Identification of novel argonaute-associated proteins. Curr Biol 15:2149–2155
27. Liu J, Valencia-Sanchez MA, Hannon GJ, Parker R (2005) MicroRNA-dependent localization of targeted mRNAs to mammalian P-bodies. Nat Cell Biol 7:719–723

28. Sen GL, Blau HM (2005) Argonaute 2/RISC resides in sites of mammalian mRNA decay known as cytoplasmic bodies. Nat Cell Biol 7:633–636
29. Jakymiw A, Lian S, Eystathioy T, Li S, Satoh M, Hamel JC, Fritzler MJ, Chan EK (2005) Disruption of GW bodies impairs mammalian RNA interference. Nat Cell Biol 7:1267–1274
30. Jonas S, Izaurralde E (2015) Towards a molecular understanding of microRNA-mediated gene silencing. Nat Rev Genet 16:421–433
31. Chen Y, Boland A, Kuzuoglu-Ozturk D, Bawankar P, Loh B, Chang CT, Weichenrieder O, Izaurralde E (2014) A DDX6-CNOT1 complex and W-binding pockets in CNOT9 reveal direct links between miRNA target recognition and silencing. Mol Cell 54:737–750
32. Mathys H, Basquin J, Ozgur S, Czarnocki-Cieciura M, Bonneau F, Aartse A, Dziembowski A, Nowotny M, Conti E, Filipowicz W (2014) Structural and biochemical insights to the role of the CCR4-NOT complex and DDX6 ATPase in MicroRNA repression. Mol Cell 54:751–765
33. Huntzinger E, Izaurralde E (2011) Gene silencing by microRNAs: contributions of translational repression and mRNA decay. Nat Rev Genet 12:99–110
34. Pfaff J, Hennig J, Herzog F, Aebersold R, Sattler M, Niessing D, Meister G (2013) Structural features of argonaute-GW182 protein interactions. Proc Natl Acad Sci U S A 110:E3770–E3779
35. Calin GA, Croce CM (2006) MicroRNA signatures in human cancers. Nat Rev Cancer 6:857–866
36. Kasinski AL, Slack FJ (2011) Epigenetics and genetics. MicroRNAs en route to the clinic: progress in validating and targeting microRNAs for cancer therapy. Nat Rev Cancer 11:849–864
37. Chen K, Rajewsky N (2007) The evolution of gene regulation by transcription factors and microRNAs. Nat Rev Genet 8:93–103
38. Lewis BP, Burge CB, Bartel DP (2005) Conserved seed pairing, often flanked by adenosines, indicates that thousands of human genes are microRNA targets. Cell 120:15–20
39. Till S, Lejeune E, Thermann R, Bortfeld M, Hothorn M, Enderle D, Heinrich C, Hentze MW, Ladurner AG (2007) A conserved motif in argonaute-interacting proteins mediates functional interactions through the Argonaute PIWI domain. Nat Struct Mol Biol 14:897–903
40. Hauptmann J, Schraivogel D, Bruckmann A, Manickavel S, Jakob L, Eichner N, Pfaff J, Urban M, Sprunck S, Hafner M et al (2015) Biochemical isolation of argonaute protein complexes by Ago-APP. Proc Natl Acad Sci U S A 112:11841–11845

# Chapter 15

# Small Molecules Targeting the miRNA-Binding Domain of Argonaute 2: From Computer-Aided Molecular Design to RNA Immunoprecipitation

Teresa Bellissimo, Silvia Masciarelli, Elena Poser, Ilaria Genovese, Alberto Del Rio, Gianni Colotti, and Francesco Fazi

## Abstract

The development of small-molecule-based target therapy design for human disease and cancer is object of growing attention. Recently, specific microRNA (miRNA) mimicking compounds able to bind the miRNA-binding domain of Argonaute 2 protein (AGO2) to inhibit miRNA loading and its functional activity were described. Computer-aided molecular design techniques and RNA immunoprecipitation represent suitable approaches to identify and experimentally determine if a compound is able to impair the loading of miRNAs on AGO2 protein. Here, we describe these two methodologies that we recently used to select a specific compound able to interfere with the AGO2 functional activity and able to improve the retinoic acid-dependent myeloid differentiation of leukemic cells.

**Key words** microRNAs, Argonaute 2, Myeloid differentiation, Small molecules, Molecular docking techniques, RNA immunoprecipitation

## 1 Introduction

MicroRNAs (miRNAs) and their protein complex are involved in several developmental and physiological processes by fine-tuning translation of specific mRNAs [1, 2]. miRNAs perform their regulatory functions by the interaction with one of the proteins belonging to the mammalian Argonaute (AGO) family of proteins, AGO1-4, into a functional complex known as the RNA-induced silencing complex (RISC) [3–5].

AGO proteins are characterized by a conserved structure containing an amino-terminal domain (N-domain), a so-called MID (middle) domain, and the PAZ (Piwi-Argonaute-Zwille) and Piwi (P-element-induced wimpy testes) domains that structurally resemble an RNase H fold [6]. The interaction with the miRNA structure is established by the PAZ and MID domains that bind to

Marco F. Schmidt (ed.), *Drug Target miRNA: Methods and Protocols*, Methods in Molecular Biology, vol. 1517, DOI 10.1007/978-1-4939-6563-2_15, 

the 3′- and the 5′-end of the miRNAs, respectively [6–8]. The miRNAs loaded in the RISC complex usually function as negative regulators of gene expression [9–11]. miRNAs can recognize partially complementary sequences in messenger RNA (mRNA) targets and lead to the degradation and/or repression of their translation establishing posttranscriptional regulatory networks relevant for the cell fate determination [12, 13].

The emerging relevance of miRNAs during hematopoietic differentiation and the revealed AGO2 contribution to differentiation of erythroid and B lymphoid cell lineages [14] prompted us to investigate the role of AGO2 in human myeloid cell fate differentiation. In a recent work, by using an acute promyelocytic leukemia (APL) cellular model, characterized by the clonal expansion of hematopoietic precursors blocked at the promyelocytic stage of differentiation, we showed that AGO2 is downregulated during RA-induced granulocyte differentiation of human APL NB4 cell line and freshly isolated blasts from APL patients [15]. Moreover, the reduction of AGO2 expression levels by short hairpin RNA (shRNAs) lentiviral vectors improved RA-induced myeloid differentiation of APL cells [15]. These results are bringing out a functional role for the downregulation of AGO2 expression during RA induction of myeloid differentiation that may be useful as molecular determinant for the improvement of RA treatment response in other leukemic subtypes.

In recent years the development of small-molecule-based target therapy design for human disease and cancer was object of growing attention [16]. In fact, there is an increasing interest in developing small molecules able to inhibit RISC loading, and recently specific mRNA-mimicking compounds able to bind the active site of AGO2 were described [17, 18]. Consistently with the increasing availability of structural data on Argonaute proteins [19] and taking advantage of the recent crystallographic structure of the human full-length AGO2 in complex with miR-20a [20], in a recent work, we carried out structure-based virtual screenings to search new ligands able to interfere with the AGO2 functional activity [21]. We identified a specific compound (BCI-137, Fig. 1)

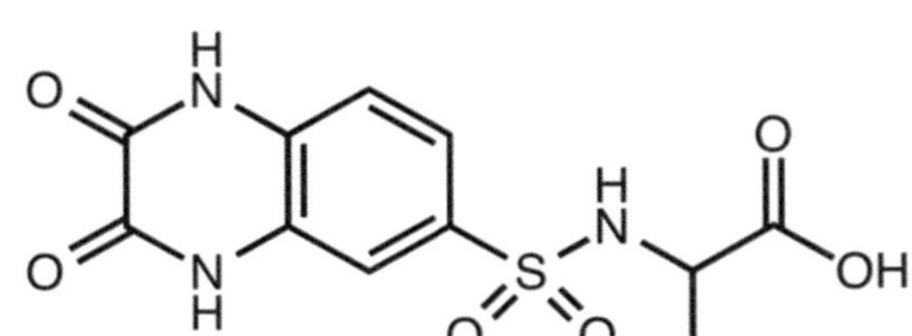


**BCI-137**

**Fig. 1** Chemical structure of the BCI-137

able to inhibit AGO2 loading, as possible alternative to the downregulation of AGO2 expression, for the improvement of RA-dependent differentiation response of APL cells [21]. This compound was identified because of its pharmacophore mimicking the structure of the uridine monophosphate that constitutes the 5′ end of the miRNAs binding into the AGO2 MID domain.

Therefore, molecular docking techniques and RNA immunoprecipitation (RIP) represent a combination of suitable methodologies to identify and experimentally determine if a compound is able to impair AGO2 loading of miRNAs. To this end, we describe here below the step-by-step molecular design and RIP experiments that we performed by using molecular docking techniques and an antibody to immunoprecipitate AGO2 in lysates from APL cell line treated or not with the selected ligand to evaluate the amount of coprecipitated miRNAs [21].

## 2 Materials

### 2.1 Instrument

1. *Workstation.* A PC workstation with the following minimum hardware requirements: x86_64 compatible processor, 4 GB memory per core, 10 GB disk space for software installation, 100 GB for databases, molecules and protein data, 60 GB minimum scratch disk space for running jobs, network card with a configured network interface, 16-bit color and a monitor with a refresh rate of 60 Hz or more and 1280 × 1024 resolution, graphics card supporting hardware-accelerated OpenGL with 1 GB onboard memory and an up-to-date vendor-supplied graphics driver, and a Linux, Windows, or Mac operating system.
2. *Molecular modeling software.* Schrödinger's small-molecule drug discovery suite (http://www.schrodinger.com/smdd/) installed on the workstation, including the following packages: Maestro, Protein Preparation Wizard, and Glide. Version should be at least the release 2015-1 (Maestro version 10.1.013, MMshare Version 2.9.013) (*see* **Note 1**).
3. *Magnetic separator* (in the absence of a magnetic separator, beads can be centrifuged at 1000 rpm for 1 min in a microfuge).

### 2.2 Buffers

All solutions are prepared by using ultrapure diethylpyrocarbonate (DEPC) water and analytical grade reagents, and all standard precautions should be taken to minimize RNase contamination. Cool buffers prior to use.

1. Ice-cold phosphate-buffered saline (PBS) buffer 1×: 137 mM NaCl, 2.7 mM KCl, 10 mM $Na_2HPO_4$, 1.8 mM $KH_2PO_4$, 1 mM $CaCl_2 \cdot 2H_2O$, 0.5 mM $MgCl_2 \cdot 6H_2O$. Store at 4 °C.
2. RIP Lysis Buffer 1×: 10 mM 2-[4-(2-hydroxyethyl)piperazin-1-yl]ethanesulfonic acid (HEPES), 100 mM KCl, 5 mM

$MgCl_2$, 0.5% NP-40, 25 mM ethylenediaminetetraacetic acid (EDTA), 1 mM 1,4-dithiothreitol (DTT), 100 U/ml RNase inhibitor, 400 mM VRC (vanadyl ribonucleoside complexes). Protease inhibitors (add fresh each time): 1 mM phenylmethylsulfonyl fluoride (PMSF), 50 mM leupeptin, 50 mM pepstatin, 0.5 mM aprotinin.

3. RIP Wash Buffer: 50 mM Tris–HCl pH 7.4, 150 mM NaCl, 1 mM $MgCl_2$, 0.05% NP40.
4. Proteinase K Buffer: 100 mM Tris–HCl pH 7.4, 10 mM EDTA, 50 nM NaCl, 1% SDS, proteinase K (100 μg/mL).
5. 0.5 M EDTA.
6. 10% sodium dodecyl sulfate (SDS).
7. 10 mg/mL proteinase K.
8. Phenol-chloroform-isoamyl alcohol (125:24:1) pH=4.5.
9. Chloroform.
10. 100% ethanol.

## 3 Methods

### 3.1 Protein and Molecular Docking Grid Preparation

1. Import the coordinates of the crystal structure of the human Argonaute 2 (AGO2) from the Protein Data Bank (PDB id: 4F3T) by means of the *protein preparation wizard* (PPW) routine as shown in Fig. 2a. Preprocess the imported structure in order to include the options indicated, e.g., assign bond orders and add hydrogens. After the preprocessing, refine the chemical structure with the module *refine* of the PPW. Optimize H-bonds through water orientation using PROPKA at pH 7.0 and perform a restrained minimization by using OPLS_2005 force field and a convergence of 0.30 Å.
2. Select and remove the miR-20a (red ribbon, Fig. 2b). This can be done through the Edit > Delete > Select menu and by selecting all the RNA sequence.
3. With the *glide* application, open the *receptor grid generation* routine and create a grid box centered in the MID domain of AGO2 as depicted in Fig. 3a. This can be done by setting the option "centroid of selected residues" in the *site* tab (Fig. 3b) and selecting the Ala859, which is a residue located in the inner binding pocket of the MID domain. Set also the option "dock ligands with length <=" to 20 Å and leave all other settings to their default values (Fig. 3b).
4. Run the grid generation and wait for the completion of the job (*see* **Note 1**).

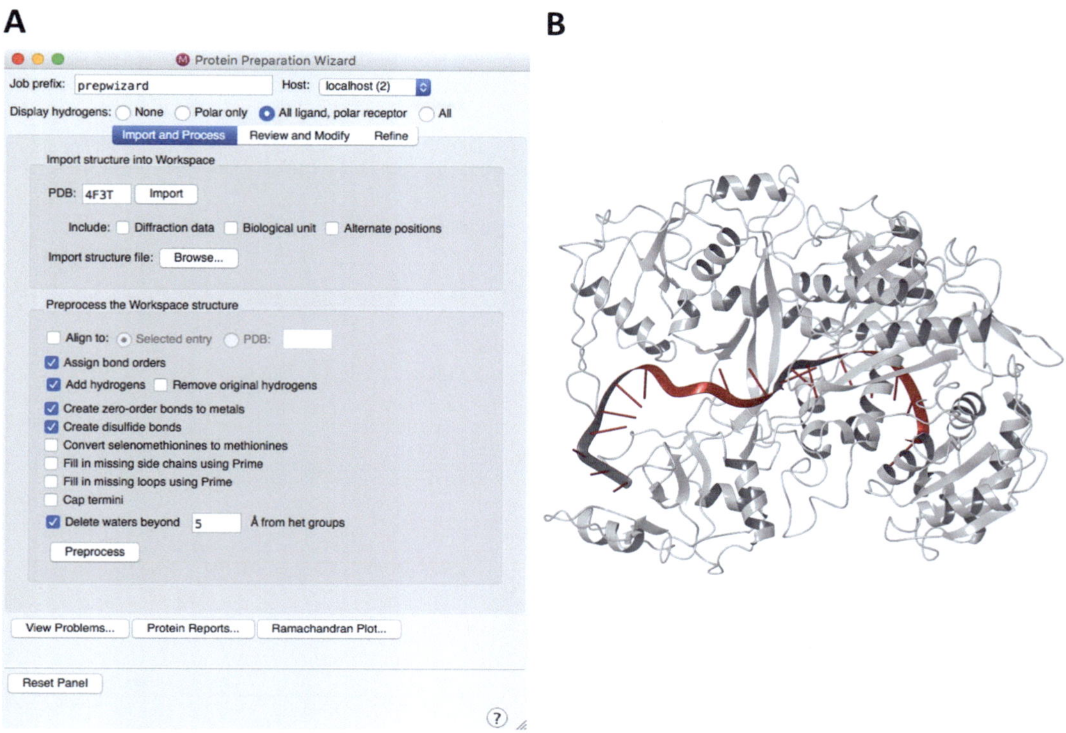


**Fig. 2** (**a**) Screenshot of the *protein preparation wizard* routine of the Schrodinger software; (**b**) Crystallographic structure of AGO2 (*white ribbon*) in complex with the miR-20a (*red ribbon*) after the preparation of the protein template with computational procedures

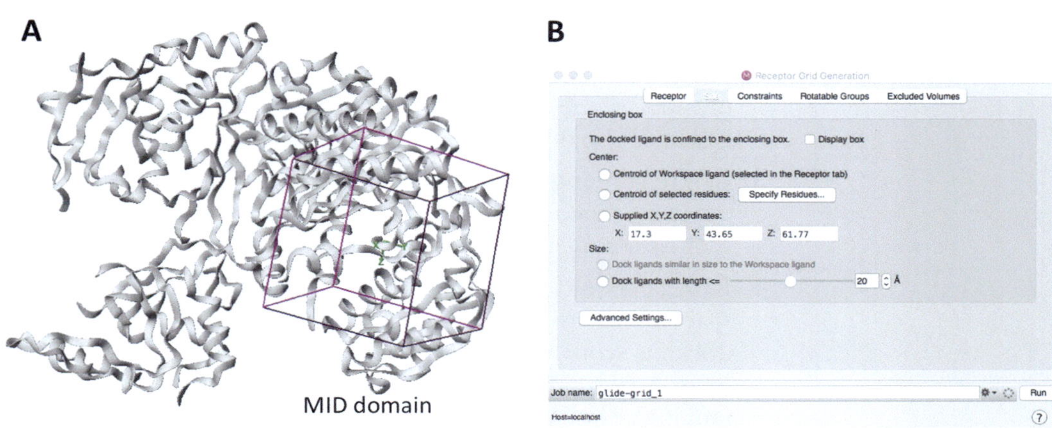


**Fig. 3** (**a**) AGO2 with receptor grid box depiction centered in the MID domain; (**b**) Screenshot of the receptor grid generation routine of the Schrodinger software

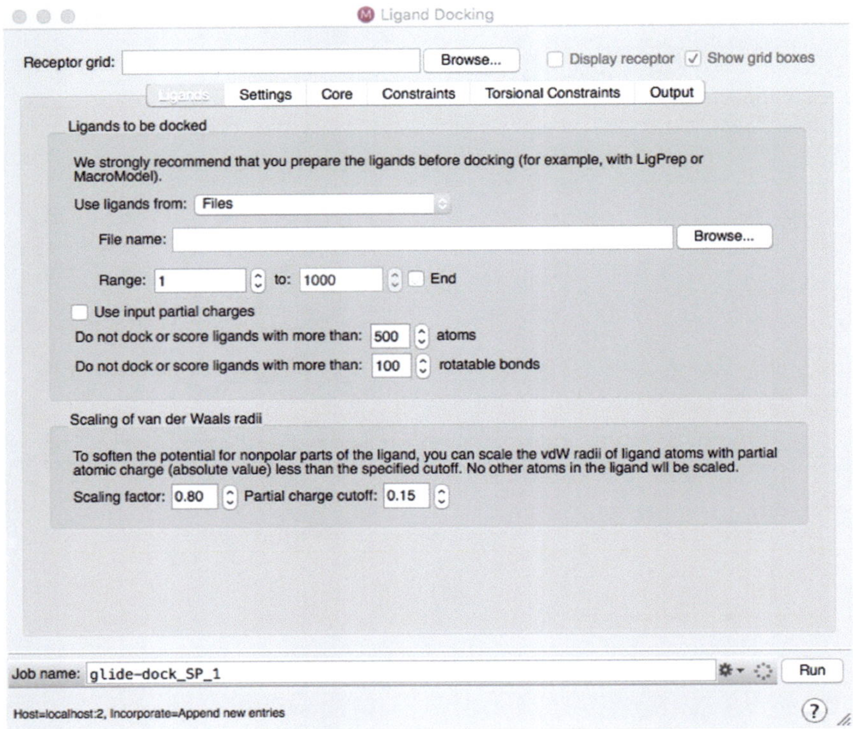


**Fig. 4** Screenshot of the ligand-docking routine of the Schrodinger software

### *3.2 Virtual Screening and Selection of New Molecules*

1. Download the CoCoCo-SC database (http://cococo.isof.cnr.it/) and follow the instructions reported on the website to uncompress and generate a local file in *sdf* format (*see* **Note 2**).
2. With the *glide* application, open the *ligand docking* routine (Fig. 4). Set the receptor grid generated as described in Subheading 3.1. Set the option "use ligands from" to *files* and browse to the *sdf* data file described in the previous point. Leave all the other settings to their default values.
3. Before running the job, check the job settings options and set the value "incorporate" to *append new entries.* Run the job and wait its completion.
4. Results should be automatically incorporated into the workspace in a new group. Molecules should be already sorted by docking score with the first entries being the most favorable ones. Analyze the binding modes by visually inspecting the top-ranking compounds and flagging those that are able to perform the best interactions within the AGO2 MID domain. A typical visual inspection should include interactions as depicted in Fig. 5 for the case of uridine monophosphate and BCI-137.
5. Once a desired set of putative AGO2 inhibitors is selected, contact the chemical vendor to check the availability of com-

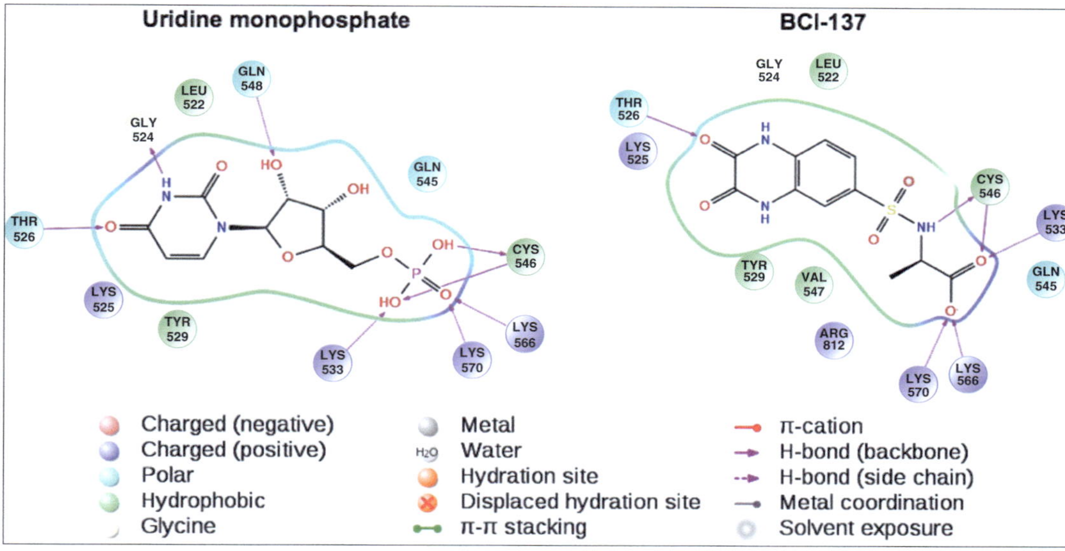


**Fig. 5** Interaction diagrams of the uridine monophosphate (**a**) and BCI-137 (**b**) in complex with AGO2

pounds and proceed with a purchase of a sufficient amount of each. Typically, 5 mg per compound should suffice to perform RIP experiments as described below.

### 3.3 Cell Cultures and Treatment

Adherent or suspension cell lines are maintained, respectively, in DMEM or RPMI 1640 medium supplemented with penicillin (50 U/mL)/streptomycin (50 μg/mL) solution, 2 mM L-glutamine, and 10% fetal bovine serum and may be treated from 48 h with increasing amounts (0.01–10 μM) of the selected compounds to start testing their dose-dependent functional and biological activity. Once assessed the optimal dose for cell response RIP methodology may be applied as described below.

### 3.4 Cell Collection and Lysate Preparation

1. Collect adherent cells at 80–90% of confluence in flask or culture dishes. Remove culture medium and wash twice the cells with PBS buffer to remove serum-containing medium. Trypsinize cells and collect them from the dishes. Centrifuge at 300×*g* for 5 min at 4 °C. For suspension cells collect cells by centrifugation at 300×*g* for 5 min at 4 °C (*see* **Note 3**).
2. Discard the supernatant and suspend cells with 5 mL of ice-cold PBS. Centrifuge at 300×*g* for 5 min at 4 °C. Discard the supernatant.
3. Suspend cell pellets in an equal pellet volume of complete RIP Lysis Buffer. Mix by pipetting up and down until cells are well resuspended. Incubate the lysate on ice for 5 min. Aliquot 220 μL of the lysate into nuclease-free microcentrifuge tubes and freeze at −80 °C (*see* **Note 4**).

### 3.5 Antibody Coating of Magnetic Beads

1. Resuspend magnetic beads by turning upside down or by pipetting.
2. Transfer 50 μL of magnetic bead suspension to nuclease-free microcentrifuge tubes for the number of desired immunoprecipitations. Each immunoprecipitation includes the antibody of interest and the negative control antibody or No Ab sample.
3. Wash magnetic beads with 0.5 ml of RIP Wash Buffer and gently resuspend beads by vortex.
4. Place the tube on a magnetic separator and discard the supernatant. Repeat **steps 3** and **4** for an additional wash.
5. Remove the tube from the magnetic separator and resuspend the beads in 100 μL of the RIP Wash Buffer. Add 5 μg of the antibody of interest or of the IgG control to the nuclease-free microcentrifuge tubes.
6. Incubate on a rotating device from 3 h until overnight at 4 °C to allow Ab to bind to the beads.
7. Centrifuge beads by brief centrifugation (at 1000 rpm at 4 °C for 1 min in a microfuge), place them on the magnetic separator, and remove the supernatant.
8. Remove the tubes from the magnetic separator and suspend the beads in 0.5 mL of the RIP Wash Buffer by a brief vortex.
9. Place the tube on the magnetic separator and discard the supernatant. Perform an additional wash.
10. For each IP resuspend the antibody-coated beads in 850 μL of the RIP Wash Buffer supplemented with 30 μL of 0.5 nM EDTA, 10 μL 0.1 M DTT, 100 U/mL RNase inhibitor, 400 mM VRC (vanadyl ribonucleoside complexes). Protease inhibitors (add fresh each time): 1 mM PMSF, 50 mM leupeptin, 50 mM pepstatin, 0.5 mM aprotinin. Suspend by inversion and cool beads on ice.

### 3.6 Immuno precipitation of Ribonucleoprotein Complexes

1. Thaw RIP lysate previously stored at −80 °C and centrifuge at 13,000 rpm for 10 min at 4 °C in a microfuge. Transfer the supernatant into a clean nuclease-free microcentrifuge tube. This is recommended to avoid co-elution of protein bound to the tube wall (*see* **Note 5**).
2. Transfer 100 μL of the supernatant to each tube with antibody-coated beads in RIP Wash Buffer. Resuspend by inversion.
3. Tumble the tubes end-over-end with rotation overnight at 4 °C.
4. Centrifuge the tubes briefly and place them on the magnetic separator (*see* **Note 6**).
5. Discard supernatant except for IgG (or No Ab)-negative controls, as it will represent the input sample (continue processing of input sample at Subheading 3.7, **step 2**).

6. Remove the tube from the magnetic separator and wash with 1 mL of ice-cold RIP Wash Buffer. Repeat this step 4–6 times to completely wash the beads (*see* **Note 7**).

### 3.7 Proteinase K Digestion and RNA Purification

1. Place the tube on the magnetic separator, discard the supernatant, and resuspend each sample in 150 μL of 1× Proteinase K Buffer.
2. Prepare input sample from Subheading 3.6, **step 5**, by mixing 75 μL of IgG (or No Ab) supernatant with 75 μL of 2× Proteinase K Buffer.
3. Heat all the tube at 55 °C for 30 min with 1000 rpm agitation.
4. Pellet beads by brief centrifugation at 1000 rpm at 4 °C for 1 min in a microfuge and place the tube on the magnetic separator and transfer the supernatant containing RNA.
5. Add 150 μL of phenol-chloroform-isoamyl alcohol to each tube, mix vigorously, and centrifuge at 13,000 rpm at RT for 15 min in a microfuge.
6. Transfer the upper phase into a new tube and add the same volume of chloroform. Vortex for 15 s and centrifuge for 10 min at 13,000 rpm at RT in a microfuge to allow phase separation.
7. Transfer carefully the top aqueous phase into a new tube and add 10 μg glycogen.
8. Add to each tube 2.5 volumes of 100% ethanol. Mix and store at −80 °C 1 h to precipitate the RNA.
9. Centrifuge for 30 min at 13,000 rpm at 4 °C in a microfuge and carefully remove the supernatant.
10. Add 500 μL of 80% ethanol to the pellet and centrifuge for 10 min at 13,000 rpm at 4 °C in a microfuge. Carefully remove the supernatant and leave the tube open at RT to evaporate the remaining ethanol.
11. Resuspend the RNA in 20 μL of RNase-free water and place the tube on ice.

### 3.8 PCR Analysis of Immunoprecipitated RNA

Specific RNAs may be detected from immunoprecipitated and input RNA samples by PCR or qRT-PCR. For RT reaction it is recommended the use of the same volume of RIP products for all samples. For the subsequent qPCR, use 1 μL of the cDNA sample as template.

### 3.9 Western Blot Analysis of Immuno precipitated Protein

Western blot control may be useful to assess the quality of RIP experiment. Total lysate (*see* **Note 5**), supernatant lysate (*see* **Note 6**), and IP lysate (*see* **Note 7**) can be used for the Western blot control to check the level of the protein of interest in the supernatant and to test if the immunoprecipitation reaction worked properly (Fig. 6).

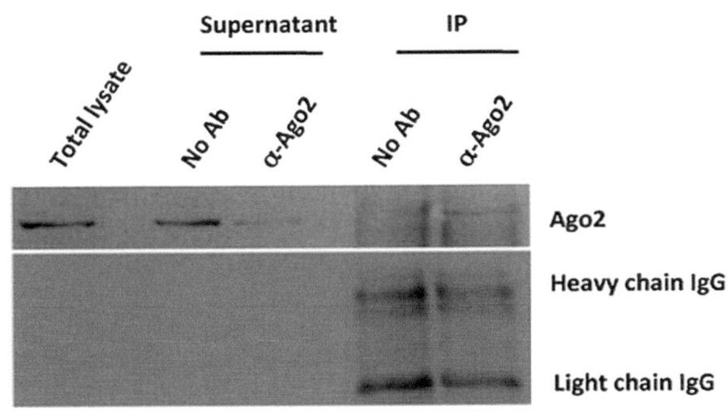


**Fig. 6** Western blot analysis to detect the presence of AGO2 protein in total lysate, supernatant lysate, and IP lysate of the RIP experiment in samples immunoprecipitated with AGO2 antibody or not (no Ab)

## 4 Notes

1. All computational procedures described in Subheadings 3.1 and 3.2 can be performed with noncommercial software like AutoDock Vina (http://vina.scripps.edu/) [22]. However, because its user-friendliness is generally lower, its usage is advised to computer science experts.
2. Virtual screening can be performed on proprietary or specific chemical libraries to replace public databases of commercial chemicals. These libraries can be prepared by means of computational tools like LigPrep (http://www.schrodinger.com/LigPrep/).
3. RIP reaction requires cell lysate from at least $2.5 \times 10^7$ cells in a volume of 100 μL. If the cells have a low level of cytoplasmic fraction, it is important to increase the amount of plated cells to ensure to have a sufficient amount of lysate.
4. This amount of lysate ensures performing RNA immunoprecipitation and Western blot total lysate control. Freeze and thaw step allows cell pellet to lyse more efficiently. Additional freeze and thaw cycles should be avoided to prevent proteins and RNA degradation. Lysate can be stored at −80 °C for 6 months.
5. Expression level of the RNA-binding protein of interest may be assessed on the whole cell lysate as RIP Lysis Buffer is compatible with Western blot analysis.
6. To test if the immunoprecipitation reaction worked properly, the supernatant from IP reactions may be used in Western blot control.
7. During the last wash step, collect 1/10 of the bead suspension to assess the efficiency of the immunoprecipitation reaction.

## Acknowledgment

The work was supported by AIRC Start-up grants 4841 and 6266.

### References

1. Bartel DP (2009) MicroRNAs: target recognition and regulatory functions. Cell 136:215–233
2. Fazi F, Nervi C (2008) MicroRNA: basic mechanisms and transcriptional regulatory networks for cell fate determination. Cardiovasc Res 79:553–561
3. Kawamata T, Tomari Y (2010) Making RISC. Trends Biochem Sci 35:368–376
4. Chendrimada TP, Gregory RI, Kumaraswamy E et al (2005) TRBP recruits the Dicer complex to Ago2 for microRNA processing and gene silencing. Nature 436:740–744
5. Su H, Trombly MI, Chen J et al (2009) Essential and overlapping functions for mammalian argonautes in microRNA silencing. Genes Dev 23:304–317
6. Meister G (2013) Argonaute proteins: functional insights and emerging roles. Nat Rev Genet 14:447–459
7. Frank F, Sonenberg N, Nagar B (2010) Structural basis for 5′-nucleotide base-specific recognition of guide RNA by human AGO2. Nature 465:818–822
8. Winter J, Jung S, Keller S et al (2009) Many roads to maturity: microRNA biogenesis pathways and their regulation. Nat Cell Biol 11:228–234
9. Friedman RC, Farh KK, Burge CB et al (2009) Most mammalian mRNAs are conserved targets of microRNAs. Genome Res 19:92–105
10. Guo H, Ingolia NT, Weissman JS et al (2010) Mammalian microRNAs predominantly act to decrease target mRNA levels. Nature 466:835–840
11. Krol J, Loedige I, Filipowicz W (2010) The widespread regulation of microRNA biogenesis, function and decay. Nat Rev Genet 11:597–610
12. Huntzinger E, Izaurralde E (2011) Gene silencing by micro-RNAs: contributions of translational repression and mRNA decay. Nat Rev Genet 12:99–110
13. Fontemaggi G, Bellissimo T, Donzelli S et al (2015) Identification of post-transcriptional regulatory networks during myeloblast-to-monocyte differentiation transition. RNA Biol 12:690–700
14. O'Carroll D, Mecklenbrauker I, Das PP et al (2007) A slicer-independent role for argonaute 2 in hematopoiesis and the microRNA pathway. Genes Dev 21:1999–2004
15. Iosue I, Quaranta R, Masciarelli S et al (2013) Argonaute 2 sustains the gene expression program driving human monocytic differentiation of acute myeloid leukemia cells. Cell Death Dis 4, e926
16. De Santa F, Iosue I, Del Rio A et al (2013) MicroRNA biogenesis pathway as therapeutic target for human disease and cancer. Curr Pharm Des 19:745–764
17. Tan GS, Chiu C, Garchow BG et al (2012) Small molecule inhibition of RISC loading. ACS Chem Biol 7:403–410
18. Schmidt MF, Korb O, Abell C (2013) MicroRNA specific argonaute 2 protein inhibitors. ACS Chem Biol 8:2122–2126
19. Schirle NT, MacRae IJ (2012) The crystal structure of human argonaute 2. Science 336:1037–1040
20. Elkayam E, Kuhn CD, Tocilj A et al (2012) The structure of human argonaute-2 in complex with miR-20a. Cell 150:100–110
21. Masciarelli S, Quaranta R, Iosue I et al (2014) A small-molecule targeting the microRNA binding domain of argonaute 2 improves the retinoic acid differentiation response of the acute promyelocytic leukemia cell line NB4. ACS Chem Biol 9:1674–1679
22. Trott O, Olson AJ (2010) AutoDock Vina: improving the speed and accuracy of docking with a new scoring function, efficient optimization and multithreading. J Comput Chem 31:455–461

# Chapter 16

# Surface Plasmon Resonance: A Useful Strategy for the Identification of Small Molecule Argonaute 2 Protein Binders

**Elena Poser, Ilaria Genovese, Silvia Masciarelli, Teresa Bellissimo, Francesco Fazi*, and Gianni Colotti***

## Abstract

Surface plasmon resonance (SPR) is one of the most important techniques for the detection and the characterization of molecular interactions. SPR technology is a label-free approach for monitoring biomolecular interactions in real time. The binding of analytes to molecules immobilized on a thin metal film (ligand) determines a change in the refractive index and, therefore in the angle of extinction of light, is reflected when polarized light hits the film, monitored in real time as a change in the position of the dip in reflected intensity. Since SPR detects mass, the technique is label-free.

Here, we describe the use of SPR techniques to study the interaction between Argonaute 2 and small molecular compounds selected by means of high-throughput docking screening.

**Key words** Surface plasmon resonance, Analyte, Ligand, Protein-inhibitor interaction, Small molecules

## 1 Introduction

Surface plasmon resonance (SPR) is an increasingly used technique for the characterization of a wide range of biomolecular interactions, such as antibody selection and screening, drug discovery, ligand fishing, binding specificity, and gene regulation [1].

SPR instruments possess three units integrated in one system: an optical unit, a liquid handling unit, and the sensor surface, which forms a physical barrier between the optical (dry) section and the flow (wet) cell (Fig. 1). The SPR phenomenon depends on the presence of oscillation of mobile electrons (plasmon) at the surface of metal (usually gold) films when incident light strikes a glass coated by the metal. The coupling of the wave vector of the incident light with the wavelength of the surface plasmon produces a loss in the intensity

*Author contributed equally with all other contributors.

Marco F. Schmidt (ed.), *Drug Target miRNA: Methods and Protocols*, Methods in Molecular Biology, vol. 1517,
DOI 10.1007/978-1-4939-6563-2_16, © Springer Science+Business Media New York 2017

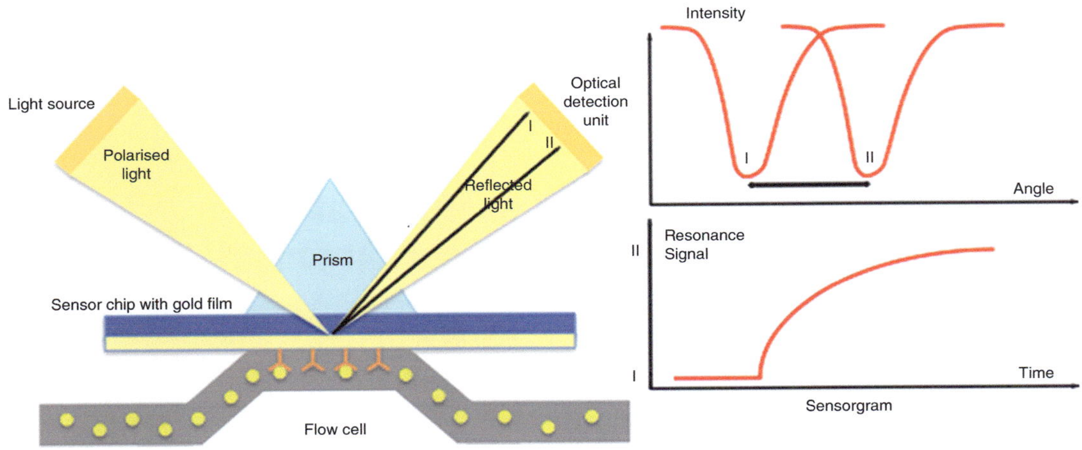


**Fig. 1** Diagram showing a SPR sensor (*left panel*), with the three units integrated in one system: an optical unit (light source, prism, detector unit), a microfluidic unit, and the sensor surface, which forms a physical barrier between the optical section and the flow cell. The detector measures small changes in the resonance frequency (dips), which can also be quantified as resonance units (*top right panel*): accumulation of biomolecules near the sensor surface increases the refractive index of the medium in a mass-dependent fashion and therefore the resonance signal (*bottom*, *right panel*)

and therefore a dip, of the reflected light, associated with an evanescent wave, which propagates into the medium from the metal film, whose resonant frequency depends on the refractive index of the medium. A detector measures small changes in this resonance frequency (dips), which are quantified in resonance units (RUs): accumulation of biomolecules near the sensor surface increases the refractive index of the medium in a mass-dependent fashion [2, 3].

SPR allows analysis of binding interactions in real time on a variety of surface chemistries and is equipped with low dead-volume microfluidics. Recent advances in SPR have improved some of the traditional drawbacks of the technique, i.e., the difficulty in performing high-throughput assays, with the evolution of single-cycle (Biacore) or dynamic injection technologies such as FastStep and OneStep (SensiQ) [4–6], and the improvement of signal/noise ratio that makes study of the binding of small analytes possible.

The Argonaute proteins (eight proteins in human) are key components of the microRNA-induced silencing complex (miRISC). The miRISC complex determines gene silencing via RNA interference (RNAi). Argonaute proteins bind different classes of small noncoding RNAs, which guide Argonaute proteins to their specific targets through sequence complementarity (base pairing), which then leads to mRNA cleavage or translation inhibition [7]. The Argonaute 2 protein (AGO2) binds to a microRNA (miRNA) or short interfering RNA (siRNA). Binding of RISC to a perfectly complementary mRNA generally results in silencing due to endonucleolytic cleavage of the mRNA specifically by AGO2. In addition, AGO2 has a key role in human myeloid cell fate determination, in LPS-induced inflammatory response of 1,25-dihydroxyvitamin D3-treated myeloid cells, and in myeloblast-to-monocyte differentiation [8–10].

Using structure-based high-throughput docking screening, by taking advantage of the crystallographic structure of the human full-length AGO2-miR-20a complex [11], we selected a compound named BCI-137 because of its marked pharmacophore mimicking the 5′ end of miRNAs in the AGO2 Mid domain [12] (Fig. 2).

For the characterization of the interaction between the AGO2 and the small molecule ligand BCI-137 [9], we have used a SensiQ Pioneer system (SensiQ, ICx Nomadics Inc.), equipped with "FastStep" method involving the injection of an analyte series from low to high concentration without buffer injections in between. However, the chapter contains a method that can be applied also to traditional SPR experiments, and can be carried out with SPR equipment of different brands, as long as they provide sufficient signal-to-noise ratio. We will not go into details about the writing of the procedures concerning instrument setup, protocol setup, operations, and analysis using the SensiQ programs (SensiQ Pioneer software, Qdat), but will present and analyze the method used as generally applicable to every SPR instrument.

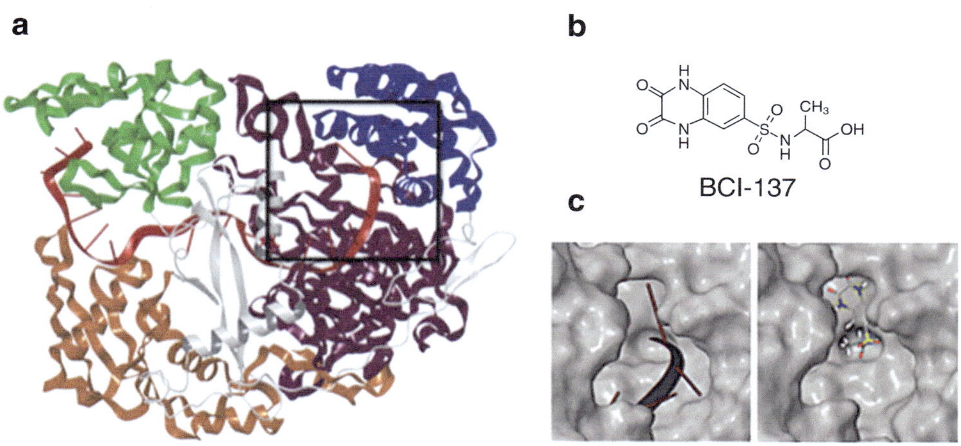


**Fig. 2** BCI-137 interacts with the Mid domain of AGO2. (**a**) Model of the human AGO2 in complex with miR-20a, based on the crystal structure (PDB ID: 4F3T, ref. 11). The N-terminal domain is shown in *orange*, the PAZ domain in *green*, the Mid domain in *blue*, the PIWI domain in *brown*, linker regions in *white*, and the miR-20a in *red*. The *black square* indicates the region of the Mid domain used to set up the high-throughput molecular docking screening [12]. (**b**) Chemical structure of the 2,3-dioxo-1,4-dihydroquinoxalin derivative BCI-137. (**c**) Molecular surfaces of the Mid domain-binding site of AGO2 in complex with the miR-20a (*left*) and the binding mode of compound BCI-137 obtained with docking simulation (*right*). Compound BCI-137 tightly binds to several residues of the Mid domain, in a mode which is similar to uridine placement at the 5′ end of miR-20a (Adapted with permission from ref. 12: Masciarelli S, Quaranta R, Iosue I, Colotti G, Padula F, Varchi G, Fazi F, Del Rio A. A small-molecule targeting the microRNA binding domain of argonaute 2 improves the retinoic acid differentiation response of the acute promyelocytic leukemia cell line NB4. ACS Chem Biol. 2014 Aug 15;9(8):1674–9. doi:10.1021/cb500286b. Copyright 2014 American Chemical Society)

## 2 Materials

Prepare all solutions using ultrapure water (prepared by purifying deionized water to attain a sensitivity of 18 M Ω cm at 25 °C) and analytical grade reagents.

### 2.1 Buffers

1. Concentrated acid and basic solutions: 2 M NaOH and 2 M HCl solutions are prepared for pH adjustments and for solution preparation.
2. Coupling buffers: dependent on isoelectric point of the ligand, either formic acid (pH 3.0–4.5), acetic acid (pH 4.0–5.5), or maleic acid (pH 5.5–7.0) is diluted in water, adjusted to proper pH with NaOH, and brought to final 20 mM concentration with water. Store at 4 °C.
3. 2× HBS. 2×4-(2-hydroxyethyl)-1-piperazineethanesulfonic acid (HEPES)-buffered saline (HBS) is a solution of 20 mM HEPES + 300 mM NaCl + 0.01 % Tween 20, pH 7.4, prepared as follows. Add about 800 mL of water to a glass cylinder. Weigh 4.77 g of HEPES, 17.53 g of NaCl and transfer to the cylinder. Add 50 μL of Tween 20, set to pH 7.4 with NaOH. Make up to 1 L with water. Degas and filter using Corning 431098 filtering units (0.22 μm polyethersulfone (PES) membrane). Store at 4 °C.
4. Running buffer 1: HEPES-buffered saline (HBS). HBS is a solution of 10 mM HEPES + 150 mM NaCl + 0.005 % Tween 20, pH 7.4, prepared as follows. Add 400 mL of 2× HBS (*see* Subheading 2.1, **item 3**) to a glass beaker. Add 300 mL of water, set to pH 7.4 with NaOH or HCl, if necessary. Make up to 800 mL with water. Degas and filter using Corning 431098 filtering units (0.22 μm PES membrane) in order to remove particles that may obstruct the microfluidics and to avoid air bubbles during the experiment (*see* **Note 1**).
5. Running buffer 2: HBS + 5 % DMSO. Add 400 mL of 2× HBS (*see* Subheading 2.1, **item 3**) to a glass beaker. Add 40 mL of DMSO (dimethyl sulfoxide), 300 mL of water, set to pH 7.4 with NaOH or HCl, if necessary. Make up to 800 mL with water. The solution has to be degased and filtered using regenerated cellulose Corning filtering units (0.2 μm) in order to remove particles that may obstruct the microfluidics and to avoid air bubbles during the experiment (*see* **Note 2**).
6. Running buffer 3: HBS + 2.4 % DMSO. Mix 480 mL of running buffer 1 (HBS) with 520 mL of running buffer 2 (HBS + 5 % DMSO).

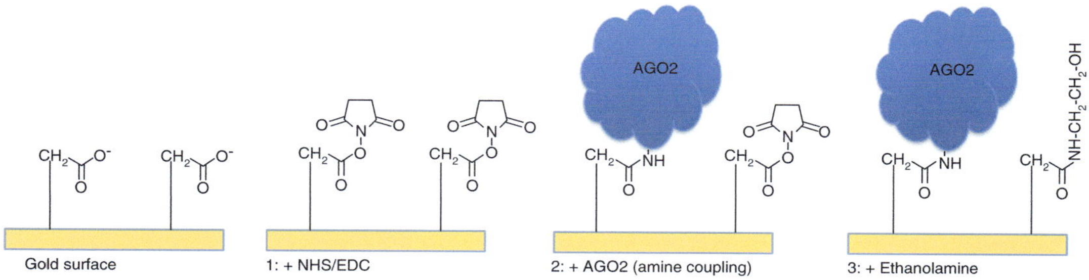


**Fig. 3** The procedure for the immobilization of AGO2. The chip surface was activated with standard amine coupling chemistry using NHS/EDC; subsequently, the amine coupling of AGO2 was carried out onto the activated surface, and the remaining activated surface groups were blocked using ethanolamine

### 2.2 Coupling Reagents

1. 0.1 M NHS: NHS (*N*-hydroxysuccinimide) is weighed, dissolved in water at a final concentration of 0.1 M, divided into 200 μL aliquots, and stored at −20 °C.
2. 0.4 M EDC: EDC (*N*-(3-dimethylaminopropyl)-*N'*-ethylcarbodiimide hydrochloride) GE Healthcare (BR-1000-50) is weighed and dissolved in water at a final concentration of 0.4 M, divided into 200 μL aliquots, and stored at −20 °C (*see* **Note 3**).
3. 1.0 M ethanolamine hydrochloride: ethanolamine hydrochloride is weighed and dissolved in water; the pH is adjusted to 9.0 with HCl (final concentration 1.0 M), divided into 200 μL aliquots, and stored at −20 °C (Fig. 3).

### 2.3 Regeneration, Cleaning, and Preparation Solutions

Mild surface preparation solutions and regeneration solutions were prepared, in order to clean the chip surface and to remove analyte traces from the immobilized ligands.

1. HCl: 10 and 50 mM solutions were prepared by diluting with water the concentrated acid solution (2 M HCl).
2. Glycine–HCl: 10 and 50 mM glycine–HCl solutions were prepared by weighting and dissolving glycine into water and adjusting the pH to 2.5.
3. NaOH: 10 and 50 mM solutions were prepared by diluting with water the concentrated basic solution (2 M NaOH).
4. SDS: 0.5% sodium dodecyl sulfate (SDS) solution was prepared by weighting and dissolving SDS into water.
5. Sodium hypochlorite: 0.4 and 1% sodium hypochloride was prepared by diluting with water concentrated (15%) sodium hypochlorite solutions.
6. NaCl: 1 M NaCl solution is prepared by weighting and dissolving sodium chloride into 10 mM final HEPES set to pH 7.4 (adjust the pH with HCl or NaOH after addition of NaCl).

## 3 Methods

We used a SensiQ Pioneer system. For this apparatus, as for most other SPR systems, including Biacore ones, many types of sensor surface exist, ranging from bare gold to many different chemically modified ones. In most chips gold is coated with three-dimensional polymers that confer thickness, density, and binding capacity. The choice of the chip depends on the immobilization chemistry optimal for ligand binding and on the amount of ligand we need to immobilize.

The study of the interaction between Argonaute 2 (AGO2) and a compound named BCI-137, selected by means of structure-based high-throughput docking screening [12], needs immobilization of high amount of protein (ligand, MW = 97.2 kDa), for the detection of the low-molecular mass (313.29 Da) compound BCI-137. We have used recombinant human AGO2 (Sino Biological Inc. # 11079-H07B), i.e., the full-length human AGO2 (NP_036286.2) (Met 1-Ala 859), expressed in baculovirus–insect cell system with a polyhistidine tag at the N-terminus, for a molecular mass of 99 kDa.

The 320:1 ratio between molecular masses of ligand vs. analyte means that we need to immobilize a reasonably high number of RUs of AGO2, in order to have a good BCI-137 signal (*see* **Note 4**). Therefore we decided to immobilize at least 5000 RUs of Ago2 by amine coupling onto a COOH5 chip, with a hydrogel-based sensing surface endowed with high binding capacity (*see* **Note 5**). We decided to immobilize AGO2 onto both Fc1 and Fc2 flow cells, leaving the empty Fc3 flow cell as control (*see* **Note 6**).

### 3.1 Determination of Coupling Conditions

Immobilization of most ligands can be obtained using 10 mM coupling buffer at one point below the isoelectric point of the protein. The theoretic isoelectric point of AGO2, calculated using the program pI tool [13], is about 5.5. However, to test for optimum coupling buffer, ligand should be injected in coupling buffers at different pH values, and electrostatic binding should be monitored for each condition (*see* **Note 7**).

1. Dilute the protein (ligand) to a final concentration of 10 μg/mL (final volume 80 μL) into pH 6.0, 5.5, 5.0, 4.5, and 4.0 coupling buffers (*see* Subheading 2.1).
2. Inject on one of the flow cells of the COOH5 chip, i.e., Fc1 (flow rate 10 μL/min), 30 μL of each sample, beginning at pH 6.0 and continuing with pH 5.5, 5.0, 4.5, and 4.0 coupling buffers, and monitor electrostatic binding (difference in RU) for each condition.
3. After each injection, inject 100 μL (flow rate 10 μL/min) of high ionic strength neutral pH buffer (1 M NaCl solution, *see* Subheading 2.3, **item 6**) onto Fc1.

4. Check that all the bound protein dissociates after the injection. If not it suggests that not all the protein was bound electrostatically and that the protein denatures irreversibly at pH values used.
5. At the end, inject 10 μL (flow rate 10 μL/min) of 10 mM NaOH solution (*see* Subheading 2.3) onto Fc1, Fc2, and Fc3 to clean the sensor surface.
6. Use the highest pH at which >10,000 RU of ligand protein binds electrostatically during the injections (in our case, pH 4.5) (*see* **Note 8**).

### 3.2 Ligand Immobilization

AGO2 was immobilized via amine coupling to the Fc1 and Fc2 of a COOH5 chip (Fig. 3). Fc3 was used as a control flow cell. To this end:

1. Combine 160 μL of 0.1 M NHS (*see* Subheading 2.2) with 160 μL of 0.1 M EDC (*see* Subheading 2.2) and inject 250 μL of this freshly prepared NHS/EDC mixture (5 min at 50 μL/min) over the surface of Fc1, Fc2, and Fc3 flow cells of the COOH5 chip (*see* **Note 9**).
2. Prepare the ligand solution: 20 μg/mL AGO2 (final volume 400 μL) into pH 4.5 coupling buffer (20 mM acetate buffer), just before use (*see* **Note 10**).
3. Inject 100 μL of the ligand solution (10 min at 10 μL/min) over Fc1 and Fc2, in order to covalently link it to the sample flow cells. Be careful not to inject ligand over Fc3.
4. Inject 100 μL of the ligand solution (10 min at 10 μL/min) over Fc1, in order to covalently link additional ligand to the sample flow cell. Be careful not to inject ligand over Fc3.
5. Inject 100 μL of 1.0 M ethanolamine hydrochloride (4 min at 25 μL/min) over the surface of Fc1, Fc2, and Fc3 flow cells of the COOH5 chip (*see* **Note 11**). Using this procedure, we were able to immobilize about 8000 RU of Ago2 on Fc1 and 5500 RU on Fc2. RU values were measured in each step for each flow cell. Immobilized ligand was calculated by subtracting the initial RU value (after **step 1**) by the final RU value (after **step 5**) for each flow cell. The RU value remained unaltered in all the experiment.

### 3.3 Regeneration

Analysis of replicates is essential when analyzing binding of an analyte to a ligand immobilized on the chip surface. Regeneration of the chip surface is needed to remove the bound analyte without affecting the immobilized ligand or the sensor surface. Ideally, for analyte–ligand interactions with fast dissociation rate, no regeneration is needed, but only extensive washing with buffer. The strategy for the choice of an efficient but non-damaging regeneration solution is to test a series of regeneration conditions, starting from the least aggressive ones. We have characterized once the regeneration conditions as follows. The following conditions described in **steps 5–8** were proved to be efficient and non-damaging. We have always used condition described in **step 6** for all the experiments, with the use of **steps 7** and **8** after a series of experiments (*see* **Note 12**).

1. Dissolve the analyte (BCI-137) at a concentration of 10 mM in 100% dimethyl sulfoxide (DMSO). To do this, weigh 10.0 mg of BCI-137 (molecular mass = 313.29) and dissolve in 3.19 mL DMSO. Mix well to allow even distribution and complete resuspension of the compound. Aliquot the compound and keep at −70 °C.
2. Take 500 μL of the BCI-137 solution and add the same amount (500 μL) of 2× HBS used for dissolution of BCI-137 to the analyte, to obtain 1 mL of 5 mM BCI-137 in HBS + 50% DMSO. Dilute the dissolved compound 20.83 times (96 μL of 5 mM BCI-137 + 1904 μL HBS (10 mM HEPES, pH 7.4; 150 mM NaCl; 0.005% surfactant P20)), to obtain a sample of 240 μM BCI-137 in HBS + 2.4% DMSO.
3. Use HBS + 2.4% DMSO (500 mL is sufficient for all the experiment) as running buffer.
4. Inject 30 μL of 240 μM BCI-137 in HBS + 2.4% DMSO (60 s at 30 μL/min) to Fc1, Fc2, and Fc3.
5. After the injection of ligand to the chip, wash by injecting running buffer 1 (*see* Subheading 2.1) (HBS). Inject 600 μL of the HBS solution (1200 s at 30 μL/min) to Fc3, Fc2, and Fc1.
6. Wash by injecting running buffer 3 (HBS + 2.4% DMSO, *see* Subheading 2.1, **item 5**). Inject 600 μL of HBS + 2.4% DMSO (1200 s at 30 μL/min) to Fc3, Fc2, and Fc1.
7. Wash by injecting (HBS—1 M NaCl, *see* Subheading 2.3, **item 6**). Inject 600 μL of HBS—1 M NaCl (1200 s at 30 μL/min) to Fc3, Fc2, and Fc1.
8. Wash by injecting (10 mM NaOH, *see* Subheading 2.3, **item 3**). Inject 10 μL of 10 mM NaOH (20 s at 30 μL/min) to Fc3, Fc2, and Fc1.

### 3.4 Experiment: FastStep Injection

We decided to use FastStep injection experiments, in order to obtain rapidly information on the binding of the analyte at different concentrations, with a single dissociation phase (*see* **Note 13**). However, similar procedures can be followed in traditional SPR experiments, where injections of single concentrations of analyte are carried out, followed by analyte dissociation and regeneration of the chip surface, and each series is repeated for the analyte concentrations used [14–17].

1. Use filtered and degased running buffer 3 (HBS + 2.4% DMSO) as running buffer. 500 mL is sufficient for all the experiment).

2. Set up a FastStep injection protocol to perform injections of buffer, bulk standard, and analyte (*see* Subheading 3.4, **step 3–5**). Either the running buffer, the bulk standard, or the analyte was automatically diluted in HBS + 2.4% DMSO and injected by seven serial doubling steps (step contact time = 15 s, nominal flow rate = 200 μL/min). The following dilutions are injected to Fc3, Fc2, and Fc1: 0–17 s: 1/64 dilution; 17–33 s: 1/32 dilution; 33–48 s: 1/16 dilution; 48–62 s: 1/8 dilution; 63–78 s: 1/4 dilution; 78–93 s: 1/2 dilution; 94–100 s: undiluted sample. After the injection, a dissociation/regeneration injection of 600 μL of HBS + 2.4% DMSO (1200 s at 30 μL/min) to Fc3, Fc2, and Fc1 (*see* Subheading 3.3, **step 2**) follows.
3. Perform FastStep injections of HBS + 2.4% DMSO. This step is needed as reference sensorgram for the experiment. Seven serial doubling dilutions are carried out using the same buffer as a diluent and are injected to Fc3, Fc2, and Fc1 (step contact time = 15 s, nominal flow rate = 200 μL/min) as in **step 2**. RU changes indicate the response of the chip surface and of the immobilized protein to small changes in buffer composition and of pressure during the experiment. RU variations were negligible. Three different FastStep injections of HBS + 2.4% DMSO must be performed as initial reference standard, plus one injection after every other experiment (*see* Subheading 3.4, **steps 4** and **5**).
4. Perform FastStep injections of HBS + 2.4% DMSO + 20% sucrose. This step is needed as a bulk reference standard and internal control for the experiment. Seven serial doubling dilutions are carried out using HBS + 2.4% DMSO buffer as a diluent and are injected to Fc3, Fc2, and Fc1 (step contact time = 15 s, nominal flow rate = 200 μL/min) as in Subheading 3.4, **step 2**.
5. Perform FastStep injections of sample prepared in **step 2** of Subheading 3.3 (240 μM BCI-137 in HBS + 2.4% DMSO): the inhibitor compound is automatically diluted in HBS + 2.4% DMSO and injected to Fc3, Fc2, and Fc1, by seven serial doubling steps (step contact time = 15 s, nominal flow rate = 200 μL/min). The following samples were injected: 0–17 s: 3.75 μM BCI-137; 17–33 s: 7.5 μM BCI-137; 33–48 s: 15 μM BCI-137; 48–62 s: 30 μM BCI-137; 63–78 s: 60 μM BCI-137; 78–93 s: 120 μM BCI-137; 94–100 s: 240 μM BCI-137 (Fig. 4). At least three different experiments have to be performed and averaged (*see* **Note 14**).

### 3.5 Data Analysis

Sensorgrams were subjected to global analysis using Qdat software 2.1 (*see* **Note 15**). Scatchard analysis of the dependence of Req on the concentration of analyte concentration was also performed to assess the equilibrium dissociation constant:

1. Check every sensorgram independently. Fc2 and Fc1 sensorgrams show the interaction (association phase, then dissociation and regeneration) of BCI-137 with the immobilized

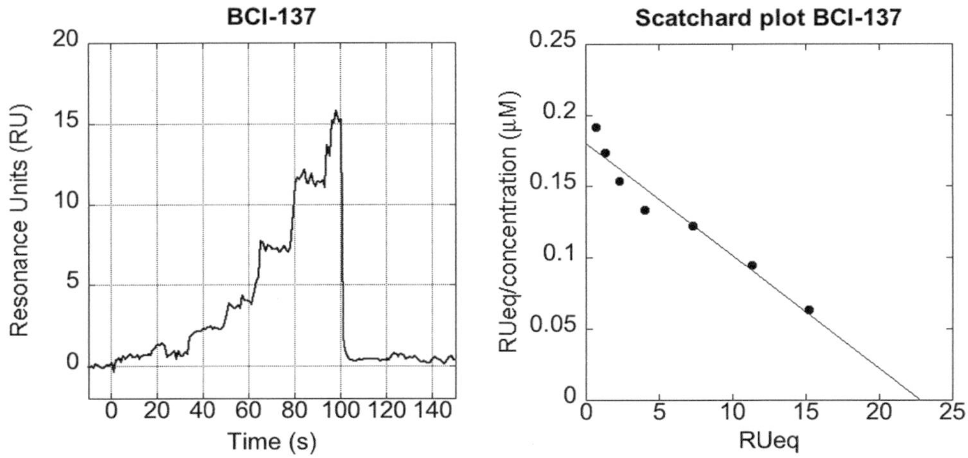


**Fig. 4** *Left panel*: sensorgram showing the binding of BCI-137 to immobilized AGO2. The association phase (0 – 100 s) shows the injection of the following samples in running buffer 3 (HBS + 2.4 % DMSO): 0 – 16 s, 3.75 µM BCI-137; 17 – 33 s, 7.5 µM BCI-137; 33 – 48 s, 15 µM BCI-137; 48 – 63 s, 30 µM BCI-137; 63 – 78 s, 60 µM BCI-137; 78 – 93 s, 120 µM BCI-137; 94 – 100 s, 240 µM BCI-137. A single dissociation phase was measured by injecting HBS at a rate of 30 µL/min, starting at 100 s. *Right panel*: Scatchard plot of the interaction in *left panel*: for each concentration of the analyte, the RUeq and RUeq/c values were plotted and fitted by linear regression (Adapted with permission from ref. 12: Masciarelli S, Quaranta R, Iosue I, Colotti G, Padula F, Varchi G, Fazi F, Del Rio A. A small-molecule targeting the microRNA binding domain of argonaute 2 improves the retinoic acid differentiation response of the acute promyelocytic leukemia cell line NB4. ACS Chem Biol. 2014 Aug 15;9(8):1674–9. doi: 10.1021/cb500286b. Copyright 2014 American Chemical Society)

AGO2. Fc3 sensorgrams represent control experiments, i.e., the interaction of BCI-137 with a flow cell in the absence of immobilized protein (*see* **Note 16**).

2. Subtract the sensorgrams Fc1–Fc3 and Fc2–Fc3, in order to eliminate the unspecific interaction of the analyte with the chip surface.
3. Analyze the Fc1–Fc3 and Fc2–Fc3 with the Qdat program (Biologic Software LTD and SensíQ Technologies, Inc.) to obtain global fitting analyses of association and dissociation constants ($k_{on}/k_{off}$), with a simple 1:1 Langmuir model, where A + B ↔ AB; A, analyte; B, ligand; AB, complex; $k_{on}$, association rate constant ($M^{-1}\ s^{-1}$); and $k_{off}$, dissociation rate constant ($s^{-1}$). For this part, refer to the Qdat tutorial.
4. A simpler analysis, which can be applied to all types of SPR experiments and to all SPR outputs, can be performed by Scatchard analysis of the sensorgrams: we prefer to use this approach for the analysis of the interaction between Ago2 and BCI-137 because it is easy and direct (*see* **Note 17**). From sensorgrams Fc1–Fc3 and Fc2–Fc3 (**step 2**), check whether for each injection of BCI-137, at each concentration used, an asymptote of RU is reached (RUeq), corresponding to the RU

that would be reached at equilibrium (theoretically, at injection time = infinite). For many small analytes, the association rate is fast enough to reach a value that approaches RUeq.

Most scientific software programs contain a linear regression calculator. A freely usable one is the linear regression calculator on QuickCalcs (http:// www.graphpad.com/quickcalcs/linear1/). The calculator yields slope, *Y*- and *X*-intercepts, 95 % confidence intervals, goodness of fit, and an analysis of significativity. The dissociation constant (−1/slope) for the interaction between AGO2 and BCI-137 is 126 μM ± 11 μM (Fig. 4). The regression coefficient ($r$ = 0.9733) is rather good (*see* **Note 18**).

5. We have also calculated an IC50 by carrying out an SPR experiment of competitive binding of miR-223 mimic (Ambion) and BCI-137 compound to the full-length AGO2 immobilized on the COOH5 sensor chip. For the experiment, a series of sensorgrams was measured by injecting mixtures containing miR-223 at a concentration of 250 nM and serial dilutions of BCI-137 (0, 31.25, 62.5, 125, 250, 500 μM). A control series was carried out by injecting BCI-137 alone, at the same concentrations. The experiment was repeated twice. The ΔRU between the two series, as a function of BCI-137 concentration, shows a reduction of ΔRU with the increase of the concentration of the compound, supporting the competition of miR-223 and BCI-137 compound for the binding to AGO2. In this experimental condition, an IC50 of 342 μM ± 52 μM was obtained (data not shown).

## 4 Notes

1. The SensiQ Pioneer is provided with a further degasing unit.
2. Filtering units have to be chosen according to their resistance to the content of the solution: regenerated cellulose Corning filtering units (0.2 μm) are resistant to DMSO.
3. Special care for the stocking of solid EDC should be taken because the compound is hygroscopic and labile.
4. In general, a total analyte response of maximal 50–200 RU when the analyte is injected is desirable. With this value in mind, and since a linear relation between the response and amount of molecule immobilized at the sensor surface, the level of ligand immobilization should depend on the ratio between molecular masses of ligand vs. analyte. Theoretically, for a ratio of 320:1 between molecular masses of Ago2 vs. BCI-137, we should immobilize 10,000 RU of AGO2 to obtain a BCI-137 signal of about 30 RU for a single binding site, provided that all ligand is fully active.

5. Polyhistidine tag can also be used for the immobilization of the ligand to HisCap sensor chips, derived from the COOH5 biosensor, modified with nitrilotriacetic acid (NTA) functional groups that chelate nickel ions for the selective capture of 6× and 10× His-tagged targets. This surface can be partially regenerated by injecting imidazole, EDTA, or other similar reagents that compete for nickel. However, we prefer to covalently immobilize the ligand on COOH5 chips, because they have a higher binding capacity and can maintain a more constant baseline during the experiment.
6. The SensiQ Pioneer has three flow-cell sensor chips. This is useful, because immobilization of the ligand at different densities on two flow cells allows improved control on the experiments. One of the flow cells has to be left empty, since it is necessary as a reference flow cell.
7. Electrostatic binding takes place in conditions where the chip matrix is negatively charged (pH > 4) and the ligand is positively charged (below its pI). Theoretical pI calculators can help, but every ligand needs to be tested.
8. Usually, the most physiological is the pH value; the highest is the possibility that the ligand is not denatured before or during immobilization.
9. This procedure activates the carboxyl groups of the sensor to give succinimide esters, which are able to react spontaneously with primary amines of the ligand, to link it covalently to the chip.
10. Rapid buffer exchange using desalting columns is preferable to dilution from stock solution, but dilution usually works well.
11. This procedure caps, and therefore deactivates, the unreacted succinimide esters.
12. Good regeneration experiments maintain the baseline RU in all flow cells (remove bound analytes but do not remove nor damage the immobilized ligand) and allow to perform replicate experiments without loss of sample binding response.
13. FastStep is a method that enables in situ dilution of the analyte and multiple consecutive injections of analyte at increasing concentrations to be performed. The dissociation of analyte can be accurately estimated from a single dissociation phase curve recorded after the step injection is complete. This eliminates the overhead associated with multiple loading, injecting, and regeneration cycles. Using this approach, we limited the number of experiments, maintaining a high level of available information from each experiment [18, 19].
14. The interaction of the immobilized protein with the analyte was detected by mass concentration-dependent changes of the

refractive index on the sensor chip surface. The changes in the observed SPR signal are expressed as resonance units (RUs). Typically, a response change of 1000 RU corresponds to a change in the surface concentration on the sensor chip of about 1 ng of protein per $mm^2$ [20, 21]. Each sensorgram is the average of three different experiments (a plot of the SPR signal against time is called sensorgram).

15. Global fitting analyzes association and dissociation data for all ligand concentrations simultaneously and, by doing so, allows for a more accurate description of the ratio between association and dissociation constants ($k_{on}/k_{off}$). A simple 1:1 Langmuir model was employed to fit the data, where $A + B \leftrightarrow AB$; A, analyte; B, ligand; and AB, complex.
16. A good experiment has on one hand complete regeneration of the chip, i.e., the RU at the end of each sensorgram has to be the same (or very similar) than at the beginning, before analyte injection. On the other hand, the ΔRU (difference between RU at the end of the analyte injection and RU at the beginning of analyte injection) of the analyte injected on Fc3 flow cell has to be negligible (or at least much less than RUmax of the analyte injected on Fc1 or Fc2 flow cells).
17. Many SPR fitting programs (including Qdat) can calculate RUeq values from the sensorgrams. For each analyte concentration, calculate the RUeq value reached and the ratio RUeq/concentration. Plot each point ($x$ = RUeq; $y$ = RUeq/concentration) and perform a linear regression, in order to calculate slope, *X*- and *Y*-axis intercepts, and regression coefficient. A Scatchard plot is a method for analyzing data for freely reversible ligand/receptor-binding interactions; it is a plot of the ratio of concentrations of bound ligand to unbound ligand versus the bound ligand concentration or in our case RUeq/analyte concentration (assuming that only a small part of it results bound to the ligand) vs. RUeq (RUeq is proportional to bound ligand. The plot yields a straight line of slope $-K$, where $K$ is the affinity constant for ligand binding, i.e., the inverse of the dissociation constant. The intercept on the *X* axis is RUmax. It is sometimes the case that binding data does not form a straight line when plotted in a Scatchard plot. Such is the case when ligand bound to substrate is not allowed to achieve equilibrium before the binding is measured or binding is cooperative.
18. Scatchard plot may distort experimental error, because the assumption of independence in linear regression model is violated since bound ligand is used in the *X* and *Y* axes. However, if the regression coefficient is >0.9, it can be used successfully.

## References

1. Schuck P (1997) Use of surface plasmon resonance to probe the equilibrium and dynamic aspects of interactions between biological macromolecules. Annu Rev Biophys Struct 26:541–566
2. Schasfoort RBM, Tudos AJ (2008) Handbook of surface plasmon resonance. RCS Publishing, London
3. van der Merwe AP (2001) Surface plasmon resonance. In: Harding SE, Chowdhry BZ (eds) Protein-ligand interactions: hydrodynamics and calorimetry. Oxford University Press, New York, NY, pp 137–184
4. Rich RL, Quinn JG, Morton T, Stepp JD, Myszka DG (2010) Biosensor-based fragment screening using FastStep injections. Anal Biochem 407(2):270–277. doi:10.1016/j.ab.2010.08.024
5. Quinn JG (2012) Modeling Taylor dispersion injections: determination of kinetic/affinity interaction constants and diffusion coefficients in label-free biosensing. Anal Biochem 421(2):391–400. doi:10.1016/j.ab.2011.11.024
6. Quinn JG (2012) Evaluation of Taylor dispersion injections: determining kinetic/affinity interaction constants and diffusion coefficients in label-free biosensing. Anal Biochem 421(2):401–410. doi:10.1016/j.ab.2011.11.023
7. Ha M, Kim VN (2014) Regulation of microRNA biogenesis. Nat Rev Mol Cell Biol 15(8):509–524. doi:10.1038/nrm3838
8. De Santa F, Iosue I, Del Rio A, Fazi F (2013) microRNA biogenesis pathway as a therapeutic target for human disease and cancer. Curr Pharm Des 19(4):745–764, Review
9. Iosue I, Quaranta R, Masciarelli S, Fontemaggi G, Batassa EM, Bertolami C, Ottone T, Divona M, Salvatori B, Padula F, Fatica A, Lo-Coco F, Nervi C, Fazi F (2013) Argonaute 2 sustains the gene expression program driving human monocytic differentiation of acute myeloid leukemia cells. Cell Death Dis 4, e926. doi:10.1038/cddis.2013.452
10. Fontemaggi G, Bellissimo T, Donzelli S, Iosue I, Benassi B, Bellotti G, Blandino G, Fazi F (2015) Identification of post-transcriptional regulatory networks during myeloblast-to-monocyte differentiation transition. RNA Biol 12(7):690–700. doi:10.1080/15476286.2015.1044194
11. Elkayam E, Kuhn CD, Tocilj A, Haase AD, Greene EM, Hannon GJ, Joshua-Tor L (2012) The structure of human argonaute-2 in complex with miR-20a. Cell 150(1):100–110. doi:10.1016/j.cell.2012.05.017
12. Masciarelli S, Quaranta R, Iosue I, Colotti G, Padula F, Varchi G, Fazi F, Del Rio A (2014) A small-molecule targeting the microRNA binding domain of argonaute 2 improves the retinoic acid differentiation response of the acute promyelocytic leukemia cell line NB4. ACS Chem Biol 9(8):1674–1679. doi:10.1021/cb500286b
13. Bjellqvist B et al (1993) Electrophoresis 14(10):1023–1031
14. Franceschini S, Ilari A, Verzili D, Zamparelli C, Antaramian A, Rueda A, Valdivia HH, Chiancone E, Colotti G (2008) Molecular basis for the impaired function of the natural F112L sorcin mutant: X-ray crystal structure, calcium affinity, and interaction with annexin VII and the ryanodine receptor. FASEB J 22(1):295–306
15. Zamparelli C, Macquaide N, Colotti G, Verzili D, Seidler T, Smith GL, Chiancone E (2010) Activation of the cardiac Na(+)-Ca(2+) exchanger by sorcin via the interaction of the respective Ca(2+)-binding domains. J Mol Cell Cardiol 49(1):132–141. doi:10.1016/j.yjmcc.2010.03.003
16. Sechi S, Colotti G, Belloni G, Mattei V, Frappaolo A, Raffa GD, Fuller MT, Giansanti MG (2014) GOLPH3 is essential for contractile ring formation and Rab11 localization to the cleavage site during cytokinesis in Drosophila melanogaster. PLoS Genet 10(5), e1004305. doi:10.1371/journal.pgen.1004305
17. Perli E, Giordano C, Pisano A, Montanari A, Campese AF, Reyes A, Ghezzi D, Nasca A, Tuppen HA, Orlandi M, Di Micco P, Poser E, Taylor RW, Colotti G, Francisci S, Morea V, Frontali L, Zeviani M, d'Amati G (2014) The isolated carboxy-terminal domain of human mitochondrial leucyl-tRNA synthetase rescues the pathological phenotype of mitochondrial tRNA mutations in human cells. EMBO Mol Med 6(2):169–182. doi:10.1002/emmm.201303198
18. Ilari A, Fiorillo A, Poser E, Lalioti VS, Sundell GN, Ivarsson Y, Genovese I, Colotti G (2015) Structural basis of Sorcin-mediated calcium-dependent signal transduction. Sci Rep 5:16828. doi:10.1038/srep16828
19. Perli E, Fiorillo A, Giordano C, Pisano A, Montanari A, Grazioli P, Campese AF, Di Micco P, Tuppen HA, Genovese I, Poser E, Preziuso C, Taylor RW, Morea V, Colotti G, d'Amati G (2015) Short peptides from leucyl-tRNA synthetase rescue disease-causing mitochondrial tRNA point mutations. Hum Mol Genet pii:ddv619

20. Colotti G, Zamparelli C, Verzili D, Mella M, Loughrey CM, Smith GL, Chiancone E (2006) The W105G and W99G sorcin mutants demonstrate the role of the D helix in the Ca(2+)-dependent interaction with annexin VII and the cardiac ryanodine receptor. Biochemistry 45(41):12519–12529

21. Fiorillo A, Colotti G, Boffi A, Baiocco P, Ilari A (2012) The crystal structures of the tryparedoxin-tryparedoxin peroxidase couple unveil the structural determinants of Leishmania detoxification pathway. PLoS Negl Trop Dis 6(8), e1781. doi:10.1371/journal.pntd.0001781

# Chapter 17

# Antagonists of the miRNA-Argonaute 2 Protein Complex: Anti-miR-AGOs

**Marco F. Schmidt, Oliver Korb, and Chris Abell**

## Abstract

microRNAs (miRNAs) have been identified as high-value drug targets. A widely applied strategy in miRNA inhibition is the use of antisense agents. However, it has been shown that oligonucleotides are poorly cell permeable because of their complex chemical structure and due to their negatively charged backbone. Consequently, the general application of oligonucleotides in therapy is limited. Since miRNAs' functions are executed exclusively by the Argonaute 2 protein, we therefore describe a protocol for the design of a novel miRNA inhibitor class: antagonists of the miRNA-Argonaute 2 protein complex, so-called anti-miR-AGOs, that not only block the crucial binding site of the target miRNA but also bind to the protein's active site. Due to their lower molecular weight and, thus, more drug-like chemical structure, the novel inhibitor class may show better pharmacokinetic properties than reported oligonucleotide inhibitors, enabling them for potential therapeutic use.

**Key words** Drug design, microRNA, miRNA-Argonaute 2 protein complex, miRNA inhibitors, miRNA seed region

## 1 Introduction

microRNAs (miRNAs), noncoding, single-stranded ribonucleic acid (RNA) molecules, on average only 22–23 nucleotides long, are posttranscriptional gene regulators [1–3]. They have been identified to play a crucial role in various human diseases and are thus regarded as high-value drug targets [4].

Enormous efforts using antisense oligonucleotides to inhibit miRNA functions have been made [5]. However, it has been shown that oligonucleotides are poorly cell permeable because of their complex chemical structure and due to their negatively charged backbone [6]. As a result, the general application of oligonucleotides in therapy is limited. In order to overcome pharmacokinetic limitations, new chemical entities with more drug-like properties are urgently needed to target miRNAs applied in therapies.

Marco F. Schmidt (ed.), *Drug Target miRNA: Methods and Protocols*, Methods in Molecular Biology, vol. 1517,
DOI 10.1007/978-1-4939-6563-2_17, © Springer Science+Business Media New York 2017

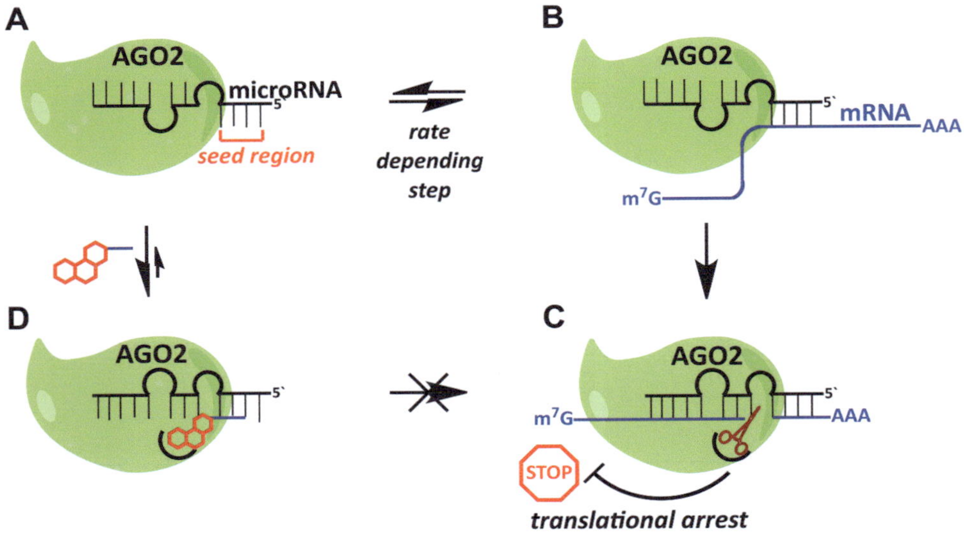


**Fig. 1** Mechanism of mRNA binding to the miRNA-Argonaute 2 protein complex and the binding mode of anti-miR-AGOs: (**a**) Only the seed region of bound miRNA to Argonaute 2 is solvent-exposed and undergoes binding to target mRNA in a rate-dependent step. (**b**) Then, full binding of mRNA to the miRNA/AGO2 complex occurs. (**c**) The target mRNA is cleaved by AGO2 followed by a translational arrest. (**d**) In contrast, an anti-miR-AGO binds via miRNA's seed region (blue part of the inhibitor) and blocks either AGO2's active site (red part of the inhibitor), thus inhibiting the silencing effect of the target mRNA (reproduced from [10] with permission from ACS Publications)

The miRNA-mediated gene silencing process is executed by a specialized family of RNA-binding proteins named Argonaute [3]. These proteins bind miRNA and silence complementary target messenger RNA (mRNA) either by direct cleavage or by recruitment of additional silencing factors as part of microRNA-induced silencing complex (miRISC) [3, 4]. Recently, it was reported that mRNA binding to the complex of target miRNA and Argonaute 2 protein occurs in two steps (Fig. 1) [7]: firstly, the solvent-exposed first eight nucleotides of miRNA's 5′-end, the so-called seed region, bind in a rate-depending step to target mRNA. Next, in the second step, full binding of mRNA to the miRNA-Argonaute 2 protein complex occurs. In conclusion, the blockage of only the miRNA's seed region totally inhibits miRNA binding to the target mRNA. Additionally, it was reported that non-RNA antisense agents such as deoxyribonucleic acid (DNA) or locked nucleic acid (LNA) [8] do not only disrupt miRNA-mRNA interaction but also cannot be cleaved by Argonaute 2. Therefore, DNA and LNA are Argonaute 2 inhibitors [9].

As miRNA functions are executed by the Argonaute 2 protein, we have recently described a novel inhibitor class that targets the complex of miRNA and the Argonaute 2 protein [10]. The so-called antagonists of the miRNA-Argonaute 2 complex (anti-miR-AGOs) consist of a short oligonucleotide sequence and a small-molecule moiety. Anti-miR-AGOs bind via their short but specific nucleotide sequence to the solvent-exposed target miRNA's seed region and with their small-molecule moiety in the active site of the Argonaute 2 protein (Fig. 1d). Consequently, anti-miR-AGOs bind to two sites, the miRNA's seed region and the protein active site, thus benefiting from cooperative ligand binding [11]. Although their nucleotide sequence is short (<10 nucleotides), anti-miR-AGOs bind to target mRNA specifically, since only approximately 2000 miRNAs exist (www.mirbase.org), and a hexamer oligonucleotide sequence potentially results in 4096 permutations (four different bases per position). In conclusion, adopting the concept of small molecule to target the AGO2 protein's active site, combined with a short but specific oligonucleotide sequence addressing the miRNA of interest, leads to the development of more hydrophobic molecules with lower molecular weight than reported oligonucleotide inhibitors. Therefore, anti-miR-AGOs may promise better pharmacokinetic properties, providing a chance of tackling delivery issues compared with reported oligonucleotide-based inhibitors and hopefully enabling them for therapeutic use.

Here, we present a protocol for the rational design of small-molecule moieties for Argonaute 2 protein's active site, the synthesis of small molecule–peptide nucleic acid (PNA) adducts, and the biological evaluation of anti-miR-AGOs in an mRNA cleavage assay. The protocol discusses exemplarily an anti-miR-AGO that targets microRNA-122 (miR-122), an essential host factor in hepatitis C virus infection [12]. However, the protocol is not limited to miR-122 and can be adapted to any other miRNA of interest.

## 2 Materials

As with any procedure involving RNAs and RNA-binding proteins, it is recommended that all buffer components are RNAse-free.

### 2.1 Molecular Modeling

1. CambridgeSoft ChemBioDraw.
2. Discovery Studio Visualizer (Accelrys Corp., now BIOVIA Dassault Systèmes SE) (www.accelrys.com/products/collaborative-science/biovia-discovery-studio/visualization-download.php).
3. PyMOL Molecular Graphics System [13].
4. CORINA [14].
5. ZINC Database (www.zinc.docking.org).
6. GOLD, version 5.1 (2006-2009) docking software (www.ccdc.cam.ac.uk/products/life_science/gold) [15].

### 2.2 Synthesis of Anti-miR- AGOs

1. Plastic syringes equipped with polyethylene (PE) filters.
2. Rink amide resin.
3. Fmoc-protected peptide nucleic acid (Fmoc-PNA) monomers (Link Technologies).
4. 20% piperidine in *N*,*N*-dimethylformamide (DMF).
5. Coupling reagent: 1-[bis(dimethylamino)methylene]-1*H*-1,2,3-triazolo[4,5-b]pyridinium 3-oxid hexafluorophosphate (HATU).
6. 2,4,6-Collidine or *N*,*N*-diisopropylethylamine (DIPEA).
7. Organic solvents: diethyl ether, *N*,*N*,-dimethylformamide (DMF); dichloromethane (DCM).
8. Kaiser test kit (Sigma Aldrich).
9. Vac-Man® Laboratory Vacuum Manifold (Promega).

### 2.3 mRNA Cleavage Assay

1. Argonaute 2 protein (AGO2) (Sino Biological, Beijing, P.R. China).
2. miR-122 (5′ pUGGAGUGUGACAAUGGUGUUUG 3′) and complementary fluorescein-labeled RNA substrate (5′ 6-FAM-AUGCAAACACCAUUG↓UCACACUCC 3′) or other miRNAs with complementary fluorescein-labeled RNA substrate (Eurogentec).
3. mRNA cleavage assay buffer: 30 mM Tris-HCl pH 7.5, 130 mM KCl, 1.1 mM $MgCl_2$, 1 mM DTT, and 0.1 mM ethylenediaminetetraacetic acid (EDTA).
4. Formamide loading/quenching buffer: 95% formamide, 18 mM EDTA, 0.025% w/v sodium dodecyl sulfate, 0.025% w/v xylene cyanol, 0.025% bromophenol blue.
5. 10× Tris/borate/EDTA (TBE) buffer for 1 L: 121.1 g Tris base, 61.8 g boric acid, 7.4 g EDTA (disodium salt).
6. 1× Tris/borate/EDTA (TBE) buffer for 1 L: dilute 100 mL to 1 mL to make gel running buffer. Store for up to 6 months at room temperature (RT).
7. 20% polyacrylamide RNA denaturating (10 M urea) gel for 20 mL: 15 mL 30% acrylamide solution, 10 g urea, 2 mL 10× Tris/borate/EDTA (TBE) buffer, 2.8 mL $H_2O$. Start polymerization with 200 μL 10% fresh solution of w/v ammonium persulfate (APS) and 20 μL *N*,*N*,*N*′,*N*′-tetramethylethylenediamine (TEMED).
8. Electrophoresis chamber: Mini-PROTEAN® Tetra Handcast Systems (Bio-Rad).
9. GE Typhoon Trio ImageQuant TL.

## 3 Methods

The methodology is comprised of three stages: molecular modeling of peptide nucleic acid–small molecule adducts, solid phase synthesis of peptide nucleic acid–small molecule adducts (so-called anti-miR-AGOs), and in vitro determination of anti-miR-AGOs in an mRNA cleavage assay.

### *3.1 Molecular Modeling*

1. A model of a peptide nucleic acid (PNA) mimicking the mRNA substrate is generated. As an Argonaute 2, crystal structure with a bound RNA substrate is only reported for *Thermus thermophilus* (pdb code: 3HJF) [16]; the RNA substrate conformation resolved in this structure is used as the template for modeling the PNA sequence onto.
2. The structure of PNA sequence 5′ $H_2N$-t-a-c-t-a-c-c-t-$CONH_2$ 3′ is drawn in CambridgeSoft ChemBioDraw and converted into an SDF file by Discovery Studio Visualizer. A one-to-one mapping of the residues in PNA sequence to the RNA substrate sequence 5′ UACUACCU 3′ in 3HJF is used (Fig. 2a).
3. For each of the side chains, distance restraints between corresponding atoms in the PNA and substrate RNA structure are defined.
4. In CORINA [14] the target distance of each distance restraint was set to 0 Å aiming at overlaying the PNA atoms onto the fixed RNA substrate ones. These distance restraints are added to a Tripos force field implementation and a Cartesian minimization is carried out. While the atoms of the PNA structure are moved during the minimization, the positions of the substrate RNA atoms are kept fixed.

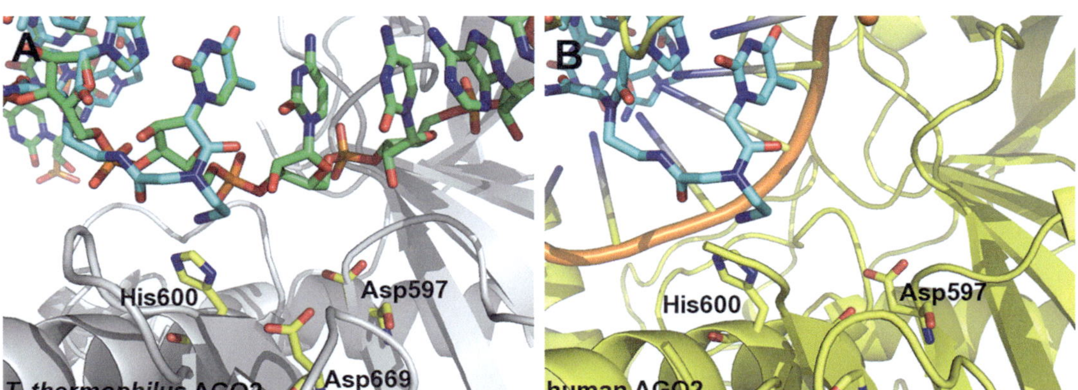


**Fig. 2** (**a**) Superposition of modeled peptide nucleic acid structure (*blue*) with substrate RNA (*green*) in the *Thermus thermophilus* Argonaute 2 protein (*gray*, pdb code: 3HJF [16]). (**b**) Superposition of *Thermus thermophilus* Argonaute 2 protein with human Argonaute 2 protein (*yellow*, pdb code: 4EI1 [17]). Molecular modeling was applied since the human Argonaute 2 protein crystal structure has no RNA substrate bound. The modeled peptide nucleic acid into the human AGO2 structure enabled the development of anti-miR-AGOs (reproduced from [10] with permission from ACS Publications)

5. Next, the human Argonaute 2 structure (pdb code: 4EI1) [17] is superimposed onto the *Thermus thermophilus* structure containing the modeled PNA conformation such that the catalytic residues in the active site are overlaid (Fig. 2b) in a PyMOL session file [13].
6. Starting from the modeled PNA conformation superimposed with the human Argonaute 2 structure (pdb code: 4EI1), covalent docking experiments are carried out to link small molecules targeting AGO's active site in the virtual screen of the ZINC fragment subset to the PNA using GOLD [15].
7. The N-terminus of the PNA is defined as the covalent link atom on the protein side. The covalent docking functionality in the GOLD docking software is used to predict the linked small-molecule binding modes. Since these calculations are not time critical, GOLD's *autoscale* parameter was set to 3.0 and ten genetic algorithm runs per fragment are performed.
8. The screening hits are ranked according to the ChemPLP scoring function, an indication of how well a ligand conformation is interacting with the binding site [18]. The top-ranked hits are analyzed by visual inspection (Fig. 3).

### 3.2 Synthesis of Anti-miR- AGOs

1. A 20 mL plastic syringe equipped with PE filter is filled with 1 g rink amide resin (0.4 mmol/g loading).
2. 10 mL DCM is added slowly to rink amide resin in the syringe for swelling.
3. DCM is removed by Vac-Man® Laboratory Vacuum Manifold.
4. Fmoc deprotection: 10 mL of 20% v/v piperidine in DMF is added. The syringe is shacked slowly for 5 min.
5. Piperidine/DMF solution is removed by Vac-Man® Laboratory Vacuum Manifold.

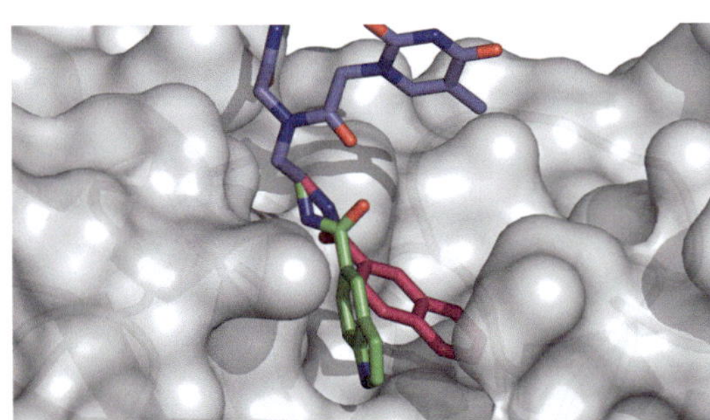

**Fig. 3** Predicted likely binding modes of naphthalene (*red*) and indole (*green*) scaffolds in the nuclease active site (reproduced from [10] with permission from ACS Publications)

6. The resin is washed three times with DMF (15 mL), followed by DCM (15 mL) using Vac-Man® Laboratory Vacuum Manifold.
7. Repeat **steps 5** and **6** two times.
8. Fmoc-protected PNA monomer (1 mmol, 2.5 eq.), HATU (379 mg, 1 mmol, 2.5 eq.), and collidine (262 μL, 2 mmol, 5 eq.) are dissolved in 10 mL DMF and added to the resin (*see* **Note 1**). The reaction is shacked slowly for 2 h.
9. Completeness of reaction is checked by Kaiser test according to manufacturer's instruction.
10. After a negative Kaiser test, the resin is washed three times with DMF (15 mL), followed by DCM (15 mL) using Vac-Man® Laboratory Vacuum Manifold.
11. Repeat **steps 4–10** *n*-times (max. ten times) to get a PNA sequence which targets the miRNA's seed region of interest.
12. Repeat **steps 4–7**.
13. The carboxylic acid to address AGO's active site (1 mmol, 2.5 eq.), HATU (379 mg, 1 mmol, 2.5 eq.), and 2,4,6-collidine (262 μL, 2 mmol, 5 eq.) are dissolved in 10 mL DMF and added to the resin. The reaction is shacked slowly for 2 h.
14. Repeat **steps 9–10**.
15. The anti-miR-AGO is cleaved off from the resin by adding 10 mL TFA/*m*-cresol v:v (95:5).
16. The anti-miR-AGO/TFA solution is moved into a flask. TFA is removed by flushing the flask with nitrogen.
17. Before the TFA is totally removed, diethyl ether (10 mL) is added and the anti-miR-AGO precipitates.
18. The precipitated anti-miR-AGO is washed several times with diethyl ether.
19. The desired anti-miR-AGO is dissolved in $H_2O$ and lyophilized to yield usually a powder and analyzed by high-resolution electrospray ionization mass spectrometry (HR-ESI-MS) and high-performance liquid chromatography (HPLC).

### 3.3 mRNA Cleavage Assay

1. 20 nM recombinant Argonaute 2 protein (*see* **Note 2**) and 200 nM single-stranded miR-122 were preincubated for 1 h to reconstitute the microRNA-induced silencing complex (miRISC) in mRNA cleavage assay buffer in a total volume of 10 μL at 30 °C.
2. Then 5 μL of inhibitor (0 nM, 40 nM, 400 nM, 4 μM, 40 μM, 400 μM, 2 mM) in mRNA cleavage buffer solved is added and further incubation for 15 min at 30 °C is followed.
3. Reaction is started by adding 5 μL 40 nM of substrate. Final concentrations are 10 nM recombinant Argonaute 2 protein, 100 nM single-stranded miR-122, inhibitor (0 nM, 10 nM,

100 nM, 1 μM, 10 μM, 100 μM, 500 μM), and 10 nM fluorogenic substrate in a total volume of 20 μL in mRNA cleavage assay buffer.

4. After 5, 10, 15, 30, 45, and 60 min, 3 μL aliquots are removed and quenched by 12 μL formamide loading/quenching buffer and can be stored at −20 °C in the dark for several days.
5. All experiments are done in triplicate.
6. Assemble the gel according to manufacturer's description and fix the gel in the gel-casting chamber.
7. Immediately after adding 200 μL 10% w/v APS and 20 μL TEMED to RNA denaturating gel, pour the gel using a serological pipette between the two glass plates. Avoid introducing air bubbles. Insert the combs into the liquid stacking gel. Let the gel polymerize at room temperature, about 30–60 min.
8. Dismount the gel from the casting chamber and assemble it to the gel apparatus according to manufacturer's instructions.
9. Fill the chamber with running buffer (1× TBE).
10. Remove the comb and rise the wells with running buffer by using a pipette.
11. Apply the samples (15 μL) carefully from the bottom of the pocket. Avoid introducing air bubbles.
12. Assemble the lid and run the gel at constant watts. Observe the migration of the marker dyes until the dye front reached the lower end of the gel. A run lasts between 45 and 60 min.
13. When the dye front reached the end of the gel, put the gel out of the buffer chamber. Remove the gel from the chamber, pull away spacers, and carefully dissemble the glass plates.
14. Transfer the gel into a dish with 1× TBE buffer. The gel is ready to be scanned.
15. The fluorescence-labeled substrate and product were visualized and quantified by GE Typhoon Trio with ImageQuant TL (fluorescein filter).
16. For kinetic analyses, the relative product formation was measured as fluorescence $\text{intensity}_{\text{product}}$/(fluorescence $\text{intensity}_{\text{product}}$ + fluorescence $\text{intensity}_{\text{substrate}}$). Data were analyzed by GraphPad Prism 5 for Mac (GraphPad, La Jolla, USA) by nonlinear regression (curve fitting) (Figs. 4 and 5).

## 4 Notes

1. Fmoc-PNA monomers dissolve slowly in DMF. Addition of some mL of *N*-methyl-2-pyrrolidone (NMP) can help.

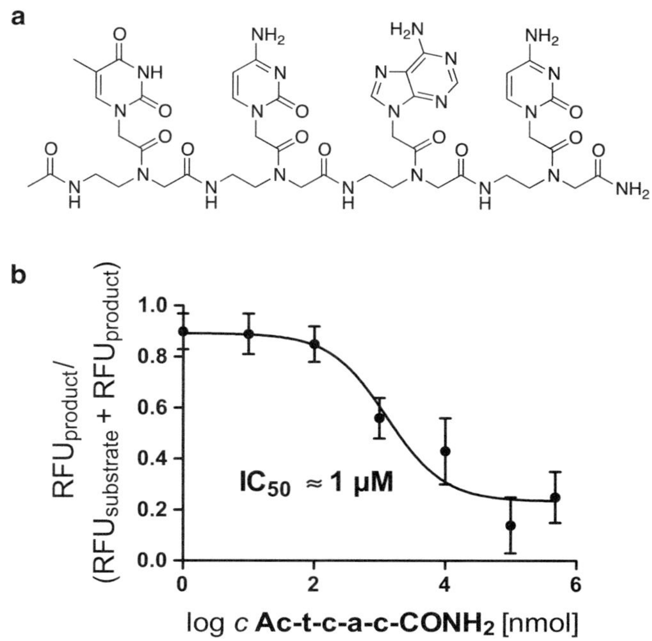


**Fig. 4** Exemplary $IC_{50}$ determination of PNA inhibitor Ac-t-c-a-c-$CONH_2$ in the Argonaute 2 activity assay: (**a**) Structure of inhibitor Ac-t-c-a-c-$CONH_2$. (**b**) The Argonaute 2 protein (10 nM) was incubated with miRNA-122 (100 nM) and the fluorogenic substrate (5′ 6-FAM-AUGCAAACACCAUUG↓UCACACUCC 3′) (10 nM) and different concentrations of inhibitor (500 μM, 100 μM, 10 μM, 1 μM, 100 nM, 10 nM). To monitor cleavage, RNAs were resolved on a denaturing polyacrylamide gel. As a negative control, 100 nM of substrate was run in the *two lanes* on the left-hand side of the gel. The fluorescence-labeled substrate and product were visualized and quantified by GE Typhoon Trio with ImageQuant TL. For kinetic analyses, the relative product formation was measured as $RFU_{product}/(RFU_{product} + RFU_{substrate})$. At these low concentrations, we used in the mRNA cleavage assay (close to reported $K_M$ value of 10 nM) the correlation between the quantified relative fluorescence, and for the human eye, visible gel bands are difficult to see. Data were analyzed by GraphPad Prism 5 for Mac (GraphPad, La Jolla, USA) by nonlinear regression (curve fitting). After considering two other independent experiments, an $IC_{50}$ of approximately 1 μM was determined (reproduced from [10] with permission from ACS Publications)

2. The detection limit of the mRNA cleavage assay is 10 nM (final concentration of Argonaute 2 protein). Potencies of high-affinity inhibitors (<10 nM, e.g., with longer oligonucleotide sequence than 7) cannot be determined! For this purpose, we recommend using the methodology described in Chapter 14 by D. G. Zisoulis.

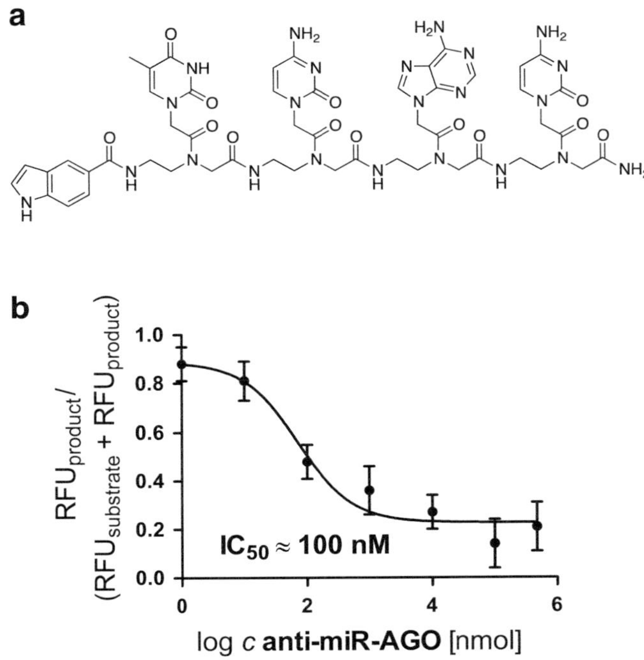


**Fig. 5** Exemplary $IC_{50}$ determination of an anti-miR-AGO in the Argonaute 2 activity assay: (**a**) Structure of the anti-miR-AGO. (**b**) The Argonaute 2 protein (10 nM) was incubated with miR-122 (100 nM) and the fluorogenic substrate (5′ 6-FAM-AUGCAAACACCAUUG↓UCACACUCC 3′) (10 nM) and different concentrations of anti-miR-AGO (500 μM, 100 μM, 10 μM, 1 μM, 100 nM, 10 nM). To monitor cleavage, RNAs were resolved on a denaturing polyacrylamide gel. The fluorescence-labeled substrate and product were visualized and quantified by GE Typhoon Trio with ImageQuant TL. For kinetic analyses, the relative product formation was measured as $RFU_{product}/(RFU_{product} + RFU_{substrate})$. (**b**) Data were analyzed by GraphPad Prism 5 for Mac (GraphPad, La Jolla, USA) by nonlinear regression (curve fitting). After considering two other independent experiments, an $IC_{50}$ for indole-based anti-miR-AGO of approximately 100 nM was determined (reproduced from [10] with permission from ACS Publications)

## Acknowledgment

We acknowledge Dr Rajavel Srinivasan for proofreading the manuscript. Work at CCDC was performed using Darwin Supercomputer of the University of Cambridge High Performance Computing Service (http://www.hpc.cam.ac.uk/), provided by Dell Inc. using Strategic Research Infrastructure Funding from the Higher Education Funding Council for England and funding from the Science and Technology Facilities Council. Work at the University Chemical Laboratory Cambridge was funded by the European Commission FP7 PEOPLE-GA-2010-275765 (Marie Curie Intra-European-Fellowship to M.F.S.).

## References


1. Dykxhoorn DM, Novina CD, Sharp PA (2003) Killing the messenger: short RNAs that silence gene expression. Nat Rev Mol Cell Biol 4:457–467
2. Bartel DP (2004) MicroRNAs: genomics, biogenesis, mechanism, and function. Cell 116:281–297
3. Fabian MR, Sonenberg N (2012) The mechanisms of miRNA-mediated gene silencing: a look under the hood of miRISC. Nat Struct Mol Biol 19:586–593
4. Schmidt MF (2014) Drug target miRNA: chances and challenges. Trends Biotechnol 32:578–585
5. Krützfeld J, Rajewsky N, Braich R, Rajeev KG, Tuschl T, Manoharan M, Stoffel M (2005) Silencing of microRNAs in vivo with antagomirs. Nature 438:685–689
6. Kole R, Krainer AR, Altman S (2012) RNA therapeutics: beyond RNA interference and antisense oligonucleotides. Nat Rev Drug Discov 11:125–140
7. Bartel DP (2009) MicroRNAs: target recognition and regulatory functions. Cell 136:215–233
8. Koshkin AA, Singh SK, Nielsen P, Rajwanshi VK, Kumar R, Meldgaard M, Olsen CE, Wengel J (1998) LNA (locked nucleic acid): synthesis of the adenine, cytosine, guanine, 5-methylcytosine, thymine and uracil bicyclonucleoside monomers, oligomerisation, and unprecedented nucleic acid recognition. Tetrahedron 54:3607–3630
9. Obad S, dos Santos CO, Petri A, Heidenblad M, Broom O, Ruse C, Fu C, Lindow M, Stenvang J, Staarup EM, Hanssen HF, Koch T, Pappin D, Hannon GJ, Kauppinen S (2011) Silencing of microRNA families by seed-targeting tiny LNAs. Nat Genet 43:371–378
10. Schmidt MF, Korb O, Abell C (2013) MicroRNA-specific argonaute 2 protein inhibitors. ACS Chem Biol 8:2122–2126
11. Schmidt MF, Rademann J (2009) Dynamic template-assisted strategies in fragment-based drug discovery. Trends Biotechnol 27:512–521
12. Jopling CL, Yi M, Lancaster AM, Lemon SM, Sarnow P (2005) Modulation of hepatitis C virus RNA abundance by a liver-specific microRNA. Science 309:1577–1581
13. DeLano WL (2006) The PyMOL molecular graphics system, v.0.99rc6. DeLano Scientific LLC, San Carlos, CA
14. Gasteiger J, Rudolph C, Sadowski J (1990) Automatic generation of 3D atomic coordinates for organic molecules. Tetrahedron Comput Methodol 3:537–547
15. Jones G, Willett P, Glen RC (1995) Molecular recognition of receptor sites using a genetic algorithm with a description of desolvation. J Mol Biol 245:43–53
16. Wang Y, Juranek S, Li H, Sheng G, Wardle GS, Tuschl T, Patel DJ (2009) Nucleation, propagation, and cleavage of target RNAs in Ago silencing complexes. Nature 461:754–761
17. Schirle NT, MacRae IJ (2012) The crystal structure of human Argonaute 2. Science 336:1037–1040
18. Korb O, Stützle T, Exner TE (2009) Empirical scoring functions for advanced protein-ligand docking with PLANTS. J Chem Inf Model 49:84–96

# Chapter 18

# Elucidating Mechanisms of Molecular Recognition Between Human Argonaute and miRNA Using Computational Approaches

**Hanlun Jiang, Lizhe Zhu, Amélie Héliou, Xin Gao, Julie Bernauer, and Xuhui Huang**

## Abstract

MicroRNA (miRNA) and Argonaute (AGO) protein together form the RNA-induced silencing complex (RISC) that plays an essential role in the regulation of gene expression. Elucidating the underlying mechanism of AGO-miRNA recognition is thus of great importance not only for the in-depth understanding of miRNA function but also for inspiring new drugs targeting miRNAs. In this chapter we introduce a combined computational approach of molecular dynamics (MD) simulations, Markov state models (MSMs), and protein-RNA docking to investigate AGO-miRNA recognition. Constructed from MD simulations, MSMs can elucidate the conformational dynamics of AGO at biologically relevant timescales. Protein-RNA docking can then efficiently identify the AGO conformations that are geometrically accessible to miRNA. Using our recent work on human AGO2 as an example, we explain the rationale and the workflow of our method in details. This combined approach holds great promise to complement experiments in unraveling the mechanisms of molecular recognition between large, flexible, and complex biomolecules.

**Key words** miRNA, Argonaute, Molecular recognition, Molecular dynamics, Markov state model, Protein-RNA docking

## 1 Introduction

MicroRNAs (miRNAs) are short, noncoding RNAs that regulate more than half of human protein-coding genes [1–5]. Because of their crucial roles in normal physiological functions and disease progression [6–8], miRNAs can greatly inspire the development of new therapeutic agents such as miRNA mimics [9] and anti-miRNA oligonucleotides [10]. Argonaute (AGO) proteins serve as the central platform of miRNA functions [11]. A mature miRNAs is loaded into AGO to form RNA-induced silencing complex (RISC) that recognizes and inhibits target messenger RNAs (mRNAs) with high specificity and efficiency [12, 13]. There are four human AGOs (hAGO1-4), among which hAGO2 has

Marco F. Schmidt (ed.), *Drug Target miRNA: Methods and Protocols*, Methods in Molecular Biology, vol. 1517, DOI 10.1007/978-1-4939-6563-2_18, 

attracted the greatest attention due to its active target-slicing function and sequence-specific interactions with miRNAs [14–17]. Therefore, hAGO2 has been recognized as a promising target for the miRNA-based drug discovery [18, 19]. Elucidating the molecular recognition between miRNA and hAGO2 is thus critical for the rational design of drugs targeting miRNAs.

Recent breakthroughs in structural biology have successfully produced the crystal structures of hAGO2-miRNA complex [15, 16]. In these structures, miRNAs are buried in the RNA-binding groove and hAGO2 adopts a partially open conformation where the miRNA loading channel is sterically hindered. Such conformation suggests that hAGO2-miRNA recognition is a multistep process involving large conformational changes of hAGO2. A recent kinetic characterization also indicates that multiple stages exist during the loading of miRNA into hAGO2 [20]. However, details of the dynamics for hAGO2-miRNA recognition at atomic level remain elusive.

Molecular dynamics (MD) simulations are key to complement experimental research because they can model the conformational dynamics of biomolecules at atomic resolution [21, 22]. Prior to our work, MD simulations have successfully investigated the conformational stability of the bacterial AGO-miRNA/DNA-mRNA complexes [23–25]. However, directly simulating the entire process of miRNA loading into hAGO2 via conventional MD simulations is prohibitively challenging. Since both hAGO2 and miRNA are large, flexible biopolymers that have extremely rugged energy landscape, there is a gap between the experimentally observed timescales (estimated to be milliseconds) and the length of conventional MD simulations (usually tens to hundreds of nanoseconds). An alternative and feasible approach to study hAGO2-miRNA recognition is to first sufficiently explore the conformational space of apo hAGO2 and then identify conformations that are available to load miRNA.

Markov state models (MSMs) are powerful tools to elucidate the conformational dynamics of apo hAGO2 as they can bridge the timescale gap between experiments and MD simulations [18, 26–39]. Based on many short MD simulations, we can construct an MSM that contains a set of conformational states and the interstate transition probabilities. Once validated, an MSM can be used not only to estimate the long-timescale dynamics with reasonable accuracy but also to investigate the underlying mechanisms of conformational changes of biomolecules. In recent years, such methodology has been successfully applied to elucidate mechanisms of protein/RNA folding [40–49], functions of molecular machines [50–54], and molecular recognitions [55–59].

Protein-RNA docking excels in efficiently assessing if an apo hAGO2 conformation can accommodate miRNA. High Ambiguity Driven protein-protein DOCKing (HADDOCK) [60, 61] is one of the best performing methods for predicting protein-protein and protein-RNA/DNA interactions, because a priori knowledge of the interface (e.g., mutagenesis experiments, crystallographic contacts, and NMR restraints) is incorporated into its flexible docking algorithms [62, 63]. Therefore, HADDOCK is particularly suited for studying hAGO2-miRNA recognition, as the binding interface is known from the existing crystal complex structure. Starting from the top ranking docking poses obtained by HADDOCK, we can perform MD simulations to further explore the conformational dynamics of hAGO2-miRNA recognition after initial binding.

Here we describe our approach combining MD simulations, MSMs, and protein-RNA docking to investigate molecular recognition between miRNA and AGO proteins. In the following part of this section, we introduce the underlying theories for each method. Next, we provide lists of software packages for the methods in Subheading 2. In Subheading 3, we present a case study of hAGO2-miRNA recognition [64] to illustrate how these methods can be combined to solve challenging biological questions.

### 1.1 MD Simulations

Molecular dynamics is a computational method to simulate the time-dependent movements of atoms and molecules [65–67]. In all-atom MD simulations, the interactions between atoms and the potential energy of the system are calculated based on a classical force field. A typical potential energy function ($U$) contains terms describing bonded (stretching, bending, and dihedrals) and nonbonded (electrostatic and van der Waals) interactions (*see* Eq. 1) [21]. After each simulation step, the force exerted on each atom is calculated by taking the negative derivatives of the potential energy function. The velocities and coordinates of the system are then updated by numerically solving Newton's equation of motion for all the atoms. Therefore, given a set of force field parameters and an initial biomolecular structure, an MD simulation produces a trajectory that displays the conformational changes of the molecule through a period of time.

$$\begin{aligned} U = & \sum_{\text{bonds}} \frac{1}{2} k_r \left( r \sum r_0 \right)^2 + \sum_{\text{angles}} \frac{1}{2} k_\theta \left( \theta \sum \theta_0 \right)^2 + \sum_{\text{dihedrals}} k_\phi \left[ 1 - \cos(n\phi + \delta) \right] \\ & + \sum_{\text{non bonded pairs}} \epsilon \left[ \left( \frac{r_0}{r} \right)^{12} - 2 \left( \frac{r_0}{r} \right)^{6} \right] + \sum_{\text{non bonded charged pairs}} k_c \frac{q_i q_j}{r} \end{aligned} \tag{1}$$

### 1.2 MSM

Straightforward MD simulations performed on state-of-the-art general-purpose computing hardware are typically limited to a short length (nano- to microseconds), orders of magnitude shorter than the biologically relevant timescale (milliseconds and beyond). Among the efforts devoted to bridge such gap between the timescale accessible by MD simulations and the biological timescale, Markov state models (MSMs) are one of the most popular computational techniques.

MSM is a kinetic network model that contains conformational states and the probabilities of transitions between the states [31,

34, 36]. The model has the Markov property that the distribution of state population in future $p(t+\tau)$ depends only on the current state $p(t)$, but not on any previous history. Therefore, the long-timescale dynamics of the system can be estimated by the master equation:

$$p(n\tau) = T(\tau)^n p(0) \quad (2)$$

where $p(0)$ and $p(n\tau)$ are the distribution of state population at the beginning and at time $n\tau$, respectively, and $T(\tau)$ is the transition probability matrix that describes the chances of transition from one state to the other after the time interval $\tau$.

To construct an MSM, the conformational space is discretized by clustering conformations from MD simulations into a group of small states. The transition probability matrix is obtained by counting the interstate transitions from the MD trajectories. However, the kinetic process described by the transition probability matrix is not necessarily Markovian, as the intrastate dynamics can no longer be distinguished and the transition probabilities become history dependent [31]. To acquire the Markov property, a lag time $\tau$ is selected so that the equilibrium in each state is reached within $\tau$. The resulting transition probability matrix $T(\tau)$ becomes history-independent and can therefore model the long-timescale dynamics by performing Markov jumps with time step $\tau$ as shown in Eq. 2.

### 1.3 Molecular Docking

Molecular docking is a computational approach to predict the three-dimensional complex structure based on the known structures of the individual partner molecules [68]. Two major steps of molecular docking are sampling and scoring. During sampling, one tries to identify as many complex conformations as possible. Since each molecule in the complex has an enormous conformational and orientational space, performing all-atom MD simulations for sampling this search space is over-expensive. In practice, more efficient approaches such as FFT-based grid search [69], geometric hashing [70], and rigid-body minimization [61] are used for the initial conformational searching. Normal mode analysis [71, 72] and Monte Carlo [73] or short MD [61] simulations are subsequently performed to consider the flexibility of the molecules. The scoring step aims to rank all the identified complex conformations by estimating their binding affinities. Like in the sampling step, accurate calculation of binding affinity is computationally demanding. A scoring function containing both basic terms in molecular mechanics (e.g., electrostatics [61, 74] and van der Waals [73]) and empirical parameters (e.g., buried surface area [61]) is used instead for fast ranking. More recently, the information-driven methods which incorporate experimental data into the prediction have become the most successful docking approaches [63, 68, 75].

## 2 Materials

### 2.1 MD Simulations

#### 2.1.1 System Setup

The starting conformations for MD simulations come from experimentally solved X-ray crystal structures, NMR structures, or homology models. The missing protein residues and nucleotides must be modeled prior to MD simulations, with software such as MODELLER [76–79] and ModeRNA [80] for proteins and RNA molecules, respectively. GROMACS [81–83] is one of the most popular packages for preparing, performing, and analyzing MD simulations (*see* **Note 1**). The following bullet points outline a typical protocol and the commands (in brackets) for preparing MD simulations with GROMACS:

1. Converting the input coordination file (e.g., PDB files) into the GROMACS format and generating the topology by choosing an appropriate force field (*see* **Note 2**) (*pdb2gmx*)
2. Defining the shape and the size of the simulation box (*editconf*)
3. Adding solvent into the box for explicit solvent simulations (*solvate*)
4. Adding ions into the simulation box to maintain the charge balance and the physiological salt concentration (*grompp* and *genion*)
5. Performing energy minimization to eliminate steric clashes and improper geometry (*grompp* and *mdrun*)
6. Performing equilibration with fixed solute to equilibrate the solvent under NVT and NPT ensembles, respectively (*grompp* and *mdrun*)
7. Performing production MD simulations under either NVT or NPT ensembles (*grompp* and *mdrun*)

#### 2.1.2 Sampling Strategy

To obtain global thermodynamic and kinetic information of the system of interest, straightforward MD simulations alone are normally insufficient, unless a single ultra-long MD simulation can be performed using special-purpose machines such as Anton [84]. Therefore, for MD simulations performed on general-purposed computing facilities, it is useful to apply methods such as Markov state models (discussed in Subheading 2.2) that estimate the global information from a large set of MD simulations of relatively short length. In such an approach, one needs to first explore the conformational space sufficiently and use the initial sampling to seed subsequent MD simulations. This can be achieved either by using enhanced sampling methods or by multiple independent MD simulations launched from the starting conformation (*see* **Note 3**). To obtain a final MSM with high statistical robustness, one usually needs to perform multiple rounds of MD simulations by iterating the following procedure:

1. Initiating MD simulations from the input structure
2. Building preliminary MSMs based on the obtained MD trajectories
3. Selecting representative conformations from the poorly sampled regions identified by the preliminary MSMs (*see* **Note 4**)
4. Launching the new round of MD simulations from the representative conformations

#### 2.1.3 Trajectory Analysis

MD trajectories can be visualized by packages such as PyMOL [85] and VMD [86] and analyzed by VMD, MDAnalysis [87], or MDTraj [88]. Most MD programs also provide tools for basic trajectory analysis. Root mean square deviation (RMSD) and root mean square fluctuation (RMSF) are two of the most frequently inspected properties of MD trajectories. The essential conformational dynamics of the system can be further elucidated with dimension reduction methods such as principal component analysis [89], multidimensional scaling [90], isomap [91], and diffusion map [92, 93].

## 2.2 MSM

#### 2.2.1 Constructing MSMs from MD Trajectories

Two frequently used tools for building and analyzing MSMs are MSMBuilder [34, 94] and EMMA [95, 96]. The general protocol for MSM construction is shown in Fig. 1. Usually two models (microstate MSM and macrostate MSM) are produced for the prediction of quantitative properties and the visualization of the important metastable states, respectively.

Since MD trajectories are separated from each other by nature, the transitions between conformations from different trajectories cannot be estimated with kinetic information alone. To solve this issue, conformations are geometrically clustered into hundreds or

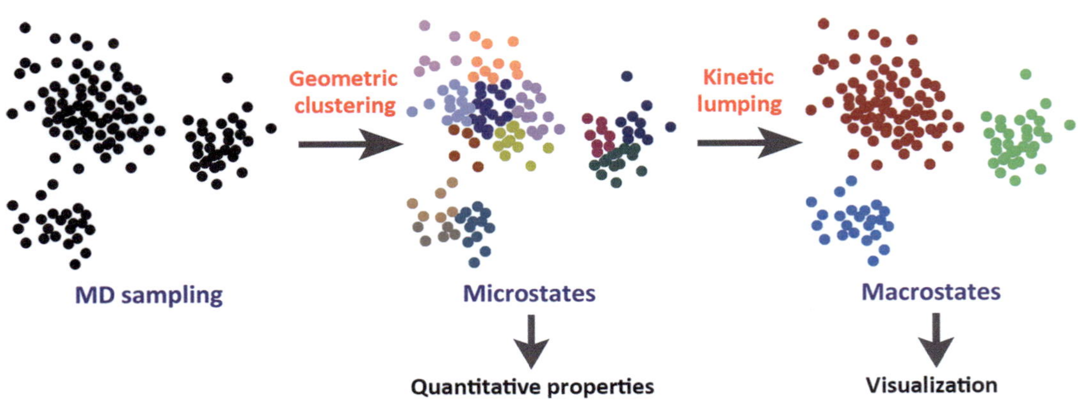


**Fig. 1** General protocol of MSM construction. Conformations obtained from MD simulations are geometrically clustered into microstates. The transition probability matrix of microstates, once validated, can be used to predict quantitative properties (e.g., equilibrium population and MFPT) of the system. To facilitate the visualization of metastable states, microstates are further grouped into several macrostates by kinetic lumping

thousands of microstates, with the assumption that conformations separated by short distances are also kinetically close to each other (*see* **Note 5**). In each of the microstates, the intrastate relaxation should be faster than the interstate transitions. Commonly used clustering algorithms for microstate generation include K-centers [97] and K-medoids [98]. The distance metric for clustering is typically measured by RMSD between pairs of conformations. In practice, some physical understanding may be needed to choose an appropriate set of atoms to be included in the RMSD calculations. Such set of atoms can also be determined by recent algorithms [18, 19, 99] such as the time-structure-based Independent Component Analysis (tICA) [19]. Since tICA identifies a set of key tICs that can sufficiently describe slowest dynamics of the system, distances between pairs of conformations can be subsequently computed in the reduced dimensional space containing these tICs. The tICA method provides a promising approach to automatically choose metrics that can best describe the conformational dynamics of interest.

A transition count matrix is first generated by counting the number of pairwise microstate transitions from all the MD trajectories. By symmetrizing and then normalizing the transition count matrix, we obtain the transition probability matrix (*see* **Note 6**). Based on the transition probability matrix of microstates, we can plot a series of implied timescales to determine the lag time $\tau$ for production MSM and the number of macrostates.

While the validated microstate MSM can be used to predict long-timescale dynamics, such model usually contains hundreds or thousands of states which cannot be easily visualized. To facilitate the illustration of the essential dynamics, we further lump the kinetically related microstates into several metastable macrostates based on the microstate transition probability matrix. Commonly used algorithms for macrostate constructions are PCCA [100, 101], PCCA+ [102, 103], SHC [104], BACE [105], and HNEG [38]. To elucidate the dynamic behaviors at different timescales, we have recently developed the APM algorithm [39] which incorporates the kinetic information into microstate- and macrostate-MSM construction.

To sum up, typical MSM construction involves the following steps:

1. Choosing a proper distance metric and geometrically clustering MD conformations into hundreds or thousands of microstates
2. Constructing transition probability matrix of microstates and plotting implied timescales to determine the lag time for MSM construction and the number of macrostates
3. Kinetically lumping microstates into several macrostates to facilitate visualization

*2.2.2 Validation of MSM*

The implied timescales serve as the primary means of MSM validation. They can be calculated by the following equation:

$$\tau_k = -\frac{\tau}{\ln \lambda_k} \tag{3}$$

where $\lambda_k$ is the *k*th largest eigenvalue of the transition probability matrix of $\tau$, and $\tau_k$ denotes the *k*th slowest implied timescales of the system. The implied timescales usually level off after the lag time reaches certain value, indicating the model is Markovian at this time or longer. This time is designated as the Markovian time and used for building the production MSM. Based on the largest gap between the slowest timescales, the plot of implied timescales can also be used for determining the number of macrostates.

Another important approach to validate an MSM is to perform the Chapman-Kolmogorov test [31]. In this test, the kinetics of inter- and intrastate transitions predicted by the MSM are compared with the actual dynamics observed by MD simulations. The MSM is validated only if the prediction is in reasonable agreement with the observation from the MD simulations.

*2.2.3 Mean First Passage Time (MFPT)*

MFPT, defined as the average time taken by the first transition from one state to the other (both direct and indirect transitions considered), is an important property to elucidate the kinetic information from an MSM. One can compute MFPT by the following equation:

$$X_{if} = \sum_j T(\tau)_{ij}\left(\tau + X_{jf}\right) \tag{4}$$

where $T(\tau)_{ij}$ is the transition probability from state *i* to state *j*, $\tau$ is the lag time, and $X_{ff} = 0$. In order to provide kinetic descriptions of macrostate transitions, MFPTs from each microstates of the initial macrostate to the finial macrostate are calculated and averaged according to their normalized equilibrium population based on the validated microstate MSM.

*2.2.4 Transition Path Theory (TPT)*

Another application of MSM is to elucidate the major transition pathways between functional states of biomolecules. Based on the framework of TPT [37, 49], we can calculate the flux of each pathway from the initial state to the final state using a greedy backtracking algorithm. The major pathway which carries the highest flux provides the direct illustration on the underlying mechanism of conformational dynamics (*see* **Note 7**).

## 2.3 Protein-RNA Docking

*2.3.1 HADDOCK Procedure*

HADDOCK [60, 61] is a docking software that utilizes the information about the binding interface known from the crystal complex (*see* **Note 8**). In particular, ambiguous interaction restraints (AIRs) can be defined based on the crystal contacts to efficiently drive the docking procedure to produce high-quality models. The molecular interactions were computed by CNS 1.3 [106, 107] using PARALLHDG5.4 [108, 109] and OPLS-AA [110] force field for protein and RNA, respectively. The HADDOCK approach consists of three stages: rigid-body minimization, semiflexible simulated annealing, and solvated refinement. The output docking poses are clustered and ranked by their HADDOCK score which includes descriptions of van der Waals, electrostatics, desolvation, buried surface area, and ambiguous interaction restraints. The docking simulations can be performed by submitting input structures to the web server [91] or running HADDOCK locally following the procedure below:

1. Preparing input structures by modeling the missing residues and nucleotides
2. Defining AIRs for the docking
3. Defining extra constraints (e.g. unambiguous distance constraints, constraints from NMR data)
4. Determining the force field parameters and docking procedures by modifying the running script (*run.cns*)

#### 2.3.2 Analysis of the Docking Poses

Since the optimal binding pose is known from the crystal complex structure, we can use the fraction of native contacts ($f_{nat}$) to evaluate the quality of the docking poses:

$$f_{nat} = \frac{q_{pose}}{q_{crystal}} \tag{5}$$

where $q_{pose}$ denotes the numbers of protein-protein or protein-RNA/DNA crystal contacts (distance smaller than 4 Å) found in the docking pose and $q_{crystal}$ is the number of observed contacts in the crystal structure.

# 3 Methods

In this section, we describe the protocol of the combined method of MD simulations, MSM, and protein-RNA docking in details with our recent work on hAGO2-miRNA recognition as an example.

### 3.1 Performing MD Simulations of Apo hAGO2

The initial conformation of apo hAGO2 was obtained from the hAGO2-miR-20a crystal complex (PDB ID: 4F3T) [16]. Residues missing in the density map were modeled with MODELLER [76–79]. The MD simulations were prepared and performed with GROMACS-4.5.4 [81–83] using Amber99SB-ILDN force field [111]. A dodecahedron box filled with 42,847 SPC water molecules was used to solvate the protein [112]. To balance the charge and maintain the physiological salt concentration, 129 $Na^+$ ions and 159 $Cl^-$ ions were added into the system. The particle mesh Ewald method [113] was applied to efficiently compute long-range electrostatic interactions. A cutoff scheme of 10 Å was applied to van der Waals interactions and short-range electrostatic interactions. The LINCS algorithm [114] was applied to constrain all the bonds. The solvated system was first energy minimized by the steepest decent algorithm for 10,000 steps. A 1-ns equilibration was subsequently performed under the NPT ensemble (310 K and 1 atm) with the temperature and the pressure controlled by velocity-rescaling thermostat [115] and Parrinello-Rahman barostat [116], respectively. The last frame from the equilibration was used for the production MD simulations under NVT ensemble at 310 K.

To sufficiently sample the conformational space of apo hAGO2, we performed three rounds of MD simulations. From the equilibrated hAGO2 system, we first initiated six MD simulations which added up to ~400 ns. The ~20,000 conformations obtained from this round of simulations were geometrically grouped into 20 clusters with the K-center algorithm [97]. For the second round of sampling, a random conformation from each of the 20 clusters was selected to seed a 150-ns MD simulation. Using over 170,000 conformations obtained from the first two rounds of simulations, we built two preliminary models with the APM algorithm [39]: a 553-microstate MSM and a 9-macrostate MSM. However, both models predict the kinetics that is inconsistent with the observation from MD simulations (*see* details of MSM construction and validation in Subheading 3.2), which suggests additional sampling is required. Therefore, we further selected conformations according to the equilibrium population predicted by the 9-macrostate MSM and launched the third round of simulations (thirty 150-ns trajectories). Taken together, we performed ~8 μs MD simulations from which over 394,000 apo hAGO2 conformations were obtained.

As shown in Fig. 2a, the PAZ domain, the N domain, and two PIWI loops (the major loop V818-D838 and the minor loop P601-P609) are the most flexible hAGO2 regions. Interestingly, the PIWI loops and the PAZ domain form extensive hydrogen bonding network, which blocks the entrance to the RNA-binding groove (*see* Fig. 2b, c). Therefore, we used these regions to define the metric for the geometric clustering during MSM construction.

### 3.2 Constructing MSMs to Elucidate Conformational Dynamics of Apo hAGO2

We constructed MSMs with the recently developed APM algorithm [39] to elucidate the conformational dynamics of apo hAGO2. To compute their pairwise distance, MD conformations were aligned against the crystal structure of hAGO2 at the PIWI Cα atoms, and the pairwise Euclidean distances of the PIWI loop Cα atoms (describing the conformations of PIWI loops) and every third Cα atoms of the PAZ domain (describing the opening motions of hAGO2) were calculated. Using APM, we obtained a

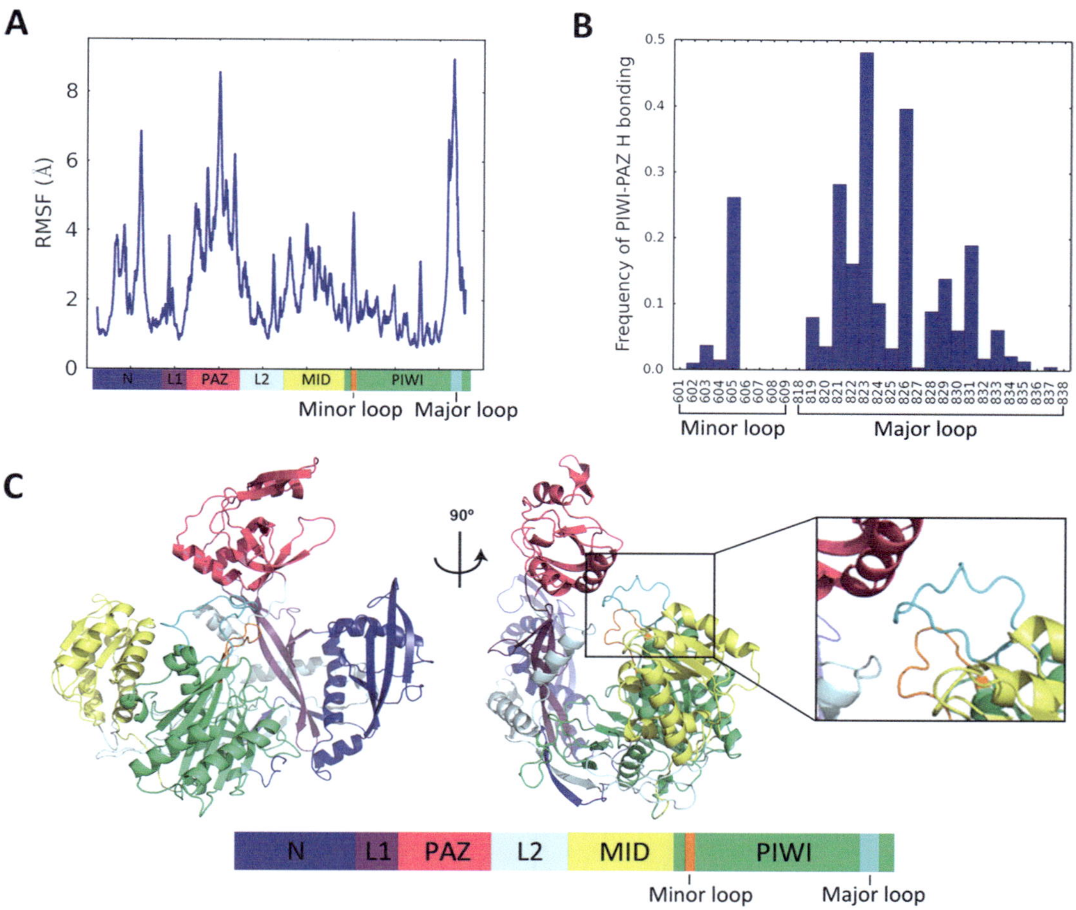


**Fig. 2** Analysis of MD trajectories of apo hAGO2. (**a**) Residue RMSF of apo hAGO2 from MD simulations. The PAZ and N domains, together with the major PIWI loop (V818-D838), are among the most flexible regions of hAGO2. (**b**) Frequency of the residues on PIWI loops for forming hydrogen bonding network with the PAZ domain. (**c**) hAGO2 is comprised of six major domains: N, L1, PAZ, L2, MID, and PIWI. Two PIWI loops are colored in *cyan* (major) and *orange* (minor). The *inset panel* on the *right* highlights the interaction between the PAZ domain and the PIWI loops. This figure was reproduced from [64]

480-microstate MSM. As shown in Fig. 3a, there is a clear gap between seventh and eight slowest timescales of the microstate MSM ($\lambda_1 = 1$ and thus $\tau_1$ was not plotted). Therefore, a seven-macrostate MSM should be constructed. The reasonable agreement between the slowest dynamics of the 480-microstate MSM and that of the seven-macrostate MSM indicates that both models capture the essential dynamics of hAGO2 (*see* Fig. 3a, c).

To systematically validate our MSMs, we applied the residence probability test [31, 47], a variant of the Chapman-Kolmogorov test. In particular, we used the MSM to compute the probability of hAGO2 staying in a certain state and compared it with the same probability obtained by counting transitions from MD trajectories.

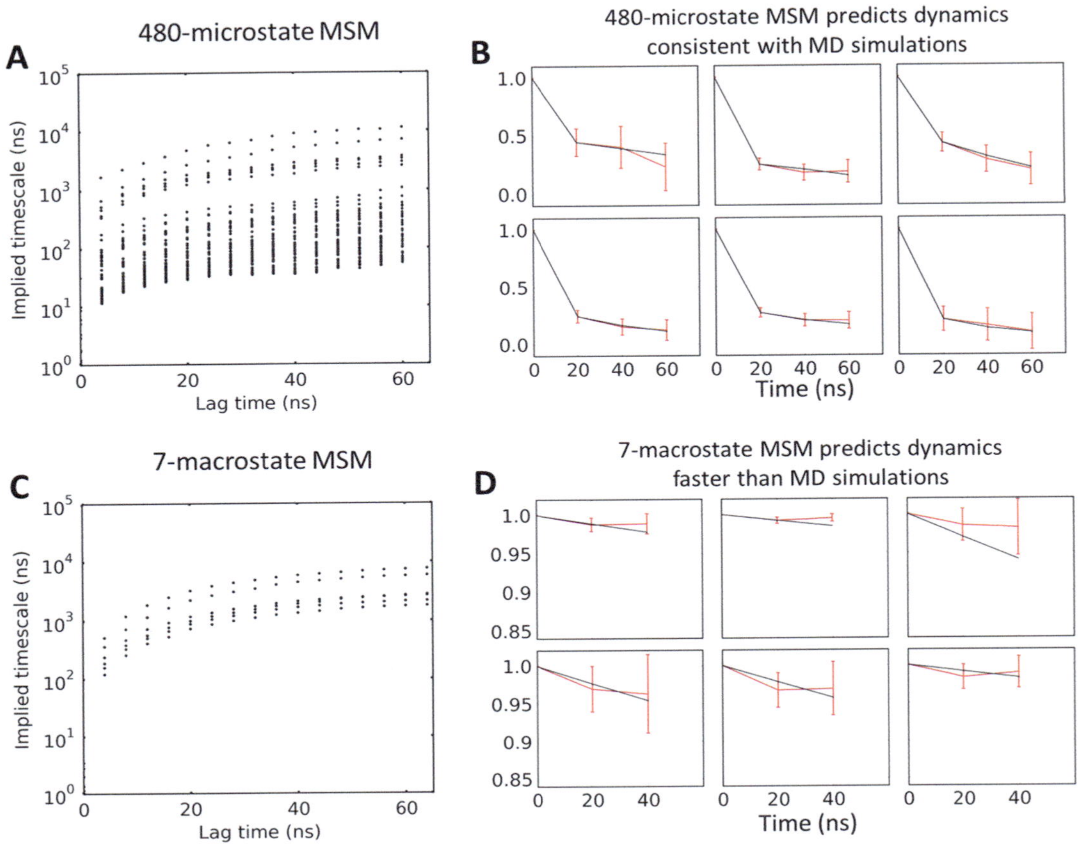


**Fig. 3** Validating the 480-microstate MSM and the 7-macrostate MSM by plotting implied timescales and performing residence probability tests. (**a**) Implied timescales plot of microstates. (**b**) Results of residence probability tests on representative microstates. The observation from MD simulations is marked in *red* and the kinetics predicted by MSMs is marked in *black*. (**c**) Implied timescale plot of macrostates. (**d**) Results of residence probability tests on the macrostates with the same coloring scheme as in (**b**). This figure was reproduced from [64]

As suggested by Fig. 3b, d, while the 480-microstate MSM is in good agreement with the MD simulations, the seven-macrostate MSM predicts faster kinetics than the observation in the simulations. Therefore, the microstate MSM was used for reporting quantitative predictions and the macrostate MSM for visualization of the metastable states.

The seven macrostates can be further grouped into three classes: the closed states, the partially open state, and the open state (*see* Fig. 4). In the closed states and the partially open state, the PAZ domain interacts with PIWI loops, blocking the entrance of RNA-binding groove (*see* Fig. 4b, c). Interestingly, conformations in the open state have fully exposed RNA-binding groove

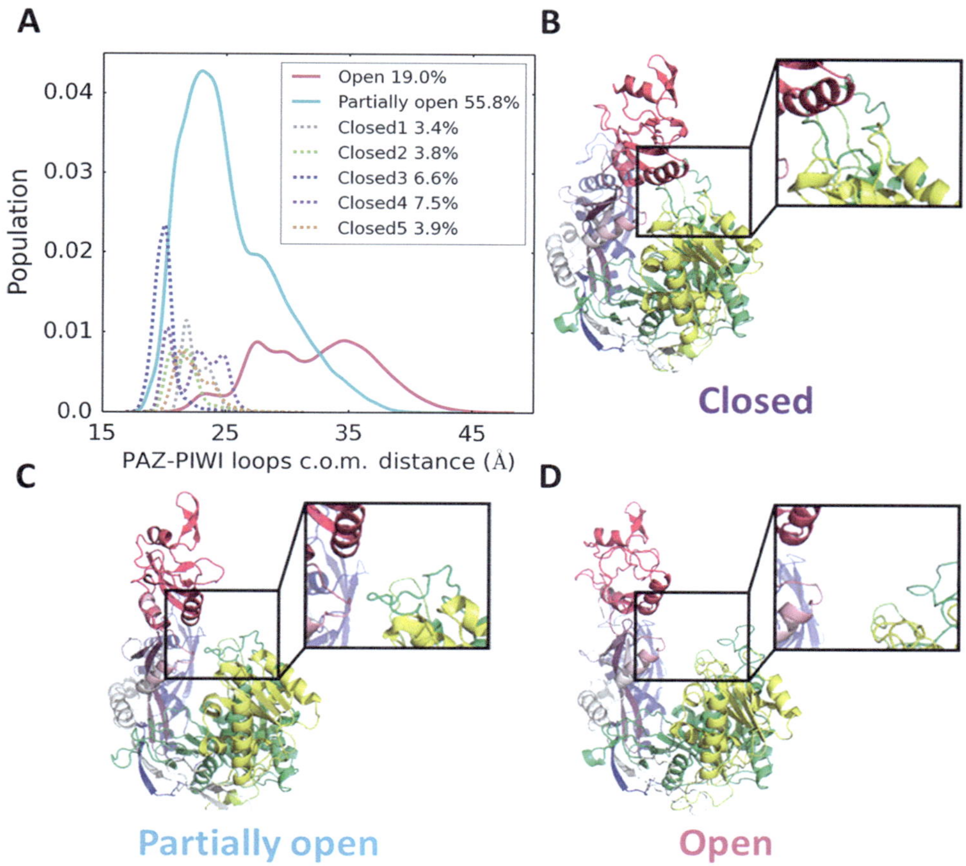


**Fig. 4** The seven macrostates of apo hAGO2 can be grouped into three classes: open, partially open, and closed states. (**a**) Projection of macrostate population onto the center-of-mass (c.o.m.) distance between PIWI loops and the PAZ domain. (**b–d**) Representative structures from the closed state, the partially open state, and open state, respectively. The *inset panel* on the *right* of each structure highlights the PAZ-PIWI loop interactions. This figure was adapted from [64]

(indicated by the large PAZ-PIWI loop c.o.m. distance), suggesting they may be available for miRNA loading (*see* Fig. 4a, d).

The major transition pathways from the closed states of hAGO2 to the open state, obtained by applying TPT, demonstrate that the most transitions involve the intermediate, partially open state (*see* Fig. 5).

### *3.3 Performing Protein-RNA Docking to Assess Open hAGO2 Conformations*

To examine if the widely open hAGO2 conformations are available for miRNA loading, we performed hAGO2-miRNA docking with HADDOCK. The input hAGO2 conformations were randomly selected from the widely open microstates (with average PAZ-PIWI loops c.o.m. distance >25Å), and the input miRNA structure was obtained from the crystal complex structure (PDB ID: 4F3T) with missing nucleotides modeled by ModeRNA [80]. The AIRs

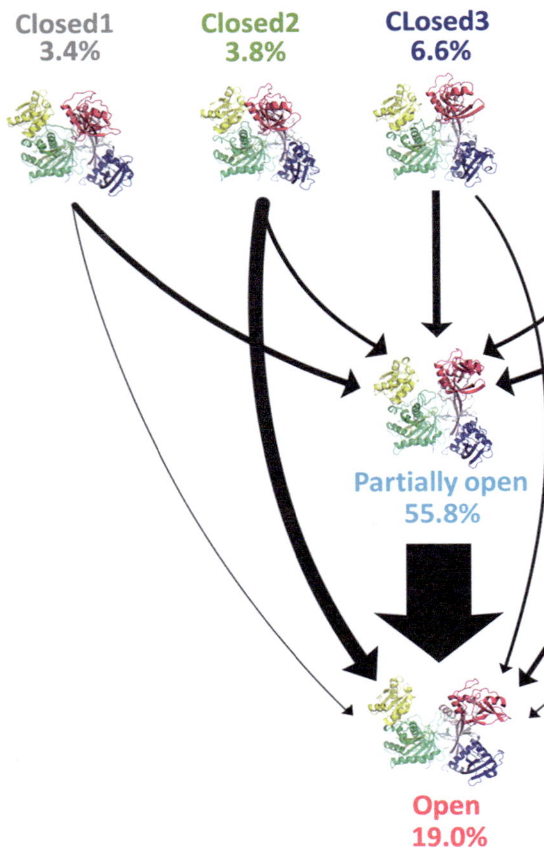


**Fig. 5** Major transition pathways from the closed states to the open state. By applying TPT, we used the validated 480-microstate MSM to compute the flux of individual pathways. All the microstate pathways were then combined into the major pathways from the five closed states to the open state. The size of the *arrows* indicates the amount of interstate flux. This figure was reproduced from [64]

were defined based on the hAGO2-miRNA crystal contacts. In addition, we defined unambiguous distance restraints between the termini of miRNA and their binding sites in hAGO2 to produce high-quality docking models. In total, we performed 150 docking simulations which generated 7500 refined docking poses.

We used the HADDOCK score to rank the high-quality docking poses. The funnel shape shown in the HADDOCK score-$f_{nat}$ plot suggest that the best scoring hAGO2-miRNA docking poses indeed adopt the native mode of intermolecular interactions (*see* Fig. 6a). We further defined the successful docking poses where both 5′ and 3′ termini of miRNA correctly locate in the corresponding binding pocket on hAGO2. As shown in Fig. 6b, all the successful docking poses were generated from conformations of the open state. Therefore, only the open state of hAGO2 can accommodate miRNA.

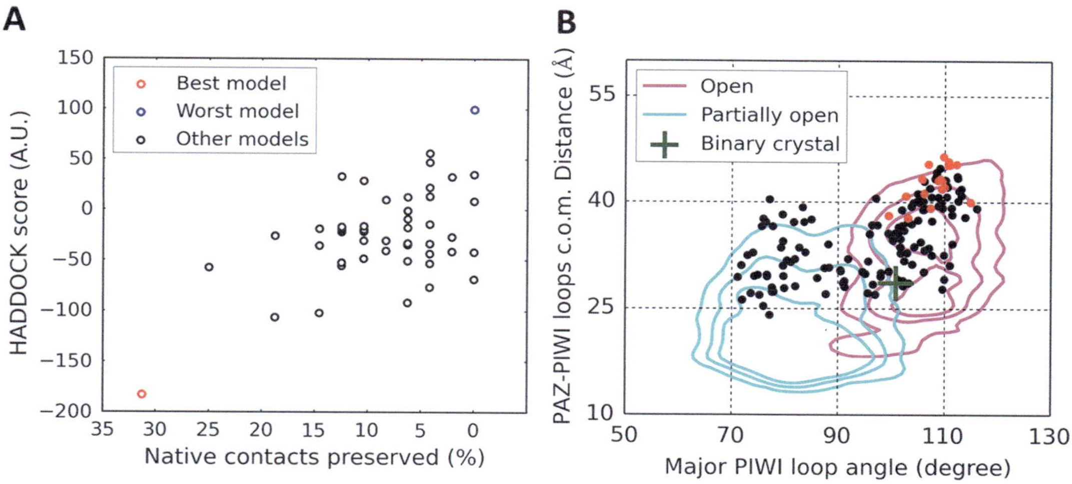


**Fig. 6** Docking miRNA onto hAGO2 with HADDOCK. (**a**) Typical results of a HADDOCK simulation: 50 hAGO2-miRNA docking poses were ranked according to the HADDOCK scores and the fraction of native hAGO2-miRNA contacts. (**b**) Projection of hAGO2-miRNA docking poses onto major PIWI loop angle (defined by Cα atoms of A596, V614, and D823) and PAZ-PIWI loops c.o.m. distance. *Red* and *black dots* indicate the successful and the unsuccessful docking models, respectively. This figure was adapted from [64]

### 3.4 Conducting MD Simulations of hAGO2-miRNA Initial Binding Complex

To investigate the impact of miRNA binding to the conformational dynamics of hAGO2, we launched MD simulations from the successful hAGO2-miRNA docking models. The system setup followed the same procedure described in Subheading 3.1. For each successful docking model, five 20-ns simulations were performed. All the simulations displayed the decreasing PAZ-PIWI loops c.o.m. distance and the interface RMSD, suggesting hAGO2 closed upon the initial loading of miRNA (*see* Fig. 7a and the top panel of Fig. 7b). The hAGO2-miRNA contacts were maintained during the conformational changes (*see* the bottom panel of Fig. 7b). The MD-refined hAGO2-miRNA docking model displays high structural similarity to the crystal structure, indicating the structural rearrangement is required to stabilize hAGO2-miRNA interactions (*see* Fig. 7c).

Taken together, our results imply a two-step hAGO2-miRNA recognition: selective binding followed by structural rearrangement (*see* Fig. 8). As suggested by the MSMs, apo hAGO2 is in fast equilibrium among open, partially open, and closed states (MFPTs are tens of microseconds). The incoming miRNA may selectively bind to the open state, the only state that is geometrically available for miRNA loading as indicated by protein-RNA docking. Further MD simulations show that the initial miRNA binding triggers the structural re-arrangement of hAGO2 to reach the most stable conformation captured by the crystal complex.

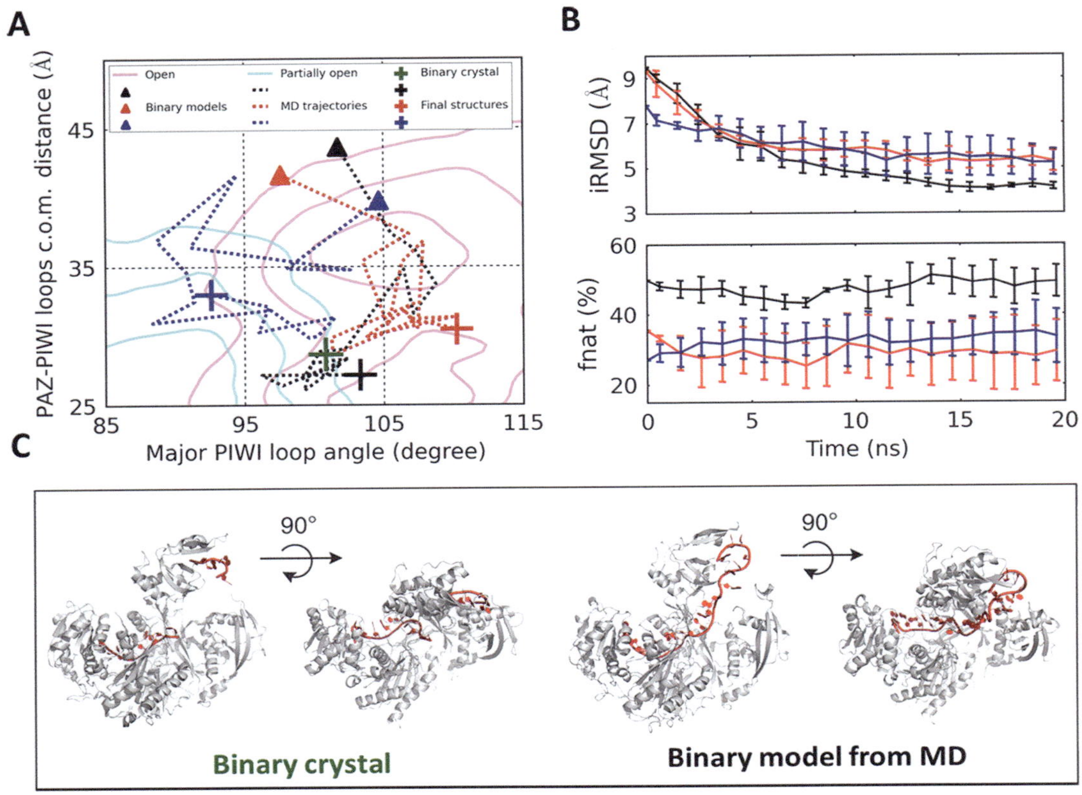


**Fig. 7** hAGO2-miRNA docking models perform significant structural rearrangement to reach the crystal conformation during short MD simulations. (**a**) MD trajectories of three selected successful docking poses projected onto major PIWI loop angle and PAZ-PIWI loop c.o.m. distance. (**b**) *Top panel*: the interface RMSD (iRMSD) of docking models against the crystal complex. *Bottom panel*: the fraction of native hAGO2-miRNA contacts (fnat). (**c**) Comparison between the crystal complex (*left*) and an MD-refined model (*right*). In these structures, hAGO2 and miRNA are colored in *gray* and *red*, respectively. This figure was reproduced from [64]

### 3.5 Limitations of the Methods and Alternative Approaches

In the previous sections, we have shown that the presented computational protocol combining MD simulations, MSMs, and protein-RNA docking successfully revealed both structural and kinetic insights at atomic resolution into the miRNA loading into hAGO2. Although this comprehensive methodology is general and can be applied to study the recognition between other proteins and nucleic acids, one shall also note its limitations.

As the construction of MSMs initiates by generating the transition count matrix from unbiased MD trajectories, it is crucial that a sufficient number of both forward and backward transitions among the states can be observed within the affordable length of MD trajectories. This, however, can be difficult to achieve, especially if the energy landscape of the system under study contains high free energy barriers separating the metastable states. Under this situation, reliable estimations of transition probabilities between pairs of

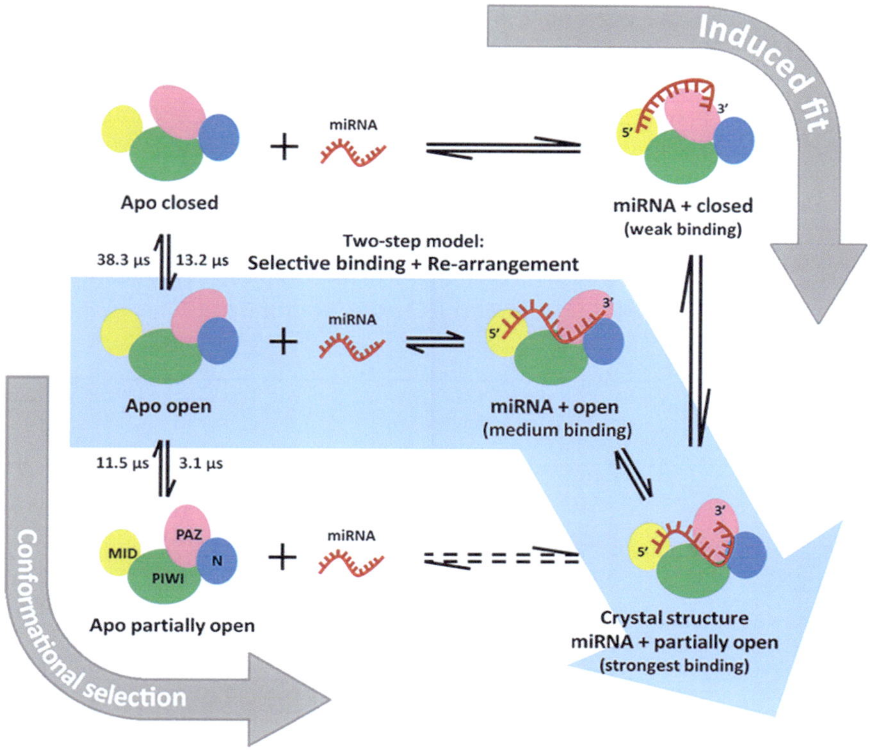


**Fig. 8** A two-step model of hAGO2-miRNA recognition: selective binding followed by structural rearrangement (the *cyan arrow*). Two classical models of molecular recognition, induced fit (the *upper right arrow* in *gray*) and conformational selection (the *lower left arrow* in *gray*), are also presented for comparison. This figure was reproduced from [64]

these metastable states are difficult based on relatively short straightforward MD simulations. Take our recent work on the guide DNA loading into the bacterium *Thermus thermophilus* Argonaute (TtAGO) [89] for an example, due to the ultrahigh flexibility of its L1-PAZ hinge, the exposure of the guide DNA-binding groove of TtAGO only occurs with very small probability. In such cases, alternative enhanced sampling techniques, such as bias-exchange metadynamics [84, 117, 118], can be applied to reveal the thermodynamic landscape of the protein. Further protein-DNA/RNA docking on the protein conformations extracted from the landscape can also measure the exposure of the binding groove and provide insights into the recognition process.

### 3.6 Concluding Remarks

In this chapter, we reviewed our recent work on the mechanism of hAGO2-miRNA recognition with the emphasis on the detailed protocol of MD simulations, MSM, and protein-RNA docking. MSM constructed from MD simulations can provide crucial insight into conformational dynamics of biomolecules. However, given the current computing power, both MSM and MD simulations might become insufficient when dealing with complex systems (e.g. hAGO2-miRNA recognition). As an alternative, one can investigate the dynamics of each molecule separately and search for the possible binding mode via molecular docking and MD refinement. This combined approach holds great promise in elucidating the essential dynamics of the molecular recognition. In addition, the important structural features of both hAGO2 and miRNA identified by this method can significantly facilitate the rational design of miRNA targeting drugs.

## 4 Notes

1. Other commonly used programs for MD simulations include AMBER [119], CHARMM [120], NAMD [121], and OpenMM [122].
2. Choosing a proper force field is crucial for the accuracy of MD simulations. For protein simulations, Amber99SB*-ILDN [111, 123] was previously reported as one of the best performing force fields [124]. More recent force fields, such as AMBER ff14SB [125], CHARM36 [126], and OPLS-AA/M [127], are expected to be more accurate but yet to be systematically tested.
3. In the circumstances where the system is trapped in the local free energy minimum, enhanced sampling strategies (e.g., generalized ensemble algorithms [128] and metadynamics [129]) are used to efficiently sample the conformational space. Based on the free energy landscape obtained by enhanced sampling algorithms, representative conformations are then selected to seed unbiased MD simulations for MSM construction.
4. We recommend the adaptive sampling strategy [130] which constructs preliminary MSMs to guide the seeding of further MD simulations to speed up the convergence.
5. One should choose the clustering metric that properly reflects the kinetic properties. A commonly used metric is pairwise RMSD of heavy atoms or Cα atoms.
6. Because all the transitions are reversible at the equilibrium, we impose the detailed balance condition by symmetrizing the transition count matrix. This approach, however, could be biased by limited MD sampling. As an alternative, one can use the maximum likelihood method to estimate the most likely transition probability matrix for the given observation from MD simulations [131].
7. In-depth discussion on the theory and the application of TPT can be found in [37, 47, 132, 133].

8. Depending on the system of study, one can choose docking approaches such HADDOCK [60, 61], ClusPro [134], SwarmDock [72], or RosettaDock [73] for protein-protein/DNA/RNA interactions and AutoDock Vina [135], GLIDE [136], GOLD [137], or DOCK [138] for protein-ligand binding.

## Acknowledgment

This work is supported by the Hong Kong Research Grant Council [grant numbers 16302214, 609813, HKUST C6009-15G, AoE/M-09/12, M-HKUST601/13, and T13-607/12R to X.H.] and the National Science Foundation of China [grant number 21273188 to X.H.]. The work is also supported by a grant from the PROCORE-France/Hong Kong Joint Research Scheme sponsored by the Research Grants Council and the Consulate General of France in Hong Kong (F-HK29/11T) (X.H. and J.B.). X.G. was supported by funding from King Abdullah University of Science and Technology. This research made use of the resources of the Supercomputing Laboratory at King Abdullah University of Science and Technology.

### References

1. Bartel DP (2004) MicroRNAs: genomics, biogenesis, mechanism, and function. Cell 116(2):281–297. doi:10.1016/S0092-8674(04)00045-5
2. Bushati N, Cohen SM (2007) MicroRNA functions. Annu Rev Cell Dev Biol 23:175–205. doi:10.1146/annurev.cellbio.23.090506.123406
3. Wilson RC, Doudna JA (2013) Molecular mechanisms of RNA interference. Annu Rev Biophys 42:217–239. doi:10.1146/annurev-biophys-083012-130404
4. Friedman RC, Farh KKH, Burge CB et al (2009) Most mammalian mRNAs are conserved targets of microRNAs. Genome Res 19(1):92–105. doi:10.1101/gr.082701.108
5. Bartel DP (2009) MicroRNAs: target recognition and regulatory functions. Cell 136(2):215–233. doi:10.1016/j.cell.2009.01.002
6. Wang XW, Heegaard NHH, Orum H (2012) MicroRNAs in liver disease. Gastroenterology 142(7):1431–1443. doi:10.1053/j.gastro.2012.04.007
7. Chivukula RR, Shi GL, Acharya A et al (2014) An essential mesenchymal function for miR-143/145 in intestinal epithelial regeneration. Cell 157(5):1104–1116. doi:10.1016/j.cell.2014.03.055
8. Jansson MD, Lund AH (2012) MicroRNA and cancer. Mol Oncol 6(6):590–610. doi:10.1016/j.molonc.2012.09.006
9. Misso G, Di Martino MT, De Rosa G et al (2014) Mir-34: a new weapon against cancer? Mol Ther Nucleic Acids 3:e194. doi:10.1038/mtna.2014.47
10. Gebert LFR, Rebhan MAE, Crivelli SEM et al (2014) Miravirsen (SPC3649) can inhibit the biogenesis of miR-122. Nucleic Acids Res 42(1):609–621. doi:10.1093/nar/gkt852
11. Meister G (2013) Argonaute proteins: functional insights and emerging roles. Nat Rev Genet 14(7):447–459. doi:10.1038/nrg3462
12. Kawamata T, Tomari Y (2010) Making RISC. Trends Biochem Sci 35(7):368–376. doi:10.1016/j.tibs.2010.03.009
13. Sasaki HM, Tomari Y (2012) The true core of RNA silencing revealed. Nat Struct Mol Biol 19(7):657–660. doi:10.1038/Nsmb.2302
14. Frank F, Sonenberg N, Nagar B (2010) Structural basis for 5′-nucleotide base-specific recognition of guide RNA by human AGO2. Nature 465(7299):818–822. doi:10.1038/nature09039
15. Schirle NT, MacRae IJ (2012) The crystal structure of human argonaute 2. Science 336(6084):1037–1040. doi:10.1126/science.1221551

16. Elkayam E, Kuhn CD, Tocilj A et al (2012) The structure of human argonaute-2 in complex with miR-20a. Cell 150(1):100–110. doi:10.1016/j.cell.2012.05.017
17. Schirle NT, Sheu-Gruttadauria J, MacRae IJ (2014) Structural basis for microRNA targeting. Science 346(6209):608–613. doi:10.1126/science.1258040
18. Pérez-Hernández G, Paul F, Giorgino T et al (2013) Identification of slow molecular order parameters for Markov model construction. J Chem Phys 139(1):015102. doi:10.1063/1.4811489
19. Schwantes CR, Pande VS (2013) Improvements in Markov State Model construction reveal many non-native interactions in the folding of NTL9. J Chem Theory Comput 9(4):2000–2009. doi:10.1021/ct300878a
20. Deerberg A, Willkomm S, Restle T (2013) Minimal mechanistic model of siRNA-dependent target RNA slicing by recombinant human argonaute 2 protein. Proc Natl Acad Sci U S A 110(44):17850–17855. doi:10.1073/pnas.1217838110
21. Levitt M (2001) The birth of computational structural biology. Nat Struct Biol 8(5):392–393. doi:10.1038/87545
22. Karplus M, McCammon JA (2002) Molecular dynamics simulations of biomolecules. Nat Struct Biol 9(9):646–652. doi:10.1038/Nsb0902-646
23. Wang YH, Li Y, Ma Z et al (2010) Mechanism of MicroRNA-target interaction: molecular dynamics simulations and thermodynamics analysis. PLoS Comput Biol 6(7):e1000866. doi:10.1371/journal.pcbi.1000866
24. Xia Z, Clark P, Huynh T et al (2012) Molecular dynamics simulations of Ago silencing complexes reveal a large repertoire of admissible 'seed-less' targets. Sci Rep 2:569. doi:10.1038/Srep00909
25. Xia Z, Huynh T, Ren PY et al (2013) Large domain motions in ago protein controlled by the guide DNA-strand seed region determine the Ago-DNA-mRNA complex recognition process. PLoS One 8(1):e54620. doi:10.1371/journal.pone.0054620
26. Noe F, Fischer S (2008) Transition networks for modeling the kinetics of conformational change in macromolecules. Curr Opin Struct Biol 18(2):154–162
27. Chodera JD, Singhal N, Pande VS et al (2007) Automatic discovery of metastable states for the construction of Markov models of macromolecular conformational dynamics. J Chem Phys 126(15):155101
28. Morcos F, Chatterjee S, McClendon CL et al (2010) Modeling conformational ensembles of slow functional motions in Pin1-WW. PLoS Comput Biol 6(12):e1001015. doi:10.1371/journal.pcbi.1001015
29. Zheng W, Andrec M, Gallicchio E et al (2007) Simulating replica exchange simulations of protein folding with a kinetic network model. Proc Natl Acad Sci U S A 104(39):15340–15345
30. Pan AC, Roux B (2008) Building Markov state models along pathways to determine free energies and rates of transitions. J Chem Phys 129(6):064107. doi:10.1063/1.2959573
31. Prinz JH, Wu H, Sarich M et al (2011) Markov models of molecular kinetics: generation and validation. J Chem Phys 134(17):174105. doi:10.1063/1.3565032
32. Schütte C, Huisinga W (2000) Biomolecular conformations as metastable sets of Markov chains. Paper presented at the proceedings of the 38th annual Allerton conference on communication, control, and computing, Monticello, IL, 4–6 Oct 2000
33. Gfeller D, De Los Rios P, Caflisch A et al (2007) Complex network analysis of free-energy landscapes. Proc Natl Acad Sci U S A 104(6):1817–1822. doi:10.1073/Pnas.0608099104
34. Bowman GR, Huang X, Pande VS (2009) Using generalized ensemble simulations and Markov state models to identify conformational states. Methods 49(2):197–201
35. Hummer G, Szabo A (2015) Optimal dimensionality reduction of multistate kinetic and Markov-state models. J Phys Chem B 119(29):9029–9037. doi:10.1021/jp508375q
36. Chodera JD, Noe F (2014) Markov state models of biomolecular conformational dynamics. Curr Opin Struct Biol 25:135–144. doi:10.1016/j.sbi.2014.04.002
37. Weinan E, Vanden-Eijnden E (2006) Towards a theory of transition paths. J Stat Phys 123(3):503–523
38. Yao Y, Cui RZ, Bowman GR et al (2013) Hierarchical Nyström methods for constructing Markov state models for conformational dynamics. J Chem Phys 138:174106. doi:10.1063/1.4802007
39. Sheong FK, Silva DA, Meng L et al (2015) Automatic state partitioning for multi-body systems (APM): an efficient algorithm for constructing Markov state models to elucidate conformational dynamics of multi-body systems. J Chem Theory Comput 11(1):17–27. doi:10.1021/ct5007168

40. Buchete NV, Hummer G (2008) Coarse master equations for peptide folding dynamics. J Phys Chem 112(19):6057–6069
41. Zheng W, Andrec M, Gallicchio E et al (2008) Simple continuous and discrete models for simulating replica exchange simulations of protein folding. J Phys Chem 112(19):6083–6093
42. Jain A, Stock G (2012) Identifying metastable states of folding proteins. J Chem Theory Comput 8(10):3810–3819. doi:10.1021/Ct300077q
43. Huang X, Yao Y, Bowman GR et al (2010) Constructing multi-resolution markov state models (msms) to elucidate RNA hairpin folding mechanisms. Pac Symp Biocomput 2010:228–239
44. Bowman GR, Voelz VA, Pande VS (2011) Taming the complexity of protein folding. Curr Opin Struct Biol 21(1):4–11. doi:10.1016/j.sbi.2010.10.006
45. Zhuang W, Cui RZ, Silva DA et al (2011) Simulating the T-Jump-Triggered Unfolding Dynamics of trpzip2 Peptide and Its Time-Resolved IR and Two-Dimensional IR Signals Using the Markov State Model Approach. J Phys Chem B 115(18):5415–5424. doi:10.1021/Jp109592b
46. Qiao Q, Bowman GR, Huang XH (2013) Dynamics of an intrinsically disordered protein reveal metastable conformations that potentially seed aggregation. J Am Chem Soc 135(43):16092–16101. doi:10.1021/Ja403147m
47. Noe F, Schutte C, Vanden-Eijnden E et al (2009) Constructing the equilibrium ensemble of folding pathways from short off-equilibrium simulations. Proc Natl Acad Sci U S A 106(45):19011–19016. doi:10.1073/pnas.0905466106
48. Razavi AM, Wuest WM, Voelz VA (2014) Computational screening and selection of cyclic peptide hairpin mimetics by molecular simulation and kinetic network models. J Chem Inf Model 54(5):1425–1432. doi:10.1021/Ci500102y
49. Voelz VA, Bowman GR, Beauchamp K et al (2010) Molecular simulation of ab initio protein folding for a millisecond folder NTL9(1-39). J Am Chem Soc 132(5):1526–1528
50. Da LT, Wang D, Huang X (2012) Dynamics of pyrophosphate ion release and its coupled trigger loop motion from closed to open state in RNA polymerase II. J Am Chem Soc 134(4):2399–2406. doi:10.1021/ja210656k
51. Silva DA, Weiss DR, Pardo Avila F et al (2014) Millisecond dynamics of RNA polymerase II translocation at atomic resolution. Proc Natl Acad Sci U S A 111(21):7665–7670. doi:10.1073/pnas.1315751111
52. Da LT, Avila FP, Wang D et al (2013) A two-state model for the dynamics of the pyrophosphate ion release in bacterial RNA polymerase. PLoS Comput Biol 9(4):e1003020. doi:10.1371/journal.pcbi.1003020
53. Kohlhoff KJ, Shukla D, Lawrenz M et al (2014) Cloud-based simulations on Google Exacycle reveal ligand modulation of GPCR activation pathways. Nat Chem 6(1):15–21. doi:10.1038/Nchem.1821
54. Shukla D, Meng YL, Roux B et al (2014) Activation pathway of Src kinase reveals intermediate states as targets for drug design. Nat Commun 5:3397. doi:10.1038/Ncomms4397
55. Held M, Metzner P, Prinz JH et al (2011) Mechanisms of protein-ligand association and its modulation by protein mutations. Biophys J 100(3):701–710. doi:10.1016/j.bpj.2010.12.3699
56. Silva DA, Bowman GR, Sosa-Peinado A et al (2011) A role for both conformational selection and induced fit in ligand binding by the LAO protein. PLoS Comput Biol 7(5):e1002054. doi:10.1371/Journal.Pcbi.1002054
57. Buch I, Giorgino T, De Fabritiis G (2011) Complete reconstruction of an enzyme-inhibitor binding process by molecular dynamics simulations. Proc Natl Acad Sci U S A 108(25):10184–10189. doi:10.1073/pnas.1103547108
58. Gu S, Silva DA, Meng L et al (2014) Quantitatively characterizing the ligand binding mechanisms of choline binding protein using Markov state model analysis. PLoS Comput Biol 10(8):e1003767. doi:10.1371/journal.pcbi.1003767
59. Plattner N, Noe F (2015) Protein conformational plasticity and complex ligand-binding kinetics explored by atomistic simulations and Markov models. Nat Commun 6:7653. doi:10.1038/Ncomms8653
60. de Vries SJ, van Dijk AD, Krzeminski M et al (2007) HADDOCK versus HADDOCK: new features and performance of HADDOCK2.0 on the CAPRI targets. Proteins 69(4):726–733. doi:10.1002/prot.21723
61. Dominguez C, Boelens R, Bonvin AM (2003) HADDOCK: a protein-protein docking approach based on biochemical or biophysical

information. J Am Chem Soc 125(7):1731–1737. doi:10.1021/ja026939x
62. Fleishman SJ, Whitehead TA, Strauch EM et al (2011) Community-wide assessment of protein-interface modeling suggests improvements to design methodology. J Mol Biol 414(2):289–302. doi:10.1016/j.jmb.2011.09.031
63. Lensink MF, Wodak SJ (2013) Docking, scoring, and affinity prediction in CAPRI. Proteins 81(12):2082–2095. doi:10.1002/prot.24428
64. Jiang HL, Sheong FK, Zhu LZ et al (2015) Markov state models reveal a two-step mechanism of miRNA loading into the human argonaute protein: selective binding followed by structural re-arrangement. PLoS Comput Biol 11(7):e1004404. doi:10.1371/journal.pcbi.1004404
65. The Journal of chemical physicsAlder BJ, Wainwright TE (1957) Phase transition for a hard sphere system. J Chem Phys 27(5):1208–1209. doi:10.1063/1.1743957
66. Rahman A, Stilling F (1971) Molecular dynamics study of liquid water. J Chem Phys 55(7):3336. doi:10.1063/1.1676585
67. Mccammon JA, Karplus M (1977) Internal motions of antibody molecules. Nature 268(5622):765–766.doi:10.1038/268765a0
68. Rodrigues JPGLM, Bonvin AMJJ (2014) Integrative computational modeling of protein interactions. FEBS J 281(8):1988–2003. doi:10.1111/febs.12771
69. Katchalskikatzir E, Shariv I, Eisenstein M et al (1992) Molecular-surface recognition – determination of geometric fit between proteins and their ligands by correlation techniques. Proc Natl Acad Sci U S A 89(6):2195–2199. doi:10.1073/pnas.89.6.2195
70. Fischer D, Bachar O, Nussinov R et al (1992) An efficient automated computer vision based technique for detection of 3-dimensional structural motifs in proteins. J Biomol Struct Dyn 9(4):769–789
71. Mashiach E, Schneidman-Duhovny D, Peri A et al (2010) An integrated suite of fast docking algorithms. Proteins 78(15):3197–3204. doi:10.1002/prot.22790
72. Moal IH, Bates PA (2010) SwarmDock and the use of normal modes in protein-protein docking. Int J Mol Sci 11(10):3623–3648. doi:10.3390/ijms11103623
73. Lyskov S, Gray JJ (2008) The RosettaDock server for local protein-protein docking. Nucleic Acids Res 36:W233–W238. doi:10.1093/nar/gkn216
74. Chen R, Li L, Weng ZP (2003) ZDOCK: an initial-stage protein-docking algorithm. Proteins 52(1):80–87. doi:10.1002/prot.10389
75. Guilhot-Gaudeffroy A, Froidevaux C, Aze J et al (2014) Protein-RNA complexes and efficient automatic docking: expanding RosettaDock possibilities. PLoS One 9(9):e108928. doi:10.1371/journal.pone.0108928
76. Sali A, Blundell TL (1993) Comparative protein modeling by satisfaction of spatial restraints. J Mol Biol 234(3):779–815. doi:10.1006/jmbi.1993.1626
77. Marti-Renom MA, Stuart AC, Fiser A et al (2000) Comparative protein structure modeling of genes and genomes. Annu Rev Biophys Biomol Struct 29:291–325. doi:10.1146/annurev.biophys.29.1.291
78. Eswar N, Webb B, Marti-Renom MA et al (2006) Comparative protein structure modeling using Modeller. Curr Protoc Bioinformatics 5:56. doi:10.1002/0471250953.bi0506s15
79. Fiser A, Do RKG, Sali A (2000) Modeling of loops in protein structures. Protein Sci 9(9):1753–1773
80. Rother M, Rother K, Puton T et al (2011) ModeRNA: a tool for comparative modeling of RNA 3D structure. Nucleic Acids Res 39(10):4007–4022. doi:10.1093/nar/gkq1320
81. Berendsen HJC, Vanderspoel D, Vandrunen R (1995) Gromacs – a message-passing parallel molecular-dynamics implementation. Comput Phys Commun 91(1-3):43–56. doi:10.1016/0010-4655(95)00042-E
82. Hess B, Kutzner C, van der Spoel D et al (2008) GROMACS 4: algorithms for highly efficient, load-balanced, and scalable molecular simulation. J Chem Theory Comput 4(3):435–447
83. Pronk S, Pall S, Schulz R et al (2013) GROMACS 4.5: a high-throughput and highly parallel open source molecular simulation toolkit. Bioinformatics 29(7):845–854. doi:10.1093/bioinformatics/btt055
84. Shaw DE, Deneroff MM, Dror RO et al (2008) Anton, a special-purpose machine for molecular dynamics simulation. Commun ACM 51(7):91–97. doi:10.1145/1364782.1364802
85. Schrodinger, LLC (2015) The PyMOL molecular graphics system, Version 18. Schrodinger, New York, NY
86. Humphrey W, Dalke A, Schulten K (1996) VMD: visual molecular dynam-

ics. J Mol Graph Model 14(1):33–38. doi:10.1016/0263-7855(96)00018-5

87. Michaud-Agrawal N, Denning EJ, Woolf TB et al (2011) Software news and updates MDAnalysis: a toolkit for the analysis of molecular dynamics simulations. J Comput Chem 32(10):2319–2327. doi:10.1002/jcc.21787
88. McGibbon RT, Beauchamp KA, Harrigan MP et al (2015) MDTraj: a modern open library for the analysis of molecular dynamics trajectories. Biophys J 109(8):1528–1532. doi:10.1016/j.bpj.2015.08.015
89. Zhu L, Jiang H, Sheong FK et al (2016) A flexible domain-domain hinge promotes an induced-fit dominant mechanism for the loading of guide-DNA into argonaute protein in Thermus Thermophilus. J Phys Chem B 20(10):2709–2720. doi:10.1021/acs.jpcb.5b12426
90. Shaw DE, Dror RO, Salmon JK et al. (2009) Millisecond-scale molecular dynamics simulations on Anton. In: High performance computing networking, storage and analysis, proceedings of the conference on, 14–20 Nov 2009. pp 1–11. doi:10.1145/1654059.1654099
91. Tenenbaum JB, Silva V, Langford JC (2000) A global geometric framework for nonlinear dimensionality reduction. Science 290(5500):2319–2323
92. Coifman RR, Lafon S, Lee AB et al (2005) Geometric diffusions as a tool for harmonic analysis and structure definition of data: diffusion maps. Proc Natl Acad Sci U S A 102(21):7426–7431. doi:10.1073/pnas.0500334102
93. Rohrdanz MA, Zheng W, Maggioni M et al (2011) Determination of reaction coordinates via locally scaled diffusion map. J Chem Phys 134(12):124116. doi:10.1063/1.3569857
94. Beauchamp KA, Bowman GR, Lane TJ et al (2011) MSMBuilder2: modeling conformational dynamics on the picosecond to millisecond scale. J Chem Theory Comput 7(10):3412–3419. doi:10.1021/ct200463m
95. Senne M, Trendelkamp-Schroer B, Mey ASJS et al (2012) EMMA: a software package for Markov model building and analysis. J Chem Theory Comput 8(7):2223–2238. doi:10.1021/ct300274u
96. Scherer MK, Trendelkamp-Schroer B, Paul F et al (2015) PyEMMA 2: a software package for estimation, validation, and analysis of Markov models. J Chem Theory Comput 11(11):5525–5542. doi:10.1021/acs.jctc.5b00743
97. Gonzalez TF (1985) Clustering to minimize the maximum intercluster distance. Theory Comput Sci 38(2-3):293–306. doi:10.1016/0304-3975(85)90224-5
98. Kaufman L, Rousseeuw PJ (2009) Finding groups in data: an introduction to cluster analysis, vol 344. John Wiley & Sons, New York, NY
99. Nüske F, Keller BG, Pérez-Hernández G et al (2014) Variational approach to molecular kinetics. J Chem Theory Comput 10(4):1739–1752. doi:10.1021/ct4009156
100. Schutte C, Fischer A, Huisinga W et al (1999) A direct approach to conformational dynamics based on hybrid Monte Carlo. J Comput Phys 151(1):146–168. doi:10.1006/jcph.1999.6231
101. Deuflhard P, Huisinga W, Fischer A et al (2000) Identification of almost invariant aggregates in reversible nearly uncoupled Markov chains. Linear Algebra Appl 315(1-3):39–59. doi:10.1016/S0024-3795(00)00095-1
102. Deuflhard P, Weber M (2005) Robust Perron cluster analysis in conformation dynamics. Linear Algebra Appl 398:161–184
103. Noe F, Horenko I, Schutte C et al (2007) Hierarchical analysis of conformational dynamics in biomolecules: transition networks of metastable states. J Chem Phys 126(15):155102. doi:10.1063/1.2714539
104. Yao Y, Sun J, Huang XH et al (2009) Topological methods for exploring low-density states in biomolecular folding pathways. J Chem Phys 130(14):144115. doi:10.1063/1.3103496
105. Bowman GR (2012) Improved coarse-graining of Markov state models via explicit consideration of statistical uncertainty. J Chem Phys 137(13):134111. doi:10.1063/1.4755751
106. Brunger AT, Adams PD, Clore GM et al (1998) Crystallography & NMR system: a new software suite for macromolecular structure determination. Acta Crystallogr Sect D Biol Crystallogr 54:905–921. doi:10.1107/S0907444998003254
107. Brunger AT (2007) Version 1.2 of the crystallography and NMR system. Nat Protoc 2(11):2728–2733. doi:10.1038/nprot.2007.406
108. Linge JP, Nilges M (1999) Influence of non-bonded parameters on the quality of NMR structures: a new force field for NMR structure calculation. J Biomol NMR 13(1):51–59. doi:10.1023/A:1008365802830
109. Linge JP, Williams MA, Spronk CAEM et al (2003) Refinement of protein structures in

explicit solvent. Proteins 50(3):496–506. doi:10.1002/Prot.10299

110. Jorgensen WL, Tiradorives J (1988) The Opls potential functions for proteins - energy minimizations for crystals of cyclic-peptides and crambin. J Am Chem Soc 110(6):1657–1666. doi:10.1021/Ja00214a001
111. Lindorff-Larsen K, Piana S, Palmo K et al (2010) Improved side-chain torsion potentials for the Amber ff99SB protein force field. Proteins 78(8):1950–1958. doi:10.1002/prot.22711
112. Berendsen H, Postma J, van Gunsteren W et al (1981) Interaction models for water in relation to protein hydration. In: Intermolecular forces. Reidel, Dordrecht, pp 331–342
113. Darden T, York D, Pedersen L (1993) Particle mesh Ewald – an N.Log(N) method for Ewald sums in large systems. J Chem Phys 98(12):10089–10092. doi:10.1063/1.464397
114. Hess B, Bekker H, Berendsen HJC et al (1997) LINCS: a linear constraint solver for molecular simulations. J Comput Chem 18(12):1463–1472. doi:10.1002/(Sici)1096-987x(199709)18:12<1463::Aid-Jcc4>3.0.Co;2-H
115. Bussi G, Donadio D, Parrinello M (2007) Canonical sampling through velocity rescaling. J Chem Phys 126(1):014101. doi:10.1063/1.2408420
116. Parrinello M, Rahman A (1981) Polymorphic transitions in single-crystals – a new molecular-dynamics method. J Appl Phys 52(12):7182–7190. doi:10.1063/1.328693
117. Todorova N, Marinelli F, Piana S et al (2009) Exploring the folding free energy landscape of insulin using bias exchange metadynamics. J Phys Chem B 113(11):3556–3564. doi:10.1021/jp809776v
118. Piana S, Laio A (2007) A bias-exchange approach to protein folding. J Phys Chem B 111(17):4553–4559. doi:10.1021/jp067873l
119. Salomon-Ferrer R, Case DA, Walker RC (2013) An overview of the Amber biomolecular simulation package. Wires Comput Mol Sci 3(2):198–210. doi:10.1002/wcms.1121
120. Brooks BR, Brooks CL, Mackerell AD et al (2009) CHARMM: the biomolecular simulation program. J Comput Chem 30(10):1545–1614. doi:10.1002/jcc.21287
121. Phillips JC, Braun R, Wang W et al (2005) Scalable molecular dynamics with NAMD. J Comput Chem 26(16):1781–1802. doi:10.1002/jcc.20289
122. Eastman P, Friedrichs MS, Chodera JD et al (2013) OpenMM 4: a reusable, extensible, hardware independent library for high performance molecular simulation. J Chem Theory Comput 9(1):461–469. doi:10.1021/ct300857j
123. Piana S, Lindorff-Larsen K, Shaw DE (2011) How robust are protein folding simulations with respect to force field parameterization? Biophys J 100(9):L47–L49. doi:10.1016/j.bpj.2011.03.051
124. Lindorff-Larsen K, Maragakis P, Piana S et al (2012) Systematic validation of protein force fields against experimental data. PLoS One 7(2):e32131. doi:10.1371/journal.pone.0032131
125. Maier JA, Martinez C, Kasavajhala K et al (2015) ff14SB: improving the accuracy of protein side chain and backbone parameters from ff99SB. J Chem Theory Comput 11(8):3696–3713. doi:10.1021/acs.jctc.5b00255
126. Huang J, MacKerell AD (2013) CHARMM36 all-atom additive protein force field: validation based on comparison to NMR data. J Comput Chem 34(25):2135–2145. doi:10.1002/jcc.23354
127. Robertson MJ, Tirado-Rives J, Jorgensen WL (2015) Improved peptide and protein torsional energetics with the OPLS-AA force field. J Chem Theory Comput 11(7):3499–3509. doi:10.1021/acs.jctc.5b00356
128. Mitsutake A, Sugita Y, Okamoto Y (2001) Generalized-ensemble algorithms for molecular simulations of biopolymers. Biopolymers 60(2):96–123. doi:10.1002/1097-282(2001)60:2<96::Aid-Bip1007>3.0.Co;2-F
129. Laio A, Parrinello M (2002) Escaping free-energy minima. Proc Natl Acad Sci U S A 99:12562–12566. doi:10.1073/pnas.202427399
130. Bowman GR, Ensign DL, Pande VS (2010) Enhanced modeling via network theory: adaptive sampling of Markov state models. J Chem Theory Comput 6(3):787–794. doi:10.1021/ct900620b
131. Noe F (2008) Probability distributions of molecular observables computed from Markov models. J Chem Phys 128(24):244103. doi:10.1063/1.2916718
132. Metzner P, Schutte C, Vanden-Eijnden E (2006) Illustration of transition path theory on a collection of simple examples. J Chem Phys 125(8):084110. doi:10.1063/1.2335447
133. Berezhkovskii A, Hummer G, Szabo A (2009) Reactive flux and folding pathways in network models of coarse-grained protein dynamics. J Chem Phys 130(20):205102. doi:10.1063/1.3139063

134. Comeau SR, Gatchell DW, Vajda S et al (2004) ClusPro: a fully automated algorithm for protein-protein docking. Nucleic Acids Res 32:W96–W99. doi:10.1093/nar/gkh354
135. Trott O, Olson AJ (2010) Software news and update AutoDock Vina: improving the speed and accuracy of docking with a new scoring function, efficient optimization, and multithreading. J Comput Chem 31(2):455–461. doi:10.1002/jcc.21334
136. Friesner RA, Banks JL, Murphy RB et al (2004) Glide: a new approach for rapid, accurate docking and scoring. 1. Method and assessment of docking accuracy. J Med Chem 47(7):1739–1749. doi:10.1021/jm0306430
137. Verdonk ML, Cole JC, Hartshorn MJ et al (2003) Improved protein-ligand docking using GOLD. Proteins 52(4):609–623. doi:10.1002/prot.10465
138. Coleman RG, Carchia M, Sterling T et al (2013) Ligand pose and orientational sampling in molecular docking. PLoS One 8(10):e75992. doi:10.1371/journal.pone.0075992

Chapter 19

# Kinetic Analysis of Target RNA Binding and Slicing by Human Argonaute 2 Protein


## Sarah Willkomm and Tobias Restle



## Abstract

Analyzing the mechanisms of Argonaute-mediated gene silencing is essential to the understanding of RNA interference (RNAi). RNAi is a process to regulate gene expression on a posttranscriptional level. Directed by single-stranded small RNA guides, Argonaute 2 binds complementary target RNAs, and if the guide displays full complementarity to the targeted sequence, Argonaute 2 slices the bound target RNA. This on the one hand is an important mechanism to regulate gene expression in the cell and on the other hand represents a powerful tool to interfere with harmful gene expression levels. Here, we present techniques to kinetically characterize recombinant Argonaute 2-mediated guide and target binding as well as target RNA slicing. We focus on fluorescence-based steady-state and in particular pre-steady-state techniques to unravel mechanistic details. Furthermore, we describe a cleavage assay to analyze Argonaute 2-mediated slicing using radioactively labeled target strands.



**Key words** RNAi, RNA interference, siRNA, Human Argonaute 2, Kinetics, Stopped flow, Pre-steady state, Steady state, microRNA, Fluorescence


## 1 Introduction

Argonaute (AGO) proteins are key players of a process called RNA interference (RNAi) [1]. In humans there are four different AGO proteins of which only Argonaute 2 (AGO2) is capable of slicing target RNAs [2, 3]. RNAi is a highly specific process to control gene expression on a posttranscriptional level. The specificity of RNAi is achieved by Watson-Crick base pairing between a target RNA and a guide strand that is bound by AGO. These guide strands are 21–22 nt in length and are generated from long double-stranded RNA precursors by the RNase III Dicer [4–6]. Dicer-mediated processing yields short double-stranded RNAs called small interfering (si)RNAs which are subsequently loaded onto AGO proteins within the so-called RNA-induced silencing complex (RISC)-loading complex (RLC) [7–9]. One of the strands is selected as a guide strand and retained in AGO to find complementary target RNAs, whereas


Marco F. Schmidt (ed.), *Drug Target miRNA: Methods and Protocols*, Methods in Molecular Biology, vol. 1517, DOI 10.1007/978-1-4939-6563-2_19, © Springer Science+Business Media New York 2017

the other, termed passenger strand, is ejected [10–13]. The complex, minimally composed of AGO2 and guide, is termed RISC and able to bind and slice target RNAs [14].

Here, we describe a method to kinetically characterize the mechanism of hAGO2-mediated silencing. Detailed characterization of hAGO2-mediated guide and target binding and subsequent target RNA slicing contributes essentially to the understanding of RNAi [15, 16]. For binding experiments we propose a fluorescence-based approach, where we use RNAs carrying a fluorophore. We selected i.a. position 14 of the guide strand (counted from the 5′-end) as attachment point and found that formation of catalytically active binary AGO2-guide as well as ternary AGO2-guide-target complexes is not disturbed [17]. For kinetic characterization of binding processes, we employ steady-state and in particular pre-steady-state methods. To characterize target slicing activity of hAGO2, we labeled target RNAs with a radioactive 5′-phosphate and analyzed cleavage products using denaturing PAGE followed by visualization via autoradiography. Altogether, information gained by these kinetic studies substantially add to our understanding how AGO binds its guide and target strands followed by target RNA slicing. Moreover, this characterization serves as a basic concept for analyzing effects of accessory proteins of RNAi which, for example, assist AGO loading and slicing as part of the RLC.

## 2 Material

All solutions are prepared using deionized water with a conductivity of 18 MΩ cm at 25 °C. Furthermore, solutions used for binding assays are filtered for sterility (pore size 0.2 μm) and are subsequently degassed. All solutions, unless indicated otherwise, can be stored at room temperature.

### 2.1 Stock Solutions for Assay Buffers (See Note 1)

1. 1 M 2-Amino-2-(hydroxymethyl)-1,3-propanediol (Tris) pH 7.4 (100 mL): Weigh 12.1 g Tris and transfer it into a 200 mL cylinder. Add water up to 80 mL. Stir until dissolved and adjust pH to 7.4. Make up with water to 100 mL.
2. 3 M KCl (50 mL): Weigh 11.2 g KCl and transfer it into a 100 mL cylinder and add water until 40 mL. Stir until dissolved. Make up with water to 50 mL.
3. 0.5 M $MgCl_2$ (25 mL): Weigh 1.2 g $MgCl_2$ and transfer it into a 100 mL cylinder. Add water until 20 mL. Stir until dissolved. Make up with water to 25 mL. Store at room temperature.
4. 10× TBE (1 L): Weigh 108 g Tris, 55 g boric acid, and 7.45 g ethylenediaminetetraacetic acid (EDTA) and transfer it to a 1 L bottle and add water until 900 mL. Stir until dissolved. Make up with water to 1 L.

5. 10% (w/v) sodium dodecyl sulfate (SDS) (10 mL) (*see* **Note 2**): Weigh 1 g SDS and add water until 9 mL. Mix until dissolved. Make up to 10 mL with water.
6. 0.5 M EDTA (10 mL): Weigh 1.46 g EDTA and dissolve in 10 mL water. To completely dissolve adjust pH to 8.

### 2.2 Oligonucleotides for Cleavage Assays, Steady-State and Pre-steady-State Measurement

All oligonucleotides should be ordered polyacrylamide gel electrophoresis (PAGE)-purified.

In principle any matching 21 nucleotide guide-target strand combination can be ordered. The guide strand should carry a phosphate at the 5′-end. Guide and target strand should display complementarity of 19 nt resulting in a 2 nt overhang at the 3′-end of both strands. For stability we prefer two deoxyribonucleotides at the 3′-end. For our studies we used i.a. a guide-target pair termed as2b/s2b [17]: guide as2b, 5′-P-UAG AGG UAC GUG CUG AGG CdTdT-3′, and target s2b, 5′-GCC UCA GCA CGU ACC UCU AdTdT-3′.

For binding studies we used a fluorescein-coupled guide strand. We found nucleotide 14 of the guide strand being a good position to study binary hAGO2-guide and ternary hAGO2-guide-target complex formation. For that purpose the uracil at position 14 of the guide strand was exchanged for a 5-C6-amino-2′-deoxythymidine. This modified thymidine enables post-synthetic labeling with the fluorophore leading to a C6 linker-coupled fluorophore. Due to its relatively small size and very intense fluorescence, the fluorescein fluorophore is well suited for binding experiments. Moreover, fluorescein is rather pH sensitive. A property often considered as drawback. However, when it comes to the analysis of macromolecular interactions, this turns into an advantage since the fluorophore reacts very sensitive to even minor changes in the local environment. As a consequence fluorescein often yields a signal where other alleged superior fluorophores fail. Then again, due to its broad emission spectrum, fluorescein is mostly limited to single color applications.

### 2.3 Cleavage Assay Components

1. 10× cleavage buffer (10 mL): 100 mM Tris (pH 7.4), 1 M KCl, and 20 mM $MgCl_2$. Transfer 1 mL 1 M Tris (pH 7.4), 3.3 mL 3 M KCl, and 400 μL 0.5 M $MgCl_2$ into a Falcon tube and add water to 10 mL.
2. 8% acrylamide/*N,N*′-methylenebisacrylamide solution with 7 M urea (500 mL) (*see* **Note 3**): Weigh 210 g urea and add 100 mL acrylamide/*N,N*′-methylenebisacrylamide solution (40%; mixing ratio 19:1) and 50 mL 10× TBE and make up to 500 mL with water. Stir until urea is dissolved. Afterward filter the solution using 0.2 μm filters, degas, and store at 4 °C (*see* **Note 4**).
3. 20% acrylamide/*N,N*′-methylenebisacrylamide solution with 7 M urea (500 mL) (*see* **Note 3**): Weigh 210 g urea and add

250 mL acrylamide/*N*,*N'*-methylenebisacrylamide solution (40%; mixing ratio 19:1) and 50 mL 10× TBE and make up to 500 mL with water. Stir until urea is dissolved. Afterward filter the solution using 0.2 μm filters, degas, and store at 4 °C (*see* **Note 4**).

4. Formamide RNA stop and loading buffer (10 mL) (*see* **Note 5**): Mix 9.25 mL deionized formamide with 250 μL 10% SDS (f.c. 0.025%), 10 μL 0.5 M EDTA (f.c. 0.5 mM), and 250 μL 10% bromophenol blue (f.c. 0.025%) and 10% xylencyanole (f.c. 0.025%) each.
5. [γ-$^{32}$P]-ATP (3000 Ci/mmol) (PerkinElmer, Boston, USA).
6. Nick columns (Sephadex G-50) (GE Healthcare, Munich, Germany).
7. Sequencing gel apparatus for cleavage assays (Sequi-Gen GT system, Bio-Rad) (*see* **Note 6**).
8. Siliconizing reagent to prepare the glass plates used for electrophoresis (Sigmacote® Sigma-Aldrich).
9. T4 polynucleotide kinase (Fermentas).
10. Imaging plates for autoradiography.
11. Phosphorimager to detect bands on the exposed image plate (Typhoon FLA-9500).
12. Program to evaluate band densities on the gel (ImageQuant TL, GE Healthcare).
13. Fitting program to evaluate cleavage kinetics (GraFit, Erithacus Software).

### 2.4 Binding Assay Components

1. 1× binding buffer 100 mL: 10 mM Tris (pH 7.4) and 100 mM KCl. Transfer 1 mL 1 M Tris (pH 7.4) and 3.3 mL 3 M KCl into a 100 mL graduated glass bottle and add water to 100 mL.

#### 2.4.1 Steady-State Binding Assay Using Fluorescence Spectrometer

1. Fluorescence cuvette (700 μL quartz cuvette from Hellma).
2. Fluorescence spectrometer suitable for fluorescence titrations (Fluoromax-3 by Horiba Jobin Yvon).
3. Circulating thermostat connected to the spectrometer (*see* **Note 7**).

#### 2.4.2 Pre-steady-State Binding Assay Using Stopped-Flow

1. Stopped-flow system (stopped-flow SX20 by Applied Photophysics).
2. Circulating thermostat connected to the stopped-flow device (*see* **Note 7**).

## 3 Methods

### 3.1 Cleavage Assay

A cleavage assay is used to determine the enzymatic activity of hAGO2. Here, we use a 5′ radioactively labeled target RNA with a matching guide RNA that is bound by hAGO2 and monitor cleavage by taking samples at different time points. These samples are analyzed by denaturing PAGE followed by autoradiography. By determining band densities, we are able to calculate the relative amount of cleavage product at each given time point. These data are then plotted against time to determine the cleavage kinetics.

1. Prepare a 20% acrylamide/*N*,*N*′-methylenebisacrylamide solution with 7 M urea (*see* **Note 4**).
2. Prepare radioactively labeled target RNA: Mix 10 pmol of dephosphorylated target RNA with 1× T4 polynucleotide kinase buffer A (supplied with T4 PNK), 20 U RiboLock, 10 pmol [$\gamma$-$^{32}$P]-ATP, and 10 U T4 polynucleotide kinase (PNK). Incubate for 60 min at 37 °C and subsequently heat-inactivate the polynucleotide kinase for 10 min at 75 °C. To remove excess ATP, purify labeled RNA oligonucleotide using a Sephadex G-50 column. The column has to be equilibrated with nuclease-free water according to manufacturer's instructions. Afterward apply the sample to the column and proceed to elution with water. The radioactively labeled target RNA can now be used for the cleavage assay.
3. For the cleavage assay, incubate 2.5 μM recombinant hAGO2 with 100 nM guide RNA and 2.5 nM radioactively labeled target RNA for 2 h at 37 °C. For a schematic representation of the experimental setup, *see* Fig. 1a. Samples of 5 μL volume are taken at different time points (*see* **Note 8**) and are immediately mixed with 5 μL 2× formamide RNA stop and loading buffer and subsequently stored on ice to block any further cleavage.
4. Prepare a sequencing gel. At first make sure the glass plates are cleaned thoroughly with water and detergent followed by a wash with 100% ethanol and dry with a fluff-free kerchief (*see* **Note 9**). Then add 350 μL siliconizing reagent to one of the plates (*see* **Note 10**) and spread it equally over the whole plate. Mount gel system according to manufacturer's manual. Prepare acrylamide/*N*,*N*′-methylenebisacrylamide gel solution. For a 38 × 50 cm sequencing gel with 0.25 mm spacers, we prepare 40 mL of the 20% acrylamide/*N*,*N*′-methylenebisacrylamide solution with 400 μL APS and 40 μL tetramethylethylenediamine (TEMED). Mix by inverting and subsequently pour the gel between the plates according to manufacturer's instructions. Degassing of the acrylamide solution will prevent the occurrence of air bubbles in the gel.

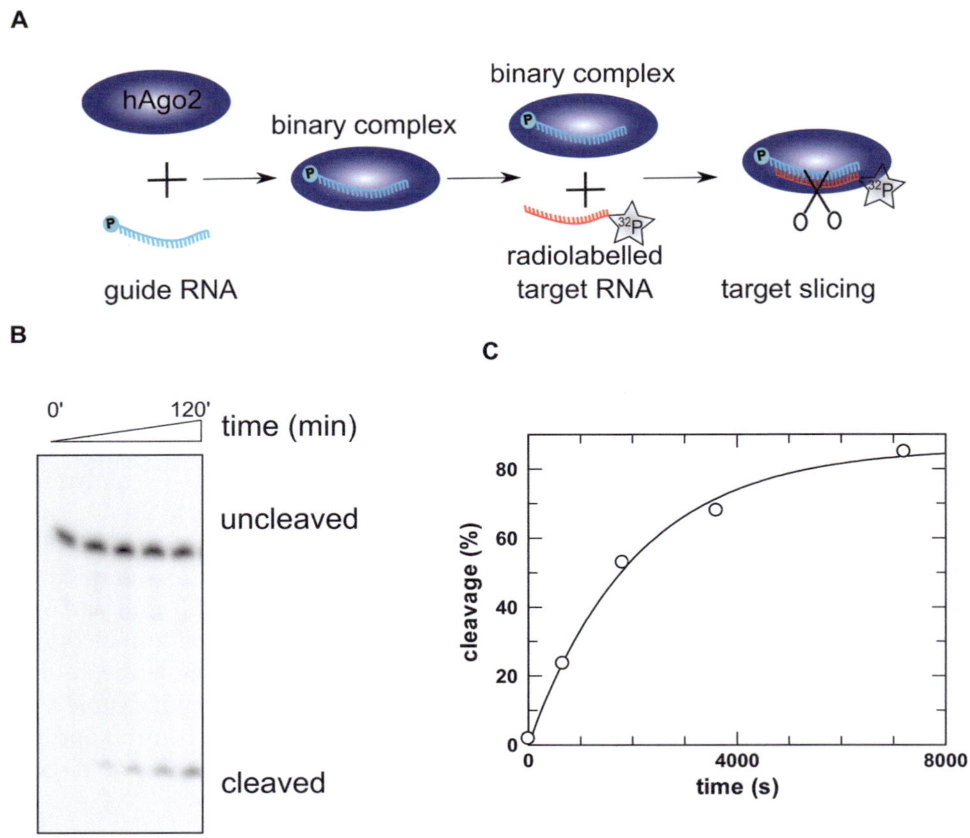


**Fig. 1** Cleavage assay to analyze hAGO2-mediated target RNA cleavage. (**a**) Schematic representation of the cleavage assay. Guide RNA is preincubated with hAGO2 to form binary complexes. The reaction is started by adding a $^{32}$P-labeled target RNA. Reaction was stopped at different time points. (**b**) Samples taken at different time points were separated using 20 %-denaturing PAGE and detected by autoradiography. (**c**) Plot of cleavage products versus time. The data were evaluated using a single exponential equation. The corresponding fit is shown as *black line*

5. Pre-run sequencing gel at 70 W until a temperature of 50 °C is reached. This takes around 1 h.
6. Load samples when the gel has reached a temperature of 50 °C and run it for around 100 min at 70 W and a constant temperature of 50 °C.
7. At the end of the run, immediately transfer the gel to a Whatman paper and cover with Saran wrap. Put on a phosphor screen for detection and incubate overnight in a −20 °C freezer (*see* **Note 11**).
8. Detect bands in the gel using a phosphorimager. For an example gel, *see* Fig. 1b.

9. Determine band intensities and calculate relative amounts of cleavage product for every time point collected.
10. Evaluate cleavage kinetics by plotting the amount of cleavage product against time and fit the data using an exponential equation. Depending on the particular setup, you can expect one or more phases. For an example, *see* Fig. 1c.

### 3.2 Steady-State Fluorescence Titrations

Steady-state fluorescence titrations enable the determination of the equilibrium dissociation constant ($K_D$) of the interaction of hAGO2 with a guide strand or a binary complex composed of hAGO2 and a guide strand with a matching target RNA. To monitor binding, one of the binding partners, in our case the guide RNA, is fluorescently labeled. The fluorophore-coupled binding partner is put in first into a cuvette. Then, increasing amounts of unlabeled binding partner are added. If binding occurs, the fluorescence signal should change. The change of fluorescence caused by the macromolecular interaction is plotted against the concentration of the unlabeled binding partner. These data are fitted using a quadratic binding equation yielding the $K_D$ value [17]. To observe larger changes in fluorescence and to minimize errors due to signal fluctuations (i.e., noise) which are not related to the macromolecular interaction of interest, an additional fluorescence quencher might be used (Fig. 2a). Since the binding and therefore the equilibrium dissociation constant is influenced by temperature changes, it is highly advisable to tightly control the cuvette temperature (*see* **Note 12**). For a schematic representation of the experimental setup, *see* Fig. 3.

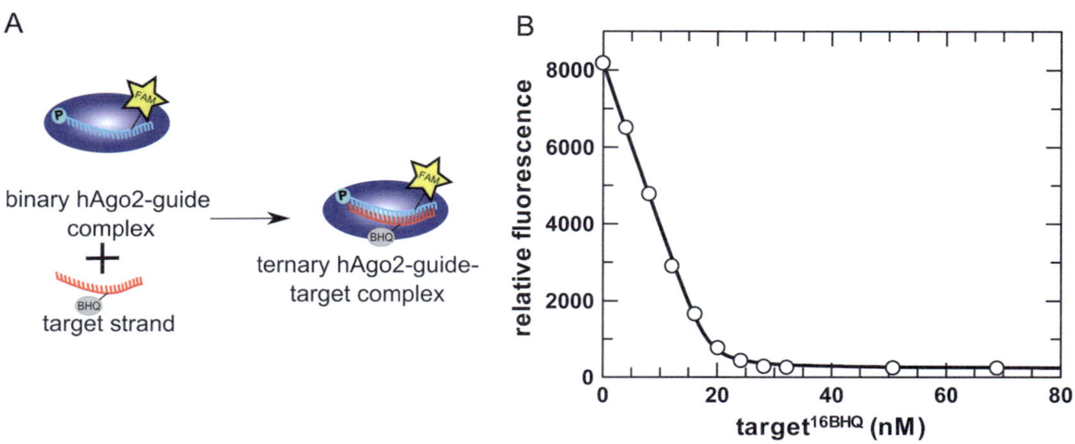


**Fig. 2** Example for steady-state fluorescence titration to analyze ternary complex assembly. (**a**) Schematic representation of formation of ternary hAGO2-guide-target complexes. A binary complex composed of hAGO2 and a fluorescently labeled guide is added into the cuvette first. A target strand with a BHQ quencher is titrated stepwise to form ternary complexes. (**b**) A representative titration experiment is shown. Data points were fitted using a quadratic binding equation. The resulting fit is depicted in black. Data taken from Deerberg et al. [17]

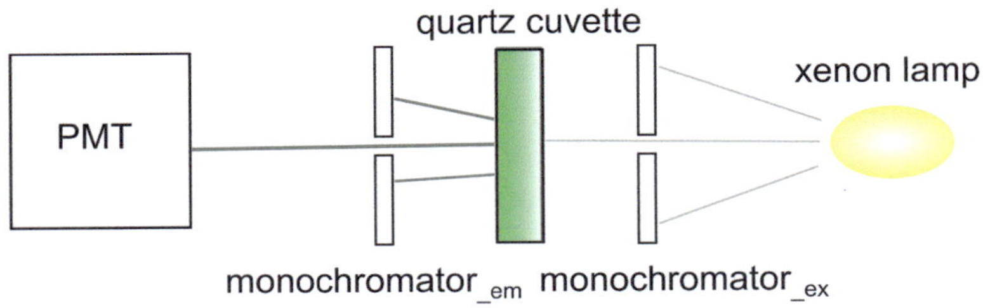


**Fig. 3** Schematic setup of the fluorescence spectrometer for steady-state titrations. The fluorescent binding partner (e.g., fluorescently labeled nucleic acid or binary AGO-fluorescently labeled guide complexes) is added into the quartz cuvette first. The non-labeled binding partner is titrated stepwise. The fluorophore is excited by a xenon lamp of which only the excitation wavelength of the guide-coupled fluorophore can pass the excitation monochromator (monochromator_ex). The emission wavelength is subsequently selected by another monochromator (monochromator_em) and detected by a photomultiplier tube (PMT)

1. Use a fluorescence cuvette, add buffer, and start the measurement. Be sure to adjust the excitation and emission monochromator to the spectral properties of the fluorophore used. For fluorescein this would be 490 nm for excitation and 516 nm for emission. Adjust the circulating thermostat so that the cuvette holder temperature matches 25 °C. It is mandatory to thoroughly clean the cuvette before each measurement. A harsh treatment with 30% $H_2O_2$ will remove any residual fluorophore that might have been left over from previous measurements. Make sure to completely remove the $H_2O_2$ by intensive washing.

   A clean cuvette will give a very low background signal. The magnitude of the corresponding background signal will depend on the particular setup and needs to be determined individually.

2. Then add the fluorescent binding partner and mix thoroughly (*see* **Note 13**). The signal observed should be at least tenfold higher than the background signal in the absence of fluorophore.

3. Subsequently, add the none-labeled binding partner in small titrations steps. The required step size and the final concentration of the binding partner will depend on the initial concentration of the fluorescent binding partner and the $K_D$ to be expected. This needs to be determined individually. Mix thoroughly after each titration step by sucking up and down with a pipette (around 200 μL for a 700 μL cuvette) while trying not to generate bubbles and note the change in fluorescence. Moreover, you will have to correct the fluorescence signal to the volume increase caused by each titration step. If you intend to measure the affinity of ternary complexes composed of hAGO2, guide RNA, and target RNA, first add the fluorescent

guide nucleic acid to the cuvette, and then form the binary complex by adding hAGO2. Mix and wait until no decrease of fluorescence can be observed any more. When a stable fluorescence signal is achieved, start with titration of the none-labeled target strand.

4. Stop the measurement when the signal reaches a plateau, which means no further change in fluorescence can be observed even at addition of large amounts of binding partner.
5. Then plot relative fluorescence values (corrected for volume increase) against binding partner concentration and evaluate the experimental data by fitting them to a quadratic binding equation. For an example, *see* Fig. 2b.

### 3.3 Pre-steady-State Stopped-Flow Measurements with AGO and Fluorescent Oligonucleotides

Stopped-flow measurements enable the analysis of a binding reaction before the binding equilibrium is reached. If two macromolecules are interacting with each other in a multistep binding reaction, these different steps of binding can be detected if they cause a decent change in fluorescence. This requires a careful placement of the fluorophore. For hAGO2 we found that position 14 (counted from the 5′-end of the guide strand) is well suited to detect different phases of binding to guide and target RNA. As for the steady-state fluorescence titration, the temperature of the measurement cell needs to be carefully controlled. The samples for the stopped-flow measurement are put into individual syringes. Using a pneumatic drive, the content of the two drive syringes is pushed into the measurement cell and thus rapidly mixed, while the content of the measurement cell is displaced into a so-called stop syringe. The plunger top of this syringe hits a trigger which on the one hand starts detection by the photomultiplier tube and on the other hand stops the flow from the drive syringes. The entire mixing process just takes around two milliseconds which is the dead time of this stopped-flow system. This enables us to monitor binding processes and accompanying conformational transitions which take place in the single digit millisecond range; i.e., rate constants of up to 500 $s^{-1}$ can be accurately determined. For a schematic representation of the experimental setup, *see* Fig. 4.

1. First be sure the stopped-flow system is well flushed with water.
2. Set the circulating thermostat so the temperature of the measurement cell matches 25 °C.
3. Before turning on the high voltage of the photomultiplier tube, insert the right filter to remove all excitation light from emission detection. For fluorescein we use a filter cutting of all wavelengths smaller than 530 nm.
4. Afterward adjust the system to the assay conditions by flushing the system with binding buffer.

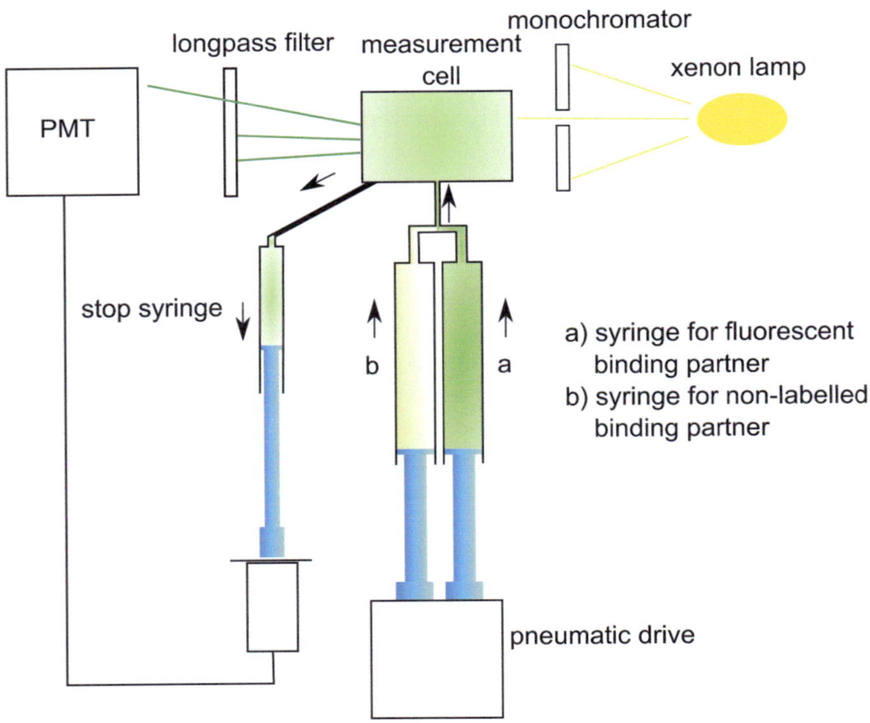


**Fig. 4** Schematic setup of the stopped-flow device. The two binding partners (e.g., AGO and fluorescently labeled guide strands or binary AGO-fluorescently labeled guide complexes and target strands) are deposited in individual syringes (**a**) and (**b**). By operating the pneumatic drive, the plungers of the two drive syringes are forcing the liquid into the measurement cell. The content of the measurement cell is thereby displaced into the stop syringe, which causes the plunger of this syringe to activate a trigger. This starts fluorescence detection by the photomultiplier tube (PMT) and at the same time stops the flow from of the two drive syringes. The fluorescent label attached to one of the binding partners is excited by a xenon lamp of which only the desirable wavelength to excite the fluorophore is transmitted by a monochromator. A cutoff filter is connected downstream to avoid excitation light entering the PMT

5. Then set up the systems to the needs of a binding measurement with hAGO2. We typically measure the fluorescence signal over 1010 s. These 1010 s are split into two time frames with different numbers of data points. To ensure detection of any fast reaction which might occur, choose 500 data points for the first 10 s. Afterward choose 2000 data points for a time period of 1000 s. Adjust the excitation monochromator to 490 nm if you use fluorescein.
6. Prepare the samples for the measurement. Since the contents of the syringes are mixed 1:1 in the measurement cell causing a dilution, use double amount of the desired final concentrations. We found a final concentration of 20 nM fluorophore-coupled nucleic acid being sufficient to monitor binding to hAGO2. However, this number is depending on the particular device and might differ for other brands.

7. Conduct a buffer control (blank) to be sure to exclude photobleaching effects and buffer-induced artifacts. Pipette hereunto the fluorophore-coupled nucleic acid in one syringe, while the other syringe is filled with buffer only. To obtain reliable data, several shots (on average at least five) have to be conducted and averaged. Per shot about 50 μL of each reactant is needed. As a result at least 500 μL (this includes the dead volume of the system) of each reactant is needed for a single run.
8. The resulting data from such a blank measurement have to be subtracted from any subsequent binding measurement. In case large signal changes are observed for the blank, the experimental setup might have to be reconsidered.
9. Having successfully fulfilled the described requirements, transient binding analysis of hAGO2 to the fluorescent guide strand can be undertaken. Typically, we use a final concentration of 400–600 nM of AGO. If monitoring of the formation of ternary hAGO2-guide-target complexes is desired, preassemble hAgo2 and the fluorescent guide strand in advance and then load one syringe with the binary complex and the other with the target RNA (*see* **Note 14**). Again larger amplitudes might be achieved by using a quencher coupled to the target strand. Furthermore, as outlined for the blank measurement, several shots have to be conducted which are averaged to yield the final binding curve.
10. To evaluate the binding curves, as mentioned earlier, subtract the blank from the binding curves that were obtained in the presence of the two binding partners. This can be easily done using Microsoft Excel. For further evaluation a data fitting program is needed. We use GraFit from Erithacus software, but global fit programs might be used as well. For an example, *see* Fig. 5.

## 4 Notes

1. Preparing stock solutions with higher concentrations minimizes weighing errors.
2. SDS irritates the skin. Avoid inhalation and therefore work under a fume hood and wear your personal protective equipment (gloves, lab goggles).
3. Preparation of acrylamide solutions as well as gel casting should be done under a fume hood, and personal protective equipment (lab goggles and gloves) should be used. Acrylamide is considered to be potentially carcinogenic and mutagenic. Furthermore, it is a neurotoxin and can cause significant irritation of the skin.

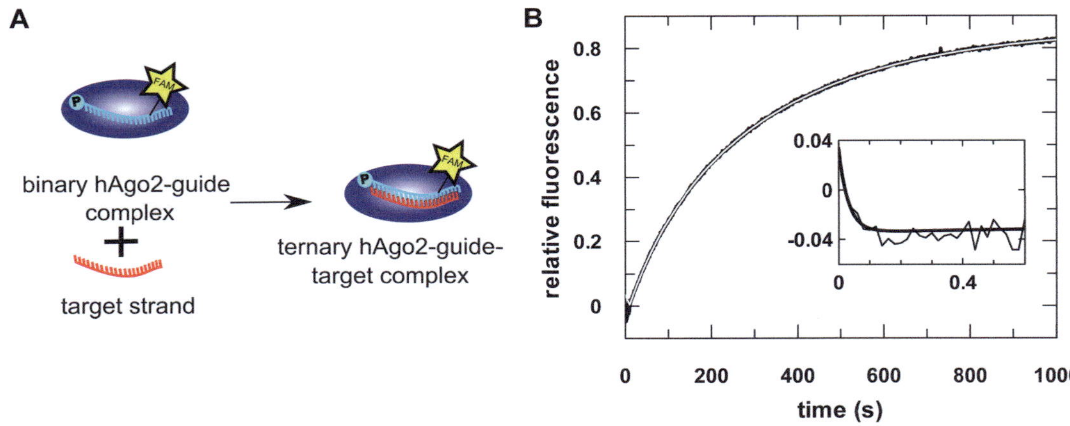


**Fig. 5** Data obtained measuring the formation of ternary hAGO2-guide-target complexes using the stopped-flow method. (**a**) Schematic representation of the experiment. Binary complexes composed of hAGO2 and a fluorescently labeled guide strand were preassembled and afterward rapidly mixed with a complementary target strand using the stopped-flow device. (**b**) Representative stopped-flow graph. The *insert* shows the reaction on a shorter time scale. Fluorescence change observed upon the formation of ternary hAGO2-guide-target complexes as depicted in part (**a**). The fluorescence data are depicted in *black*. Data were fitted using a triple exponential equation. The fit is shown in white or rather *light gray*. Data taken from Deerberg et al. [17]

4. Acrylamide/*N*,*N*′-methylenebisacrylamide solution containing 7 M urea is stable for several weeks if stored at 4 °C. The occasional appearance of white crystals is due to precipitation of urea. Such crystals can usually be easily removed by stirring the solution at room temperature. Do not use acrylamide/*N*,*N*′-methylenebisacrylamide solutions older than 6 weeks. These will not polymerize properly and cause greasy bands.
5. Formamide is teratogenic. Personal protective equipment (gloves, lab goggles) should be used.
6. Midsized gel systems are also suited to separate hAGO2 cleavage products. Though, sequencing gels (at least 20 × 40 cm in combination with thin spacers) are the preferred solution for us because they offer a single-nucleotide resolution which enables determination of the exact cleavage position.
7. We use a mixture of 70 % water and 30 % isopropanol to keep the liquid in the circulating thermostat free of mold. Alternatively, you might use regular antifreeze for automotive radiators.
8. Useful time points to take samples for hAGO2-mediated cleavage reactions for determination of multiple turnover parameters are 5′, 15′, 35′, 65′, and 125′.
9. If the polymerized gel starts migrating/moving between the glass plates while chromatography is running, the plates have not been cleaned appropriately. Even tiny amounts of residual

polyacrylamide from previous runs might lead to detachment of the gel matrix from the glass plates. Moreover, inappropriate polymerization caused by old reagents (especially APS, TEMED) can lead to such problems as well.

10. Always use the same glass plate for adding the siliconizing reagent because it is hard to thoroughly remove this reagent by just washing, and having both plates repelling the gel can also lead to migration/movement of the gel matrix inside the two glass plates.
11. Transfer of the gel to a Whatman paper and freezing at −20 °C has to be conducted as fast as possible. The gel is extremely thin and therefore tends to dry out quickly. If not frozen immediately, the gel starts curling. Furthermore, ensure that the gel does not thaw when exposing it to the phosphor screen, because this might lead to a ruptured gel.
12. Be careful if you choose temperatures above 30 °C for your titration experiments. Even if you seal your cuvette using a special lid or a Parafilm sheet, liquid evaporates from the cuvette each time you open it for adding new binding partner. Albeit the loss of liquid in your cuvette might seem very small, the fluorescence signal will be affected and in turn the measurement might not be reliable any more.
13. Be sure the fluorescence signal is stable before starting the titration. Depending on the fluorophore, the binding buffer, the degree of purity, and age of the cuvette, this might take up to 30 min.
14. Depending on the experimental setup, you might observe first-order as well as second-order reactions. The latter are usually characterized by the observed rate constant being dependent on the concentration of the binding partners and represent the initial event of collision complex formation between the two macromolecules. First-order reactions usually can be attributed to structural transition during the binding process. How many of such transitions to be observed largely depend on the sensitivity and position of the fluorophore label and the complexity of the system under investigation. For a comprehensive discussion of the analysis of kinetic data, the reader is referred to books by A. Fersht [18], H. Gutfreund [19], and a review by K.A. Johnson [20].

## References


1. Fire A, Xu SQ, Montgomery MK, Kostas SA, Driver SE, Mello CC (1998) Potent and specific genetic interference by double-stranded RNA in Caenorhabditis elegans. Nature 391:806–811. doi:10.1038/35888
2. Meister G, Landthaler M, Patkaniowska A, Dorsett Y, Teng G, Tuschl T (2004) Human Argonaute2 mediates RNA cleavage targeted by miRNAs and siRNAs. Mol Cell 15:185–197. doi:10.1016/j.molcel.2004.07.007

3. Liu J, Carmell M, Rivas FV, Marsden CG, Thomson JM, Song J-J et al (2004) Argonaute2 is the catalytic engine of mammalian RNAi. Science 305:1437–1441. doi:10.1126/science.1102513
4. Bernstein E, Caudy AA, Hammond SM, Hannon GJ (2001) Role for a bidentate ribonuclease in the initiation step of RNA interference. Nature 409:363–366. doi:10.1038/35053110
5. MacRae IJ, Zhou K, Li F, Repic A, Brooks AN, Cande WZ et al (2006) Structural basis for double-stranded RNA processing by Dicer. Science 311:195–198. doi:10.1126/science.1121638
6. Elbashir SM, Lendeckel W, Tuschl T (2001) RNA interference is mediated by 21- and 22-nucleotide RNAs. Genes Dev 15:188–200. doi:10.1101/gad.862301
7. Maniataki E, Mourelatos Z (2005) A human, ATP-independent, RISC assembly machine fueled by pre-miRNA. Genes Dev 19:2979–2990. doi:10.1101/gad.1384005
8. MacRae IJ, Ma E, Zhou M, Robinson CV, Doudna JA (2008) In vitro reconstitution of the human RISC-loading complex. Proc Natl Acad Sci U S A 105:512–517. doi:10.1073/pnas.0710869105
9. Hutvagner G, Simard MJ (2008) Argonaute proteins: key players in RNA silencing. Nat Rev Mol Cell Biol 9:22–32. doi:10.1038/nrm2321
10. Leuschner PJ, Ameres SL, Kueng S, Martinez J (2006) Cleavage of the siRNA passenger strand during RISC assembly in human cells. EMBO Rep 7:314–320. doi:10.1038/sj.embor.7400637
11. Rand TA, Petersen S, Du F, Wang X (2005) Argonaute2 cleaves the anti-guide strand of siRNA during RISC activation. Cell 123:621–629. doi:10.1016/j.cell.2005.10.020
12. Matranga C, Tomari Y, Shin C, Bartel DP, Zamore PD (2005) Passenger-strand cleavage facilitates assembly of siRNA into Ago2-containing RNAi enzyme complexes. Cell 123:607–620. doi:10.1016/j.cell.2005.08.044
13. Kim K, Lee YS, Carthew RW (2007) Conversion of pre-RISC to holo-RISC by Ago2 during assembly of RNAi complexes. RNA 13:22–29. doi:10.1261/rna.283207
14. Siomi H, Siomi MC (2009) On the road to reading the RNA-interference code. Nature 457:396–404. doi:10.1038/nature07754
15. Willkomm S, Restle T (2015) Conformational dynamics of Ago-mediated silencing processes. Int J Mol Sci 16:14769–14785. doi:10.3390/ijms160714769
16. Dornseifer S, Willkomm S, Kretschmer-Kazemi Far R, Liebschwager J, Beltsiou F, Frank K et al (2015) RNAi revised – target mRNA-dependent enhancement of gene silencing. Nucleic Acids Res 43:10623–10632. doi:10.1093/nar/gkv1200
17. Deerberg A, Willkomm S, Restle T (2013) Minimal mechanistic model of siRNA-dependent target RNA slicing by recombinant human Argonaute 2 protein. Proc Natl Acad Sci U S A 110:17850–17855. doi:10.1073/pnas.1217838110
18. Fersht A (1985) Enzyme structure and mechanism, 2nd edn. W.H. Freeman & Co Ltd., New York, NY
19. Gutfreund H (1995) Kinetics for the life sciences: receptors, transmitters and catalysts. Cambridge University Press, Cambridge
20. Johnson KA (1992) Transient-state kinetic analysis of enzyme reaction pathways. Enzymes 20:1–61. doi:10.1016/S1874-6047(08)60019-0

# Chapter 20

# Site-Specific Fluorescent Labeling of Argonaute for FRET-Based Bio-Assays

**Sarah Willkomm, Adrian Zander, and Dina Grohmann**

## Abstract

Deciphering the molecular mechanisms of eukaryotic Argonaute proteins is crucial for the understanding of RNA interference (RNAi), a posttranscriptional gene silencing process. Fluorescence-based single-molecule studies like single-molecule Förster resonance energy transfer (FRET) between a donor and acceptor dye represent a versatile tool to gain a mechanistic understanding of the structural dynamics of a biomolecular complex. Until today it was not possible to site-specifically introduce fluorophores into eukaryotic Argonaute. Using an archaeal Argonaute variant from *Methanocaldococcus jannaschii* that closely resembles its eukaryotic counterpart, we site-specifically incorporated fluorescent probes into Argonaute. In this chapter, we first describe how to express archaeal Argonaute with the site-specifically engineered unnatural amino acid *para*-azido-L-phenylalanine (pAzF) and subsequently describe the coupling of a fluorophore exploiting the unique chemistry of the azide group of pAzF. In the second part of the chapter, we present a methodological approach that probes complex formation between acceptor-labeled archaeal Argonaute and guide and target nucleic acids equipped with a donor fluorophore which ultimately allows single-molecule FRET measurements. Furthermore we describe binding and cleavage assays that report on the functionality of Argonaute–nucleic acid complexes.

**Key words** Argonaute, Gene silencing, *Methanocaldococcus jannaschii*, Archaea, Unnatural amino acid incorporation

## 1 Introduction

Argonaute (AGO) proteins are found in all three domains of life [1–3]. The biological function of eukaryotic Argonaute 2 as key player of a posttranscriptional regulation process termed RNA interference (RNAi) is well defined [4], but many mechanistic details remain elusive. Some of the prokaryotic homologues of Argonaute (pAGOs) closely resemble their eukaryotic counterpart and structural and functional studies of pAGOs provided valuable insights into the molecular mechanisms and conformational dynamics of the Argonaute protein family. Studying prokaryotic Argonaute variants furthermore informs about the evolutionary journey of Argonaute [1]. However, little is known about the biological role of prokaryotic

Marco F. Schmidt (ed.), *Drug Target miRNA: Methods and Protocols*, Methods in Molecular Biology, vol. 1517, DOI 10.1007/978-1-4939-6563-2_20, © Springer Science+Business Media New York 2017

Argonaute proteins. Recent studies revealed that prokaryotic AGOs may be involved in the defense against foreign genetic elements [3, 5, 6]. Interestingly, in contrast to eukaryotic AGOs, most prokaryotic AGOs prefer DNA over RNA substrates [1, 7–11]. This holds also true for the Argonaute protein of the hyperthermophilic archaeal organism *Methanocaldococcus jannaschii* (*M. jannaschii*; MjAGO) [12]. Nonetheless, functionally diverse, prokaryotic, and eukaryotic AGOs share a high degree of structural homology [1, 13]. Like human Argonaute 2 (hAGO2), which is the catalytic engine of RNAi [14, 15], MjAGO is capable to catalyze guide-directed cleavage of a target [12]. This close relationship to eukaryotic Argonaute proteins and the possibility to site-specifically modify the protein predestines MjAGO as a model system for mechanistic studies on AGO-mediated silencing processes.

Here, we provide a detailed description of MjAGO preparation and modification for fluorescence-based assays. MjAGO differs from eukaryotic Argonaute proteins mainly by the strict use of DNA substrates instead of RNA substrates. This issue can be neglected since it could be shown that DNA as well as RNA hybrids can be found in the same A-form like helix conformation when bound to AGO [11]. Site-specific fluorescent labeling of MjAGO is achieved via a bio-orthogonal reaction. In order to avoid perturbation of the protein structure, labeling sites within the protein are located in flexible linker regions at amino acid positions that are not highly conserved [12]. Our studies showed that these positions do not impair the activity of the protein. Likewise, different dye-coupling sites in the guide DNA strand were tested to identify positions that do not interfere with AGO binding. Having fluorescently labeled Argonaute and DNA guide and target strands available, we developed fluorescence-based assays that shed light on the substrate binding and nucleolytic cleavage properties of MjAGO.

## 2 Materials

All buffers are prepared using deionized ultrapure water and analytical grade reagents. All buffers are filtered using 0.45 μm filters unless indicated otherwise. Buffers used for chromatography purposes are additionally degassed using ultrasound in combination with vacuum.

### 2.1 Cell Growth, Protein Expression, and Cell Lysis

1. Rich medium: 2% (w/v) tryptone, 1.5% (w/v) yeast extract, 0.8% (w/v) NaCl, and 0.8% (v/v) glycerol. For 1 L media add 100 mL water and a magnetic stirrer to a 1 L glass beaker or cylinder (*see* **Note 1**). Weigh 20 g tryptone, 15 g yeast extract, and 8 g NaCl and add to the water. Add 9.3 mL 86% glycerol and water to a volume of 900 mL. Mix and when the chemicals are dissolved make up to 1 L with water.

2. M9 minimal media supplemented with minerals and vitamins: 0.4% (w/v) glucose, 2 mM $MgCl_2$, 100 mM $CaCl_2$, 3 nM $(NH_4)_6Mo_7O_{24}$, 400 nM $H_3BO_3$, 30 nM $CoCl_2$, 10 nM $CuSO_4$, 80 nM $MnCl_2$, 20 nM $ZnSO_4$, 33.9 g/L $Na_2HPO_4$, 15 g/L $KH_2PO_4$, 5 g/L $NH_4Cl$, and 2.5 g/L NaCl. The media with these components is autoclaved for sterilization. Afterward the media is supplemented with the vitamins: 2 mg/mL thiamine, 0.4 mg/mL choline chloride, 0.5 mg/mL folic acid, 0.5 mg/mL nicotinamide, 1 mg/mL myoinositol, 1 mg/mL pyridoxal, 0.05 mg/mL riboflavin, and 1 mg/mL biotin. These have to be filtered for sterilization with a 0.2 μm filter before added to the autoclaved media. The media is supplemented with appropriate antibiotics which are determined by the plasmid used. In our case, we used 25 μg/mL chloramphenicol (chloramphenicol resistance is conveyed by the pEvol-Az plasmid [16] coding for a mutant tyrosyl synthetase and the amber suppressor tRNA ($tRNA^{Tyr}{}_{CUA}$)) and 100 μg/mL ampicillin which is dictated by the pET vector system used as expression plasmid for the MjAGO gene with the amber stop codon mutation. For 1 L minimal media, weigh 33.9 g $Na_2HPO_4$, 15 g $KH_2PO_4$, 5 g $NH_4Cl$, 2.5 g NaCl, 4 g glucose, and 11.1 g $CaCl_2$, and add to a bottle with 100 mL water and a magnet inside. Subsequently, add 4 mL of a 500 mM solution of $MgCl_2$, 100 μL of a 30 μM solution of $(NH_4)_6Mo_7O_{24}$, 1 mL of a 400 μM solution of $H_3BO_3$, 1 mL of a 30 μM solution of $CoCl_2$, 1 mL of a 80 μM solution of $MnCl_2$, and 1 mL of a 20 μM solution of $ZnSO_4$ (*see* **Note 2**). Add water up to 900 mL and stir until dissolved. After autoclaving the medium, add the filtered vitamin solution composed of 2 g thiamine, 0.4 g choline chloride, 0.5 g folic acid, 0.5 g nicotinamide, 1 g myoinositol, 1 g pyridoxal, 0.05 g riboflavin, and 1 g biotin dissolved in 10 mL water. Make up to 1 L with sterile water.
3. Isopropyl-β-D-1 thiogalactopyranoside (IPTG) (1 M stock solution). Weigh 2.39 g of IPTG and prepare a 10 mL solution with water.
4. L-Arabinose (20% (w/v) solution): Weigh 2 g of L-arabinose and prepare a 10 mL solution with water.
5. *Para*-Azido-L-phenylalanine (Chem-Impex International).
6. High-performance centrifuge with capacities up to 3 L and minimal speed of 8000 × *g* (Beckmann Avanti™ J-25 with rotor JA-10, Beckmann Coulter).
7. Lysis buffer: 50 mM Tris–HCl, 100 mM NaCl, 10% (w/v) glycerol, 1 mM $MgCl_2$, and 20 mM imidazole (pH 7.4). For 1 L weigh 7.88 g Tris–HCl, 5.84 g NaCl, and 1.36 g imidazole and add 116.28 mL 86% glycerol and 2 mL of a 500 mM $MgCl_2$ stock solution. Add water up to 900 mL and mix until dissolved. Adjust the pH to 7.4 using HCl (*see* **Note 3**). Subsequently, make up to 1 L with water.

8. Ultrasound homogenizer with a small tip for volumes between 5 and 500 mL (Branson Sonifier 250, Branson Ultrasonic Corporation).

### 2.2 Protein Purification

1. High-speed centrifuge capable to centrifuge up to 200 mL at a minimal speed of 16.000×*g* (Beckmann Avanti™ J-25 with rotor JA-25.50, Beckmann Coulter).
2. Wash buffer: 1× lysis buffer.
3. Elution buffer: 1× lysis buffer supplemented with 250 mM imidazole. For 1 L prepare lysis buffer as described above with 17.02 g imidazole instead of 1.36 g imidazole.
4. Chromatography column (1 mL HisTrap Fast Flow column, GE Healthcare).
5. Fast protein liquid chromatography (FPLC) system (ÄKTA purifier, GE Healthcare).

### 2.3 Protein Labeling via Staudinger Ligation

1. Phosphine-derivatized fluorophore: DyLight fluorophores (Pierce). Choice of dye type is determined by adequate FRET donor/acceptor pairs (DyLight650) (*see* **Note 4**). Dissolve the lyophilized reagent in water-free dimethyl sulfoxide (DMSO).
2. Dithiothreitol (DTT).
3. PAGE system (Mini-PROTEAN Tetra Cell, Bio-Rad).
4. 2× SDS-PAGE loading buffer: 125 mM Tris–HCl, pH 6.8, 20% (v/v) glycerol, 4% (w/v) sodium dodecyl sulfate (SDS), 4% (v/v) 2-mercaptoethanol, and 0.02% (w/v) bromophenol blue. For 10 mL weigh 197 mg Tris–HCl and 40 mg SDS (*see* **Note 5**) and add water up to 9 mL. Adjust pH to 6.8 with HCl. Subsequently, add 40 μL 2-mercaptoethanol and 2 mg bromophenol blue and make up with water to 10 mL. This buffer does not have to be filtered.
5. Laemmli buffer for SDS-PAGE (10×): 240 mM Tris–HCl, pH 8.3, 1.92 M glycine, and 35 mM sodium dodecyl sulfate (SDS). For 1 L weigh 37.8 g Tris–HCl, 144.2 g glycine, and 10.1 g SDS. Adjustment of pH and filtration is not required.
6. Fluorescence scanner. Scanner should excite the chosen fluorophore and measure its emission (Typhoon FLA 9500, GE Healthcare).

### 2.4 MjAGO–DNA Complex Formation and Purification

1. Binding buffer: lysis buffer without imidazole.
   (a) Liquid chromatography system (*see* Subheading 2.2, **item 12**).
2. Chromatography columns: size exclusion column (Superose 6 10/300 GL, GE Healthcare).
2. Elution buffer: lysis buffer without imidazole.

### *2.5 Activity Test: Binding and Cleavage*

1. 10× TBE: 890 mM Tris, 890 mM boric acid, and 20 mM EDTA. For 1 L weigh 108 g Tris, 55 g boric acid, and 7.45 g EDTA and add to a bottle with 100 mL water and a magnet. Subsequently, add water up to 900 mL and stir until dissolved. Then make up with water to 1 L.
2. 10× running buffer for non-denaturating Tris-Glycine polyacrylamide gels: 240 mM Tris–HCl, pH 8.3, and 1.92 M glycine. For 1 L weigh 37.8 g Tris–HCl and 144.2 g glycine. Adjustment of pH and filtration is not required.
3. Fluorescently labeled oligonucleotides: To visualize binary MjAGO-guide or ternary MjAGO-guide-target complexes and cleavage fragments produced by MjAGO, we use fluorescently labeled DNA oligonucleotides (MWG Eurofins). It is also possible to use radioactively $^{32}$P-labeled oligonucleotides (*see* **Note 6**).
4. *Binding buffer*: wash buffer without imidazole.
5. *Gel solution for non-denaturing Tris-Glycine polyacrylamide gels*: 10% (v/v) acrylamide/bis-acrylamide solution. For 500 mL mix 125 mL 40% acrylamide/*N,N'*-methylenebisacrylamide (19:1) with 50 mL 10× Tris-Glycine running buffer and make up with water to 500 mL.
6. *2× EMSA loading buffer*: 125 mM Tris–HCl pH 6.8; 5% (w/v) Ficoll 400. For 10 mL weigh 197 mg Tris–HCl and 500 mg Ficoll 400 and add water up to 9 mL and dissolve. Subsequently, make up with water to 10 mL.
7. *Cleavage buffer*: wash buffer without imidazole.
8. *Gel apparatus for non-denaturing Tris-Glycine polyacrylamide gels* (Mini-PROTEAN Tetra Cell System, Bio-Rad).
9. *15% acrylamide/N,N'-methylenebisacrylamide, 6 M urea gel solution for sequencing gels*: For 500 mL mix 187.5 mL 40% acrylamide/*N,N'*-methylenebisacrylamide (19:1) with 50 mL 10× TBE and 180 g urea (*see* **Note 7**) and fill up to 500 mL with water.
10. *Running buffer for sequencing gels*: 1× TBE.
11. *2× stop buffer*: 95% formamide (v/v), 0.02% (w/v) SDS, 0.02% (w/v) bromophenol blue, and 1 mM EDTA. For 10 mL weigh 2 mg SDS, 2 mg bromophenol blue, and 3 mg EDTA and mix with 9.5 mL formamide. Afterward make up to 10 mL with water.
12. *Sequencing gel apparatus for cleavage assays* (Sequi-Gen GT System, Bio-Rad) (*see* **Note 8**).

## 3 Methods

Here, we describe a method to prepare and purify the Argonaute protein from the archaeal organism *Methanocaldococcus jannaschii* (*M. jannaschii*), followed by site-specific labeling with fluorescent dyes to conduct fluorescence-based assays including single-molecule measurements. The protein is expressed in *Escherichia coli* (*E. coli*) BL21 (DE3) cells carrying an additional plasmid coding for a mutant tyrosyl synthetase and the amber suppressor tRNA ($tRNA^{Tyr}{}_{CUA}$) derived from *M. jannaschii* [16]. Upon expression of the orthogonal tyrosyl synthetase/$tRNA^{Tyr}{}_{CUA}$ pair, the translational machinery of *E. coli* is able to recognize the amber stop codon as a sense codon and incorporates the unnatural amino acid *para*-azido-phenylalanine into the growing polypeptide chain at the site of the amber stop

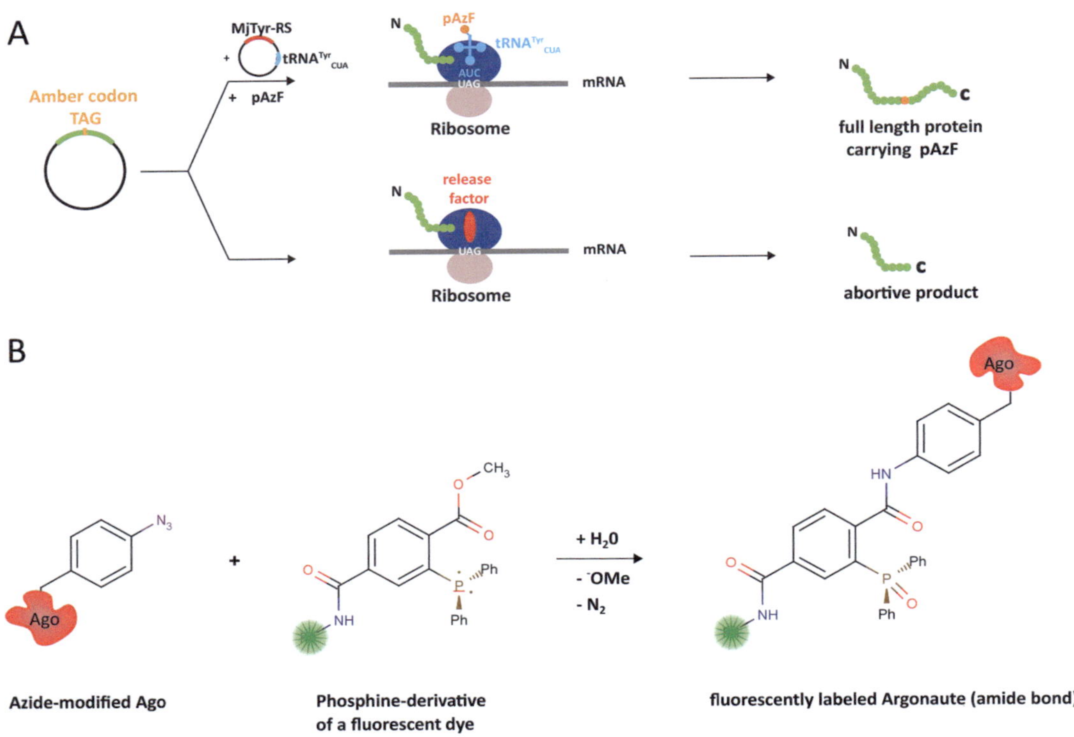


**Fig. 1** Incorporation of an unnatural amino acid into a protein using the amber suppressor strategy and subsequent protein labeling via the bio-orthogonal Staudinger–Bertozzi ligation. (**a**) Site-specific introduction of the amber stop codon (TAG) into the gene of interest usually leads to the abortion of translation at this site and consequently results in a shortened protein of interest. Co-transformation of an additional plasmid harboring an engineered orthogonal aminoacyl-tRNA synthetase/tyrosyl-tRNA pair derived from the archaeal organism *Methanocaldococcus jannaschii* specifically charges the additional tRNA with the unnatural amino acid (shown here *para*-azido-L-phenylalanine). The tRNA is optimized to work efficiently in bacterial translation leading to the incorporation of *para*-azido-L-phenylalanine into the protein strand and allows expression of the full-length protein. (**b**) Staudinger–Bertozzi ligation between a phosphine and an organic azide as reactive moiety of the unnatural amino acid *para*-azido-L-phenylalanine. The *green star* symbolizes the fluorescent dye (drawings not to scale)

codon introduced into the coding sequence of the desired protein (here MjAGO) instead of terminating translation at this site (Fig. 1a). Following expression, MjAGO is purified via its C-terminal His-tag using affinity chromatography. Since MjAGO is derived from a hyperthermophilic organism, a heat treatment of the *E. coli* cell extract at 65 °C already removes most of the endogenous proteins in the *E. coli* extract yielding a highly pure protein after affinity chromatography. The azide group of the unnatural amino acid specifically couples to the phosphine group of the fluorescent dye in a mild bio-orthogonal reaction in aqueous conditions, the so-called Staudinger–Bertozzi ligation [17]. We chose asparagine 76, serine 221, and isoleucine 410 for labeling because these positions do not affect the functionality of the protein and, according to our homology model of the protein, are most likely surface-exposed. MjAGO specifically binds short DNA guide strands (binary MjAGO-guide complex) to recognize a complementary target strand (ternary MjAGO-guide/target complex). Successful complex formation can be controlled using electromobility shift assays (EMSA) (*see* Subheading 3.5.1). Binary and ternary complexes can be formed using fluorescently labeled MjAGO even if the excessive dye from the Staudinger–Bertozzi ligation is not removed prior to complex formation. We tested positions 13, 14, and 18 (counted from the 5′-end) in the DNA guide strand as fluorophore coupling sites and found efficient binary MjAGO-guide and ternary MjAGO-guide-target complex formation. However, complex formation was most efficient when using a guide DNA modified at position 18. After complex formation, the excess of the fluorophore from the protein labeling reaction is removed by size exclusion chromatography.

### 3.1 Cell Growth, Protein Expression, and Cell Lysis

MjAGO is expressed with a $His_6$-tag using a pET101-based expression plasmid in *E. coli* BL21 (DE3), which additional carried the pEvol-AzF plasmid.

1. *E. coli* cells are grown in 5 mL LB medium with 100 μg/mL ampicillin and 25 μg/mL chloramphenicol at 37 °C and 120 rpm (Infors HT Multitron Pro) for 10–14 h. Pellet cells at 5000 × *g* and subsequently carefully resuspend the cells in 100 mL minimal medium and incubate for another 10 h. Again, pellet the cells at 5000 × *g* and subsequently carefully resuspend in 50 mL minimal medium. The resuspended cells are used to inoculate 1 L minimal medium to yield a final $OD_{600}$ of 0.2. Incubate at 120 rpm (Infors HT Multitron Pro) and 37 °C until an $OD_{600}$ of 1.2 is reached. Protein expression is induced using 1 mM IPTG and cells are grown for another 10–14 h. At the same time, expression of the orthogonal tRNA synthetase/tRNA pair is induced using 0.02% (w/v) L-arabinose. The unnatural amino acid is added at an $OD_{600}$ of 1.2 to yield a final concentration of 0.2 mg/mL.
2. Harvest cells by centrifugation at 8000 × *g* for 20 min at 4 °C and resuspended in 30 mL lysis buffer.

3. Lyse cells by sonication. Power was adjusted to 60% and the sample was sonified for 3×5 min.

### 3.2 Protein Purification

MjAGO is purified via a C-terminal His-tag using affinity chromatography after most of the *E. coli* proteins are removed by heat denaturation.

1. Separate soluble proteins from insoluble aggregates and cell debris by centrifugation at 15,000×*g* for 30 min at room temperature.
2. Incubate the supernatant for 30 min at 65 °C. Approximately 90% of the heat labile soluble proteins from the *E. coli* extract are denatured. Another centrifugation step for 45 min at 15,557×*g* removes these denatured proteins from the extract.
3. Further purification of MjAGO is achieved using a Nickel-NTA column for affinity chromatography. Before loading the supernatant, the column is equilibrated using 10 column volumes wash buffer. Subsequently, apply the supernatant to the column allowing the His-tagged MjAGO to bind to the column material. The column is washed with 20 column volumes of wash buffer to remove nonspecifically attached proteins. Afterward, elute MjAGO applying wash buffer supplemented with 250 mM imidazole to the column. Collect 0.5 mL elution fractions. Analyze the elution fractions on a 10% SDS-PAGE. Elution fractions that contain concentrated MjAGO are shock-frozen in liquid nitrogen and stored at −80 °C until use.

### 3.3 Labeling of Purified MjAGO by Staudinger Ligation

The unnatural amino acid *para*-azido-L-phenylalanine incorporated in MjAGO carries an azide group that reacts with the phosphine group conjugated to one of the commercially available DyLight fluorophores (Fig. 1b). Labeling success can be controlled using, for example, SDS-PAGE.

1. Mix 50 μL of 1–5 μM purified MjAGO with 0.5 μL of 10 mM DyLight fluorophore and incubate for 30 min at 37 °C. Stop the reaction with 1.5 mM DTT.
2. In order to check for the successful labeling of the protein, a sample of labeled MjAGO is separated on 10% SDS polyacrylamide gel (*see* **Note 9**). Detection of the fluorescently labeled MjAGO is conducted using a fluorescence scanner specifically exciting the protein-coupled fluorophore and detecting its specific emission. For an example gel, *see* Fig. 2.

## 4 MjAGO–DNA Complex Formation and Purification

Complexes between MjAGO and DNA guide and target strands are formed by incubating freshly prepared fluorescently labeled MjAGO (1–5 μM) and the DNA strands (666 nM) for 20 min at

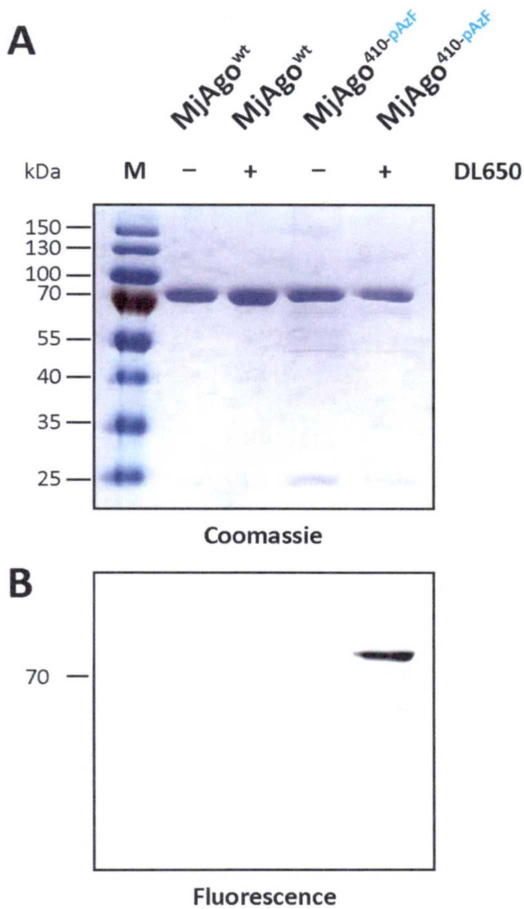


**Fig. 2** Site-specific fluorescent labeling of MjAGO. Full-length MjAGO carrying the unnatural amino acid *para*-azido-L-phenylalanine (pAzF) is purified using a genetically encoded His6-tag at the C-terminus of the protein. (**a**) Shown is the wild-type (wt) MjAGO and the MjAGO$^{I410pAzf}$ mutant separated on a 12% SDS polyacrylamide gel. (**b**) Fluorescence scan of the SDS-PAGE gel shown in (**a**) detecting the fluorescence of the DyLight650 dye (excitation, 635 nm; emission, 670 nm). Addition of the fluorescent probe DyLight650 that carries a phosphine group specifically couples the dye to the azide moiety of pAzF via the Staudinger–Bertozzi ligation but not to the wt protein

65 °C in binding buffer. In case of binary complexes, MjAGO is only incubated with the DNA guide strand, whereas in case of ternary complexes a DNA target complementary to the guide strand was added. For FRET measurements either guide or target strand were labeled with a fluorophore that is a FRET partner for the fluorophore coupled to MjAGO.

1. The excess of fluorophore from the MjAGO labeling reaction and unbound nucleic acids can be separated from the MjAGO-DNA complex by chromatography using a Superose 6 column. The complex elutes at around 17 mL.

2. The complex can be directly used for subsequent fluorescence-based analysis like single-molecule FRET measurements.

### 4.1 Activity Tests: Binding and Cleavage Activity

Binding and cleavage activity of MjAGO can be checked by electromobility shift assays (EMSA) and cleavage assays.

#### 4.1.1 Electromobility Shift Assay (EMSA)

Complexes consisting of MjAGO and guide or guide/target DNA are separated according to their size and charge by native PAGE.

1. Prepare a 10% native PAGE gel.
2. Form the complex using 2.8 μM MjAGO and 333 nM fluorescently labeled guide DNA (binary complex) or 2.8 μM MjAGO, 333 nM non-labeled guide DNA, and 333 nM fluorescently labeled target DNA (ternary complex). Incubate for 20 min at 65 °C in binding buffer. Suitable fluorophores to be coupled to the nucleic acids are, for example, Atto550 or Alexa647 (*see* Table 1).
3. Mix the sample with 1 volume of (v/v) 2× EMSA loading buffer, apply sample on the native PAGE gel and separate at 200 V for 50 min at room temperature.
4. For complex detection the gel is scanned using a fluorescence scanner, exciting the fluorophore coupled to the guide or target DNA and detecting its emission. For an example gel, *see* Fig. 3.

**Table 1**
**Positions we used to introduce a fluorescent dye in the 21 nt guide and target DNAs**

| Position of fluorophore | Fluorophores tested | Sequences |
|---|---|---|
| *Binary complexes* | | |
| Position 13-guide | Atto550 | 5′-p-TGAGGTAGTAGGTTGTATAGT-3′ |
| Position 14-guide | Fluorescein, Atto550 | 5′-p-TAGAGGTACGTGCTGAGGCTT-3′<br>5′-p-TGAGGTAGTAGGTTGTATAGT-3′ |
| Position 18-guide | Fluorescein, Atto550 | 5′-p-TGAGGTAGTAGGTTGTATAGT-3′ |
| *Ternary complexes* | | |
| Position 13-guide | Atto550 | 5′-p-TGAGGTAGTAGGTTGTATAGT-3′ |
| Position 14-guide | Fluorescein, Atto550 | 5′-p-TGAGGTAGTAGGTTGTATAGT-3′<br>5′-p-TAGAGGTACGTGCTGAGGCTT-3′ |
| Position 18-guide | Fluorescein, Atto550 | 5′-p-TGAGGTAGTAGGTTGTATAGT-3′ |
| Position 3′-end guide | Atto550 | 5′ p-TGAGGTAGTAGGTTGTATAGT-3′ |
| Position 3-target | AlexaFluor647 | 5′-TATACAACCTACTACCTCGT-3′ |
| Position 17-target | AlexaFluor647 | 5′-TATACAACCTACTACCTCGT-3′ |

Positions of fluorophores are determined counted from the 5′-end of the oligonucleotide. Denotation of guide or target indicates at which of the strands the fluorophore is positioned

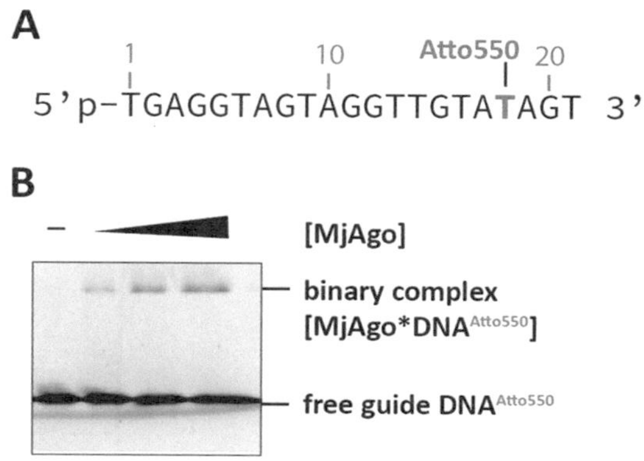


**Fig. 3** Interaction of the DNA guide strand with MjAGO. Electromobility shift assay showing the complex formation of MjAGO (0, 1, 3, 5 μM) and the fluorescently labeled DNA guide strand (333 nM). (**a**) Sequence of the guide DNA strand modified with a 5′ phosphate group and labeled with the fluorescent dye Atto550 at position 18. (**b**) Binary MjAGO-guide DNA complexes were formed at 65 °C and separated from free DNA on a 10% native polyacrylamide gel

#### 4.1.2 Cleavage Assay

Using a cleavage assay, the enzymatic activity of MjAGO can be tested.

1. Prepare a 15% acrylamide sequencing gel containing 6 M urea (*see* **Note 7**).
2. Incubate 1 μM MjAGO with 333 nM guide DNA and 666 nM fluorescently labeled target DNA in cleavage buffer for 15 min at 85 °C. Take samples at different time points (*see* **Note 10**) and stop reactions immediately by adding 1 volume of 2× stop buffer.
3. In order to ensure denaturating conditions during the sequencing gel run, the gel is preheated to 50 °C. Pre-run the sequencing gel at 70 W for 30–40 min (*see* **Note 11**).
4. Load samples when the final running temperature of 40–50 °C is reached.
5. Run the gel for 90 min at 70 W keeping the temperature of the gel constant at 40–50 °C.
6. Detection of the cleavage products is achieved using a fluorescence scanner, specifically exciting the fluorophore coupled to the target DNA and measuring its emission. For an example gel, *see* Fig. 4.

## 5 Notes

1. Adding water to the beaker or measurement cylinder before adding the other ingredients facilitates dissolving the reagents.
2. Prepare stock solutions and dilutions for the small amounts of ingredients you need for the M9 minimal media with vitamins

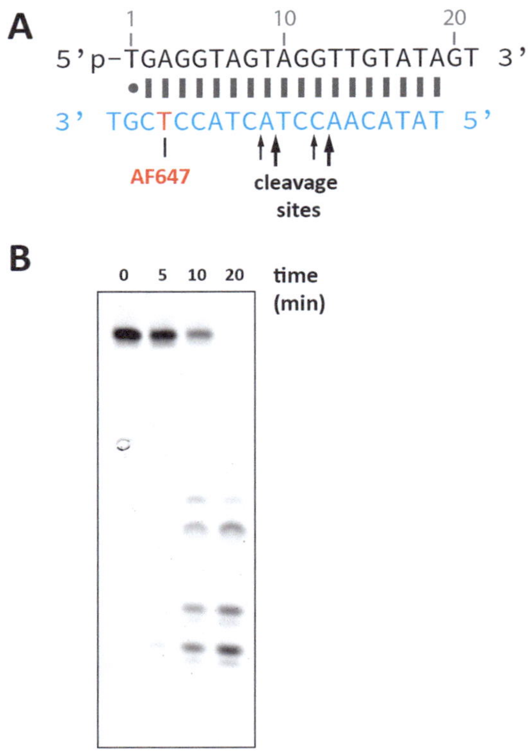


**Fig. 4** Catalytic activity of MjAGO. (**a**) The guide and target strand sequences used for the binding and cleavage experiments are derived from the human let-7 miRNA and shown as DNA duplex, which is efficiently cleaved by MjAGO. The Alexa647 (AF647) modification site in the target strand is highlighted in *red* and the cleavage sites are indicated with *arrows*. (**b**) The cleavage reactions were carried out using 1 μM MjAGO, 333 nM guide, and 666 nM target strand at 85 °C. Reactions were stopped at the indicated time points. The cleavage products were resolved on a 12 % denaturing urea polyacrylamide gel

and minerals. This prevents pipetting/weighing of tiny amounts and minimizes the pipetting/weighing error.

3. Concentrated HCl (12 M) can be used at first to narrow the gap from the starting pH to the required pH. From then on it would be better to use a series of HCl (e.g., 6 and 1 M) with lower ionic strengths to avoid a sudden drop in pH below the required pH.

4. For FRET measurements a suitable donor–acceptor dye pair must be selected. One prerequisite for FRET is that the donor's emission spectrum and the acceptor excitation spectrum overlap. Each dye pair has a characteristic Förster radius ($R_0$) which gives the distance between donor and acceptor at which the energy transfer is 50 %. Only the range that is centered near the Förster radius grants exact distance resolution. Accordingly, a FRET pair should be chosen that matches well the distance

and distance chances expected in the respective biological system. Commonly used FRET pairs are, for example, Cy3B–Atto647N ($R_0$ = 5.5 nm) and Cy3–Cy5 ($R_0$ = 5.6 nm).

5. SDS is allergy-causing and irritates the skin. Furthermore, it is harmful upon inhalation or digestion. Therefore wear your protective clothes, gloves, and lab goggles and work under the fume hood.
6. Radioactive labeling enhances sensitivity of the assays as very small amounts of a radiolabeled molecule can be detected. However, permission for the work with radioactive isotopes is required and disposal and storage of radioactive waste is regulated by specific safety rules.
7. Since acrylamide/*N,N'*-methylenebisacrylamide is possibly carcinogenic and displays neurotoxicity, preparation of the gel solution must be conducted under the fume hood. To accelerate dissolution of urea, it is possible to heat the solution. Be careful to open the lid of the bottle and work under the fume hood!
8. A midsized gel system is suited to separate the cleavage products of MjAGO. However, we found sequencing gels to show the best results because in some cases more than one cleavage product is expected and sequencing gels provide a resolution down to one nucleotide allowing a detailed analysis of cleavage products.
9. MjAGO has a size of 89 kDa including its His-tag. Therefore, a 10% SDS-PAGE gel is best suited to analyze the purity of the labeled protein.
10. Best suited time points to take sample of MjAGO-mediated cleavage: 0, 7.5, 15 min.
11. Pre-running a gel ensures to heat the gel to 50 °C ensures denaturating conditions at the start of the gel and increases its resolution. Furthermore an equilibration of the gel with the running buffer is achieved.

## References


1. Swarts DC, Makarova K, Wang Y, Nakanishi K, Ketting RF, Koonin EV, Patel DJ, van der Oost J (2014) The evolutionary journey of Argonaute proteins. Nat Struct Mol Biol 21(9):743–753
2. Willkomm S, Zander A, Gust A, Grohmann D (2015) A prokaryotic twist on Argonaute function. Life 5:538–553
3. Makarova KS, Wolf YI, van der Oost J, Koonin EV (2009) Prokaryotic homologs of Argonaute proteins are predicted to function as key components of a novel system of defense against mobile genetic elements. Biol Direct 4:29
4. Fire A, Xu SQ, Montgomery MK, Kostas SA, Driver SE, Mello CC (1998) Potent and specific genetic interference by double-stranded RNA in Caenorhabditis elegans. Nature 391(6669):806–811
5. Swarts DC, Jore MM, Westra ER, Zhu Y, Janssen JH, Snijders AP, Wang Y, Patel DJ, Berenguer J, Brouns SJJ, van der Oost J (2014) DNA-guided DNA interference by a prokaryotic Argonaute. Nature 507(7491):258–261
6. Olovnikov I, Chan K, Sachidanandam R, Newman DK, Aravin A (2013) Bacterial argonaute samples the transcriptome to identify foreign DNA. Mol Cell 51(5):594–605
7. Ma J-B, Yuan Y-R, Meister G, Pei Y, Tuschl T, Patel DJ (2005) Structural basis for 5′-end-specific recognition of guide RNA by the A. fulgidus Piwi protein. Nature 434(7033):666–670

8. Rashid UJ, Paterok D, Koglin A, Gohlke H, Piehler J, Chen J (2007) Structure of Aquifex aeolicus argonaute highlights conformational flexibility of the PAZ domain as a potential regulator of RNA-induced silencing complex function. J Biol Chem 282(18):13824–13832
9. Wang Y, Juranek S, Li H, Sheng G, Tuschl T, Patel DJ (2008) Structure of the guide-strand-containing argonaute silencing complex. Nature 456(7219):209–213
10. Wang Y, Juranek S, Li H, Sheng G, Tuschl T, Patel DJDJ (2008) Structure of an argonaute silencing complex with a seed-containing guide DNA and target RNA duplex. Nature 456(7224):921–926
11. Sheng G, Zhao H, Wang J, Rao Y, Tian W, Swarts DC, van der Oost J, Patel DJ, Wang Y (2014) Structure-based cleavage mechanism of Thermus thermophilus Argonaute DNA guide strand-mediated DNA target cleavage. Proc Natl Acad Sci U S A 111(2):652–657
12. Zander A, Holzmeister P, Klose D, Tinnefeld P, Grohmann D (2014) Single-molecule FRET supports the two-state model of Argonaute action. RNA Biol 11(1):45–56
13. Elkayam E, Kuhn CD, Tocilj A, Haase AD, Greene EM, Hannon GJ, Joshua-Tor L (2012) The structure of human argonaute-2 in complex with miR-20a. Cell 150(1):100–110
14. Meister G, Landthaler M, Patkaniowska A, Dorsett Y, Teng G, Tuschl T (2004) Human Argonaute2 mediates RNA cleavage targeted by miRNAs and siRNAs. Mol Cell 15(2):185–197
15. Liu J, Carmell M, Rivas FV, Marsden CG, Thomson JM, Song J-J, Hammond SM, Joshua-Tor L, Hannon GJ (2004) Argonaute2 is the catalytic engine of mammalian RNAi. Science 305(5689):1437–1441
16. Chin JW, Santoro SW, Martin AB, King DS, Wang L, Schultz PG (2002) Addition of p-Azido-l-phenylalanine to the genetic code of Escherichia coli. J Am Chem Soc 124(31):9026–9027
17. Kiick KL, Saxon E, Tirrell DA, Bertozzi CR (2002) Incorporation of azides into recombinant proteins for chemoselective modification by the Staudinger ligation. Proc Natl Acad Sci U S A 99(1):19–24

# Chapter 21

# Single-Molecule Fluorescence Energy Transfer Assays for the Characterization of Reaction Pathways of miRNA-Argonaute Complex

**Myung Hyun Jo and Sungchul Hohng**


## Abstract

Argonaute proteins are key components of the microRNA-induced silencing complexes (miRISCs) that mediate the posttranscriptional gene silencing of microRNAs and small interfering RNA (siRNAs). The complex reaction mechanism of miRISC is expected to be characterized by tracing the reaction pathways of miRISC at the single-molecule level in real time. In this chapter, we describe single-molecule fluorescence resonance energy transfer (FRET) assays to observe the target binding and reaction pathways of miRISC composed of a recombinant Argonaute and a small RNA.


**Key words** Argonaute, miRNA, siRNA, Single-molecule FRET

## 1 Introduction

Small RNAs are short noncoding RNA molecules, ~19–30 nucleotides in length [1, 2]. They play crucial roles in eukaryotic gene regulation via well-conserved RNA interference (RNAi) pathways [3–7]. microRNA (miRNA) and small interfering RNA (siRNA) are two mostly studied small RNAs. They are loaded into Argonaute proteins to form an effector complex, so-called miRNA-induced silencing complex (miRISC), that regulates various target messenger RNAs (mRNAs) [8, 9]. Some members of Argonaute family have slicer activity that cleaves highly complementary target RNAs and initiates their degradation [10–12]. Gene regulation via the slicer-dependent silencing pathway is conceptually simple, but most animal miRNAs seem to regulate their target genes via the slicer-independent silencing pathway [13]. It is still unclear how various miRNAs select their gene regulation pathways between the slicer-dependent and slicer-independent pathways.

Single-molecule fluorescence techniques allow us to monitor the reaction pathways of individual molecules, enabling us to

Marco F. Schmidt (ed.), *Drug Target miRNA: Methods and Protocols*, Methods in Molecular Biology, vol. 1517, DOI 10.1007/978-1-4939-6563-2_21, © Springer Science+Business Media New York 2017

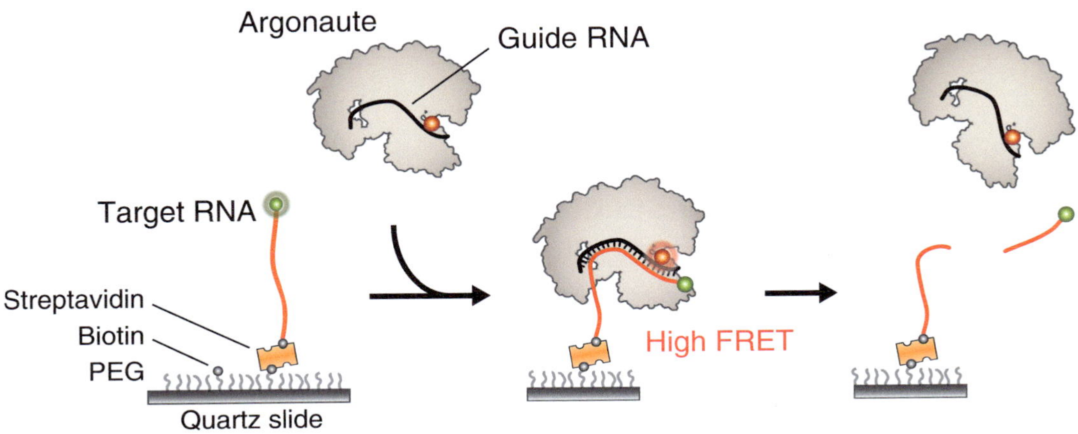


**Fig. 1** Schematics of single-molecule FRET experiments for Argonaute target binding and reaction. After target RNA immobilization, preassembled core-miRISC is added to a reaction channel while single-molecule fluorescence signals are being monitored

clearly delineate and quantitatively characterize heterogeneous biomolecular reactions [14–16]. In addition, fundamental kinetic parameters such as binding and dissociation rates can be directly determined using single-molecule fluorescence measurements [17]. Especially, single-molecule fluorescence resonance energy transfer (FRET) technique provides more accurate and detailed distance information between two fluorophores than other single-molecule fluorescence techniques based on single-molecule co-localization [14, 18–20].

We recently characterized the reaction pathways of core-miRISC composed of a small RNA and human Argonaute 2 by using single-molecule FRET assays (*see* Fig 1) [21]. We showed that target binding of core-miRISC starts at the forepart of seed region (2–5 nt). Four distinct reaction pathways followed the target binding: target cleavage, transient binding, stable binding, and Argonaute unloading. In this chapter, we describe in detail the protocols for the single-molecule FRET experiments.

## 2 Materials

### 2.1 RNA Oligonucleotides

#### 2.1.1 Guide RNA

For single-molecule FRET experiments, guide RNAs need to be labeled with a FRET probe. It is known that several regions of miRNA play important roles for Argonaute loading, target recognition, or target cleavage. Therefore, the dye-labeling position of the guide strand should be carefully selected not to hinder the Argonaute activities in miRISC. We selected 16th–18th nucleotides of the guide RNA as a dye-labeling position because they are not organized in binary complexes of Argonaute and guide RNA [22]. For internal labeling of the guide RNA, an amine-modified uracil is used. The amine residue can be labeled with amine-reactive dyes that have an NHS ester reaction group [16]. In our case, Cy5 mono-reactive NHS ester is used. The formation of secondary structures in the guide RNA can hinder the formation of miRISC. Therefore, RNA sequences that can form stable secondary structures should be avoided when designing guide strands. An example of a guide miRNA (let-7a) that we used is shown below.

let-7a: 5′-/5Phos/UGA GGU AGU AGG UUG UA/iAmMC6U/ AGU-3′ (/iAmMC6U/represents amine-modified Uracil).

#### 2.1.2 Target RNA

Target RNAs are designed to have a target sequence on the 5′-end side and a poly-U spacer on the 3′-end side. The poly-U spacer is included to minimize the steric hindrance due to surface immobilization. The 3′-end of target RNA is biotinylated for surface immobilization. The 5′ end of the target RNA is labeled with a dye (Cy3) for FRET measurement. A target RNA fully complementary to let-7a guide RNA is shown below.

Target RNA fully complementary to let-7a: 5′-/Cy3/ACU AUA CAA CCU ACU ACC UCG $(U)_{16}$ -/biotin/-3′.

### 2.2 Reagents, Buffers, and Materials

1. Methanol.
2. 1 M KOH.
3. Sulfuric acid.
4. Hydrogen peroxide.
5. Acetic acid.
6. Piranha solution: 3:1 mixture of concentrated sulfuric acid and 30% (v/v) hydrogen peroxide.
7. Amino-silane(*N*-(2-aminoethyl)-3-aminopropyltrimethoxysilane).
8. Biotin-PEG-NHS ester (Bio-PEG-SC; MW 5000).
9. PEG-NHS ester (mPEG-SVA; MW 5000).
10. 100 mM sodium bicarbonate.
11. Diamond drill bits (0.75 mm).
12. Rectangular glass cover slips (24 × 40 mm).
13. Quartz microscope slides (1 mm thick).
14. Polyethylene tubing (Becton Dickinson; PE50).
15. Scotch permanent double-sided tape (3 M).
16. Epoxy glue (Devcon; 5 min® Epoxy).
17. Custom RNA oligonucleotides (ST Pharm, PAGE purified).
18. RNA labeling buffer: 0.1 M Sodium tetraborate, pH 8.5.
19. T50: 10 mM Trizma hydrochloride, pH 8.0, 50 mM NaCl.

20. Streptavidin.
21. Saturated Trolox (*see* **Note 1**).
22. Glucose solution: 2% (w/v) glucose, 100 mM Tris–HCl, pH 8.0.
23. 100× gloxy solution: 10,000 U/mL glucose oxidase, 200,000 U/mL catalase, 10 mM Tris–HCl, pH 8.0, 2000 U/mL RNase inhibitor (*see* **Note 2**).
24. Pre-imaging buffer: 20 mM Tris–HCl, pH 8.0, 0.8% (w/v) glucose, ~2 mM Trolox, and indicated amounts of KCl and $MgCl_2$ (*see* **Note 3**).
25. Imaging buffer: pre-imaging buffer, 1× gloxy solution (*see* **Note 4**).
26. miRISC loading buffer: 135 mM KCl, 20 mM Tris–HCl, pH 8.0.
27. RNase inhibitor.
28. RNase III.
29. Catalase (Sigma; C40).

### 2.3 TIRF Microscope

A homebuilt prism-type total internal reflection fluorescence (TIRF) microscope equipped with an electron-multiplying charge-coupled device (EMCCD) can be used for single-molecule florescence imaging. Donor (Cy3) and acceptor (Cy5) dyes are excited using 532- and 635-nm lasers. Alternating laser excitation (ALEX) technique [23] should be used to identify the guide RNA binding and dissociation events without FRET signal. The Cy3 and Cy5 signals are separated using a 540-nm dichroic mirror. The other details of the microscope can be found elsewhere [16, 19].

## 3 Methods

### 3.1 Preparation of PEGylated Surface

#### 3.1.1 Drilling

1. For convenient buffer exchange, make holes in a quartz slide using a diamond drill bit (Fig. 2) (*see* **Notes 5** and **6**).

#### 3.1.2 Cleaning

1. Put quartz slides and cover slips into heat-resistant glass containers.
2. Fill the containers with piranha solution and incubate them for 30 min (*see* **Note 7**).
3. Pour out piranha solution carefully.
4. Rinse thoroughly the slide glasses and cover slips in the glass containers with distilled water.
5. Rinse the slide glasses and cover slips in the glass containers one more time with methanol.

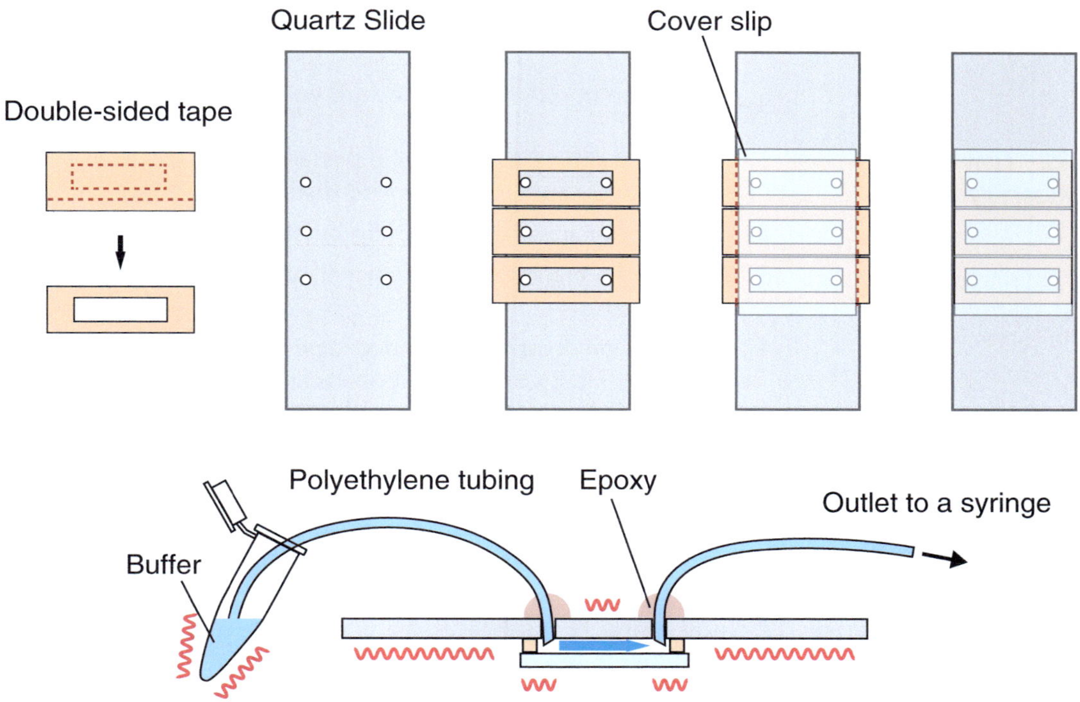


**Fig. 2** Flow cell assembly. A procedure to make a three-channel flow cell (*top*) and a scheme to connect the inlet and outlet tubings to a flow cell are shown. During single-molecule fluorescence imaging, buffer exchange can be done. The *red tildes* indicate the regions whose temperature are maintained using a temperature controller (Live Cell Instrument)

#### *3.1.3 Silanization*

1. Add 5 mL of acetic acid and 1 mL of amino-silane into 100 mL of methanol, and mix the solution well.
2. Fill the glass containers so that the slide glasses and cover slips are submerged, and incubate them for 20 min.
3. Rinse the slide glasses and cover slips with methanol.
4. Rinse the slide glasses and cover slips with distilled water thoroughly.
5. Dry slide glasses and cover slips one by one by blowing nitrogen gas, and keep the dried slide glasses and cover slips on a clean surface.

#### *3.1.4 PEGylation*

1. Dissolve 2 mg of biotin-PEG-SC and 80 mg of mPEG-SVA in 640 mL of 100 mM sodium bicarbonate solution. This amount of solution is enough for the PEGylation of nine pairs of slides and cover slips.
2. Centrifuge the solution at 10,000 × *g* for 1 min.
3. Drop 70 mL of PEG solution on a slide glass, and lay a cover slip on it carefully not to make air bubbles (*see* **Note 8**).

4. Incubate them for 4 h in a dark room at room temperature (*see* **Note 9**).
5. Store them in −20 °C freezer until you assemble a flow cell.

### 3.2 Flow Cell Assembly

1. Take out a slide glass-cover slip pair from the freezer and rinse the slide glass and cover slip with distilled water.
2. Dry the slide glass and cover slip by blowing nitrogen gas.
3. Place the slide glass on a clean paper so that the PEGylated side faces upward.
4. Prepare a piece of double-sided tape whose middle region is removed (Fig. 2), and place it on each channel of the slide glass (*see* **Note 10**). Be careful not to block the holes.
5. Place the cover slip on the double-sided tape so that the PEGylated side faces downward.
6. Make the flow channels tight by carefully rubbing the region of the cover slip on the double-sided tape. A pipette tip is good for the purpose.
7. Insert tubings into the holes in the slide glass. Inlet tubings should be long enough so that the other ends of inlet tubings can be dipped into buffers (Fig. 2) (*see* **Note 11**).
8. Fix the tubings with epoxy.

### 3.3 Preparation of Dye-Labeled RNA

1. Make 20 mM Cy5 NHS ester solution in DMSO.
2. Add 6 μL of 500 μM amine-modified RNA to 25 μL of RNA labeling buffer.
3. Add 5 μL of 20 mM Cy5 solution to the mixture.
4. Incubate the mixture for 4 h at 4 °C.
5. Add 4 μL of 5 M NaCl into the mixture.
6. Add 100 μL of 100% ethanol.
7. Incubate the mixture for 20 min at −20 °C freezer.
8. Centrifuge at >12,000 × *g* for 20 min at 4 °C.
9. Remove supernatant carefully.
10. Rinse the pellet with 75% ethanol.
11. Rinse the pellet with 100% ethanol, and dry the pellet.
12. Dissolve the pellet with T50, and check the dye-labeling efficiency by measuring the absorbance.

### 3.4 Core-miRISC Formation

For accurate estimation of binding rates and reaction pathways, it is important to minimize guide miRNA molecules that are not loaded in Argonaute. To do that, we incubated guide miRNAs with excessive Argonaute proteins (5–25× for human Argonaute 2). It is highly recommended to confirm that miRISC formation is complete using native gel electrophoresis [21, 24].

1. Add 1 μL of 200 nM guide RNA to 2 μL of miRISC loading buffer.
2. Add 2 μL of 2.5 μM human Argonaut 2 to the mixture.
3. Incubate the mixture at 23 °C for 30 min.

#### 3.5 Single-Molecule Fluorescence Measurement

1. Place a flow cell on a microscope.
2. Connect the outlet tubing to a syringe pump (*see* **Note 12**).
3. Put the end of the inlet tubing in the Eppendorf tube filled with T50 buffer (Fig. 2).
4. Flush a flow channel with T50 buffer by pulling a syringe (*see* **Note 13**).
5. Infuse 80 μL of 0.2 mg/mL streptavidin solution into the channel as described in the **steps 3** and **4**, and incubate for 2 min.
6. Remove unbound streptavidin by infusing 80 μL of T50 into the channel.
7. Infuse 80 μL of ~50 pM biotinylated target RNA, and incubate for 2 min.
8. Infuse 80 μL of imaging buffer, and check the number of target RNA molecules immobilized on the surface.
9. Add 5 μL of 40 nM miRISC solution to 95 μL of imaging buffer (*see* **Note 14**).
10. Start single-molecule imaging, and infuse 80 μL of RISC solution into the detection chamber. RISC binding is monitored via the appearance of Cy5 signal at Cy5 excitation. Guide-target annealing is monitored via FRET between Cy3 and Cy5.
11. To discriminate Argonaute unloading from stable binding of miRISC on target RNAs, RNase III treatment can be used; molecules that disappear under RNase III treatment can be regarded as free RNA duplex without Argonaute.

#### 3.6 Drift Correction and Autofocusing

Sample drift and defocusing hinder long-time fluorescence imaging. The lateral drift can be corrected after experiments by using 2D translation image registration algorithm [25]. The defocusing problem, however, should be solved in real time. Autofocusing method based on optical astigmatism analysis is a handy way that can be used for the purpose [26].

#### 3.7 Data Analysis

Target binding of miRISC is monitored via the Cy5 signal appearance at Cy5 excitation. The time delay between miRISC injection and the target binding is analyzed to estimate the binding rate of miRISC. High FRET appearance reports the full annealing of guide and target RNAs. FRET efficiency is determined as the acceptor (Cy5) signal divided by the sum of the donor (Cy3) and

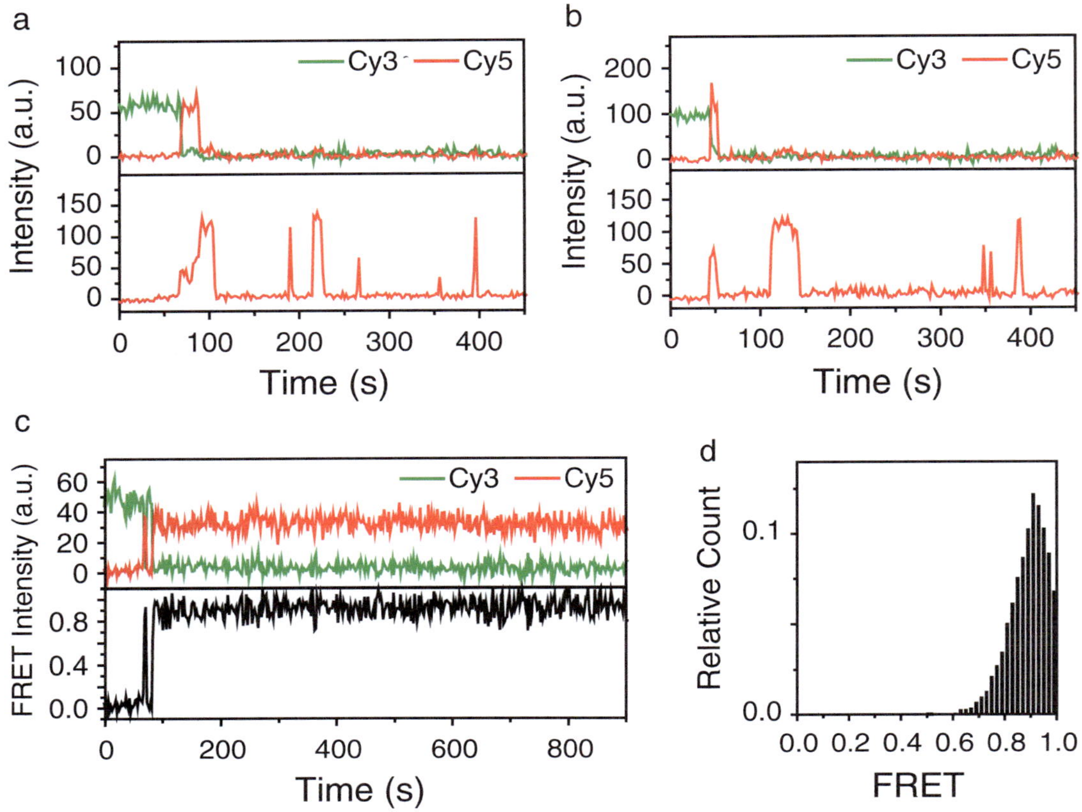


**Fig. 3** Representative data. (**a**, **b**) Representative single-molecule fluorescence time traces showing the cleavage reaction. miRISC binding induces both high FRET for Cy3 excitation (*upper panel*) and Cy5 signal appearance for Cy5 direction excitation (*lower panel*). Cy3 signal disappears first leaving Cy5 signal when 5′ end part of target with Cy3 dissociates earlier than 3′ end part (**a**). Cy3 and Cy5 signal disappear simultaneously in case of (**b**). miRISC rebinding events on truncated target RNA are observed for both cases. (**c**) Transient and long binding of miRISCs are shown in a trace. (**d**) FRET distribution for the miRISC-bound state is shown. miRISC solution was injected at 40 s for all the traces shown

acceptor signals at donor excitation. The reaction pathways of miRISC upon target binding can be identified by observing FRET time traces (Fig. 3). For instance, the cleavage reaction resulted in two different types of traces: simultaneous disappearance of Cy3 and Cy5 signals (*see* **Note 15**) and sequential disappearance of Cy3 and Cy5 signals. Repetitive miRISC rebinding events were observed for both cases. Transient miRISC binding events could be kinetically distinguished from long binding events that include both Argonaute unloading and stable miRISC binding. Argonaute unloading events could be distinguished from stable miRISC binding events using RNase III treatment.

## 4 Notes

1. Add 25 mg of Trolox into 50 mL of distilled water, and incubate on rotator at room temperature under room light for a day. Filter the buffer with 0.2-μm membrane filter.
2. We found that catalase products of some companies are contaminated with RNases [27]. Because RNase contamination is lethal for single-stranded target RNAs, the catalase product should be chosen carefully. RNase inhibitors can be added on a need. To remove the impurities, centrifuge the gloxy solution for 20 min at >12,000 × *g*, and get the supernatant.
3. It is recommended to prepare daily the pre-imaging buffer by mixing the glucose solution and saturated Trolox.
4. It is highly recommended to add 1 μL of gloxy solution into 99 μL of pre-imaging buffer just before the injection of imaging buffer into the flow cell.
5. It is important to make right-size holes. If a hole is too large, epoxy leaks into the flow cell and block the channel. If a hole is too small, tubing cannot be fitted into the hole.
6. Drilled quartz slides can be reused after experiments. In that case, separate quartz slides from cover slips by boiling used flow cells in a microwave oven, and remove visible impurities from the quartz slide using dishwashing detergent and clean water. Storing the used flow cells in methanol and adding some detergent for boiling facilitate this procedure.
7. The piranha solution should be treated with great care. Hot and boiling solution can break the glass container. It is recommended not to sonicate the containers or jars to avoid an accumulation of fatigue. The procedure should be done on an acid-resistant tray. Be aware of how to deal with liquid waste.
8. It is recommended to finish this step within 20 min after fresh PEG solution is prepared.
9. It is important to prevent PEG solution from drying during the reaction. To maintain a proper humidity level, we make the reaction happen inside a pipette tip case with small amount of water added at the bottom. Slides and cover slips are placed on top of a rack.
10. Cut a thin guide groove on a plastic surface (e.g., the cover of a used pipette tip case) with a razor or a laser engraver. Use this pattern to make the procedure fast.
11. The end part of tubing should be cut obliquely not to block the buffer flow.

12. Tubing can be connected to other tubing or a syringe by using a syringe needle. For example, a 23 G needle nicely fits into PE50 tubing (Becton Dickinson).
13. The end of the inlet tubing should be kept inside buffer to prevent air from coming into the tubing even after the buffer infusion.
14. Temperature has a major effect on reaction kinetics of miRISC. Therefore, the temperature of a flow cell and a buffer container should be maintained at the same temperature.
15. Even though the probability of simultaneous photobleaching of Cy3 and Cy5 is low, it can sometimes be observed for dye pairs with high FRET efficiency. The probability can be measured by using a guide-target duplex without Argonaute. miRISC rebinding events on truncated target RNA can be used to make sure that the cleavage reaction actually occurred.

## Acknowledgment

This work was supported by Creative Research Initiatives (Physical Genetics Laboratory, 2009-0081562) to S.H.

### References

1. Bartel DP (2004) MicroRNAs: genomics, biogenesis, mechanism, and function. Cell 116(2): 281–297
2. Kim VN (2005) Small RNAs: classification, biogenesis, and function. Mol Cells 19(1):1–15
3. Lee RC, Feinbaum RL, Ambros V (1993) The C. elegans heterochronic gene lin-4 encodes small RNAs with antisense complementarity to lin-14. Cell 75(5):843–854
4. Vagin VV et al (2006) A distinct small RNA pathway silences selfish genetic elements in the germline. Science 313(5785):320–324
5. Tam OH et al (2008) Pseudogene-derived small interfering RNAs regulate gene expression in mouse oocytes. Nature 453(7194):534–538
6. Watanabe T et al (2008) Endogenous siRNAs from naturally formed dsRNAs regulate transcripts in mouse oocytes. Nature 453(7194): 539–543
7. Wightman B, Ha I, Ruvkun G (1993) Posttranscriptional regulation of the heterochronic gene lin-14 by lin-4 mediates temporal pattern formation in C. elegans. Cell 75(5): 855–862
8. Hammond SM, Bernstein E, Beach D, Hannon GJ (2000) An RNA-directed nuclease mediates post-transcriptional gene silencing in Drosophila cells. Nature 404(6775): 293–296
9. Rivas FV et al (2005) Purified Argonaute2 and an siRNA form recombinant human RISC. Nat Struct Mol Biol 12(4):340–349
10. Elbashir SM, Martinez J, Patkaniowska A, Lendeckel W, Tuschl T (2001) Functional anatomy of siRNAs for mediating efficient RNAi in Drosophila melanogaster embryo lysate. EMBO J 20(23):6877–6888
11. Yekta S, Shih IH, Bartel DP (2004) MicroRNA-directed cleavage of HOXB8 mRNA. Science 304(5670):594–596
12. Liu J et al (2004) Argonaute2 is the catalytic engine of mammalian RNAi. Science 305(5689):1437–1441
13. Iwakawa HO, Tomari Y (2015) The functions of MicroRNAs: mRNA decay and translational repression. Trends Cell Biol 25(11):651–665
14. Ha T (2001) Single-molecule fluorescence resonance energy transfer. Methods 25(1): 78–86
15. Ha T (2001) Single-molecule fluorescence methods for the study of nucleic acids. Curr Opin Struct Biol 11(3):287–292

16. Roy R, Hohng S, Ha T (2008) A practical guide to single-molecule FRET. Nat Methods 5(6):507–516
17. Joo C, Balci H, Ishitsuka Y, Buranachai C, Ha T (2008) Advances in single-molecule fluorescence methods for molecular biology. Annu Rev Biochem 77:51–76
18. Ha T et al (1996) Probing the interaction between two single molecules: fluorescence resonance energy transfer between a single donor and a single acceptor. Proc Natl Acad Sci U S A 93(13):6264–6268
19. Hohng S, Lee S, Lee J, Jo MH (2014) Maximizing information content of single-molecule FRET experiments: multi-color FRET and FRET combined with force or torque. Chem Soc Rev 43(4):1007–1013
20. Lee S, Lee J, Hohng S (2010) Single-molecule three-color FRET with both negligible spectral overlap and long observation time. PLoS One 5(8), e12270
21. Jo MH et al (2015) Human Argonaute 2 has diverse reaction pathways on target RNAs. Mol Cell 59(1):117–124
22. Schirle NT, Sheu-Gruttadauria J, MacRae IJ (2014) Structural basis for microRNA targeting. Science 346(6209):608–613
23. Kapanidis AN et al (2004) Fluorescence-aided molecule sorting: analysis of structure and interactions by alternating-laser excitation of single molecules. Proc Natl Acad Sci U S A 101(24):8936–8941
24. Jung SR et al (2013) Dynamic anchoring of the 3′-end of the guide strand controls the target dissociation of Argonaute-guide complex. J Am Chem Soc 135(45): 16865–16871
25. Guizar-Sicairos M, Thurman ST, Fienup JR (2008) Efficient subpixel image registration algorithms. Opt Lett 33(2):156–158
26. Hwang W, Bae S, Hohng S (2012) Autofocusing system based on optical astigmatism analysis of single-molecule images. Opt Express 20(28): 29353–29360
27. Senavirathne G et al (2015) Widespread nuclease contamination in commonly used oxygen-scavenging systems. Nat Methods 12(10): 901–902

# Index

## A



## B



## C



## D



## E



## F



Marco F. Schmidt (ed.), *Drug Target miRNA: Methods and Protocols*, Methods in Molecular Biology, vol. 1517,
DOI 10.1007/978-1-4939-6563-2, © Springer Science+Business Media New York 2017

## G



## H



## I



## K



## L



## M



## N



## O

## P



## R



## S



## T



## U



## W



## Z

MIX
Papier aus verantwortungsvollen Quellen
Paper from responsible sources
FSC® C105338

If you have any concerns about our products,
you can contact us on
**ProductSafety@springernature.com**

In case Publisher is established outside the EU,
the EU authorized representative is:
**Springer Nature Customer Service Center GmbH**
**Europaplatz 3, 69115 Heidelberg, Germany**

Printed by Libri Plureos GmbH
in Hamburg, Germany